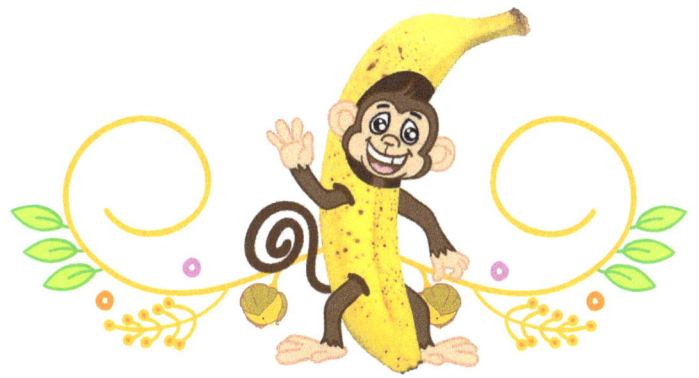

This book belongs to:

_____

experience delicious

Experience Delicious LLC

All Rights Reserved. This book or any portion thereof may not be reproduced or used in any manner whatsoever without the express written permission of the publisher except for the use of brief quotations in a book review.

Copyright 2016; 2019 Experience Delicious, LLC.
ISBN: 978-1-947001-18-3
www.experiencedeliciousnow.com

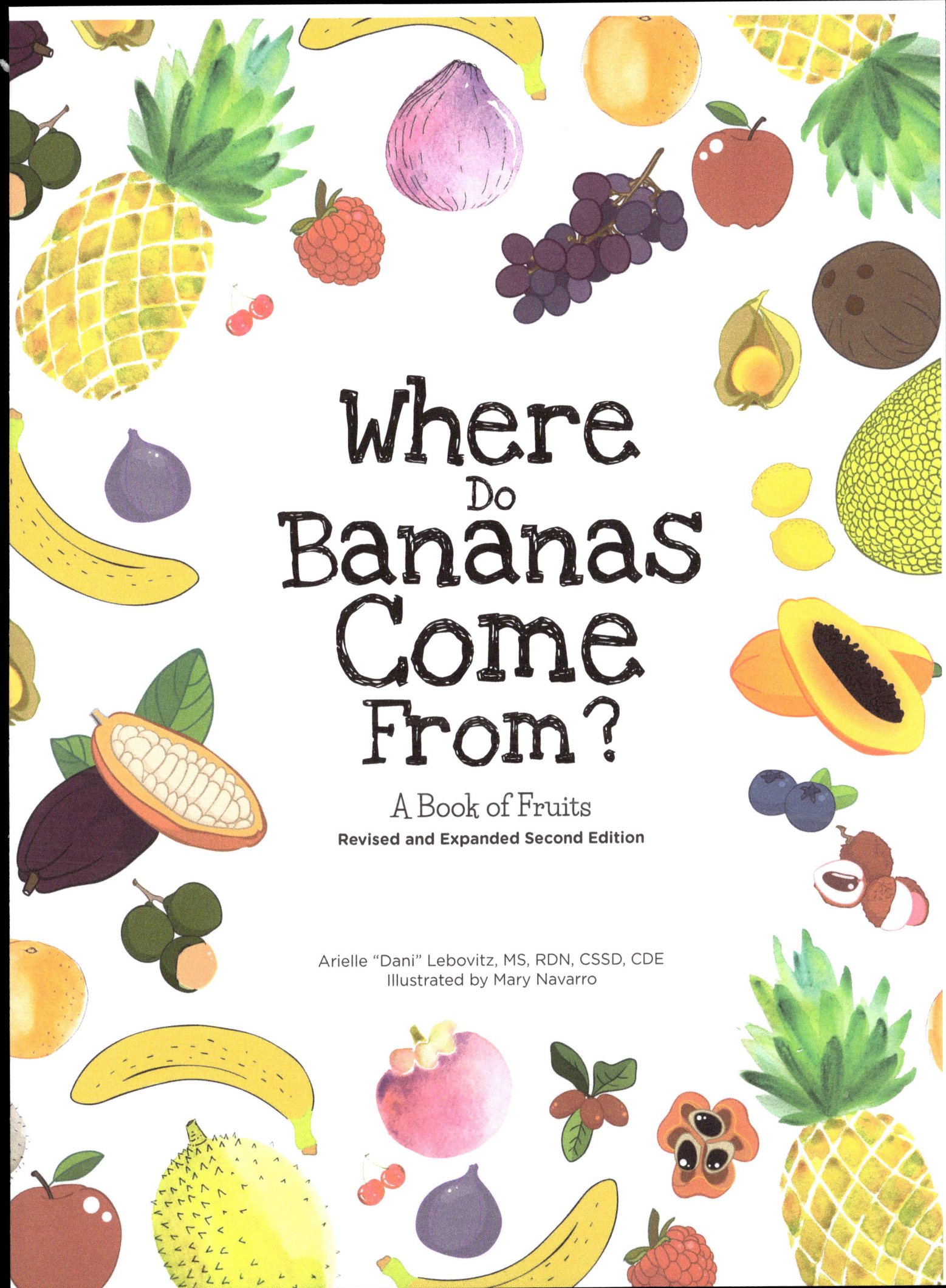

Where Do Bananas Come From?

A Book of Fruits

Revised and Expanded Second Edition

Arielle "Dani" Lebovitz, MS, RDN, CSSD, CDE
Illustrated by Mary Navarro

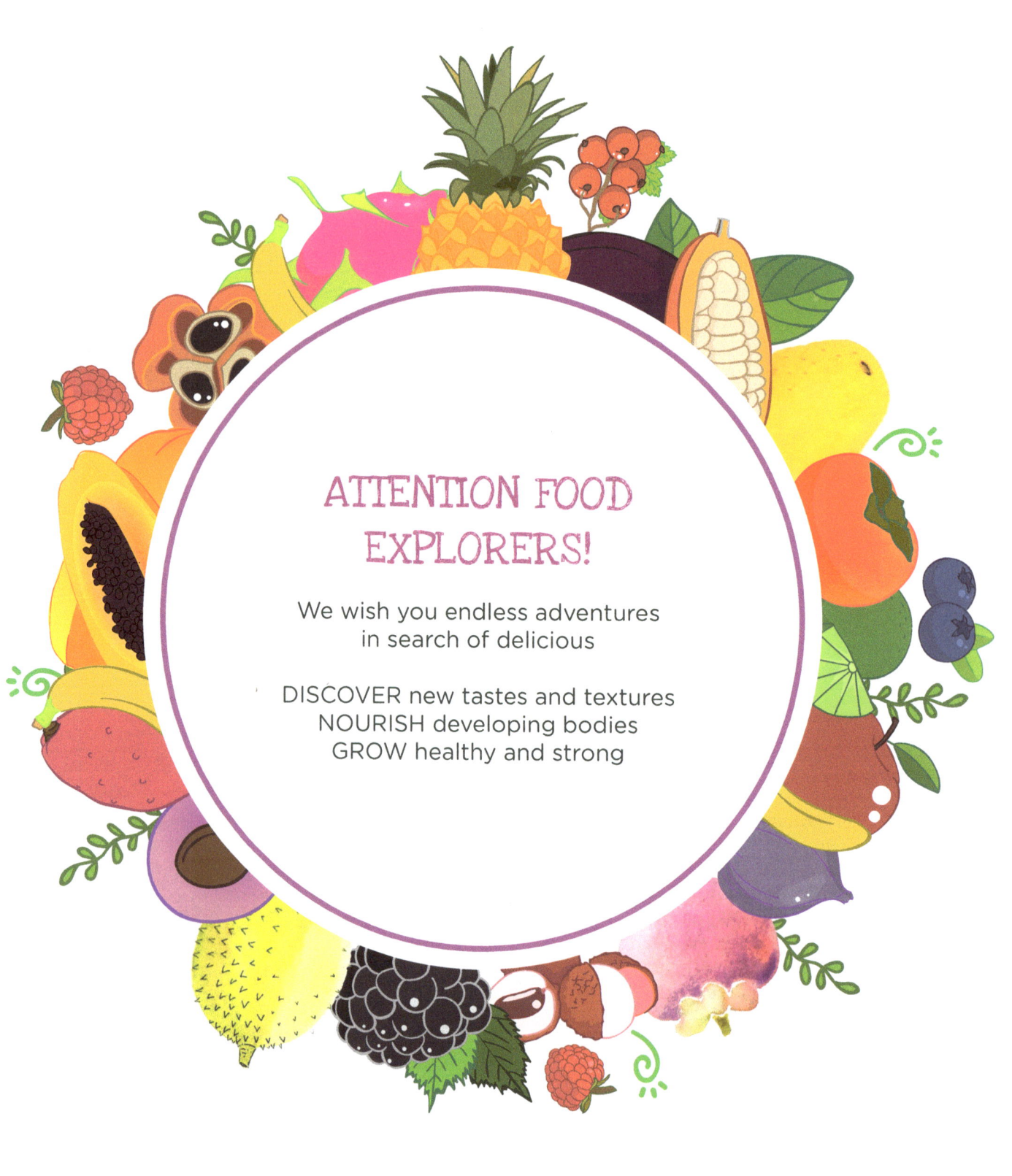

ATTENTION FOOD EXPLORERS!

We wish you endless adventures in search of delicious

DISCOVER new tastes and textures
NOURISH developing bodies
GROW healthy and strong

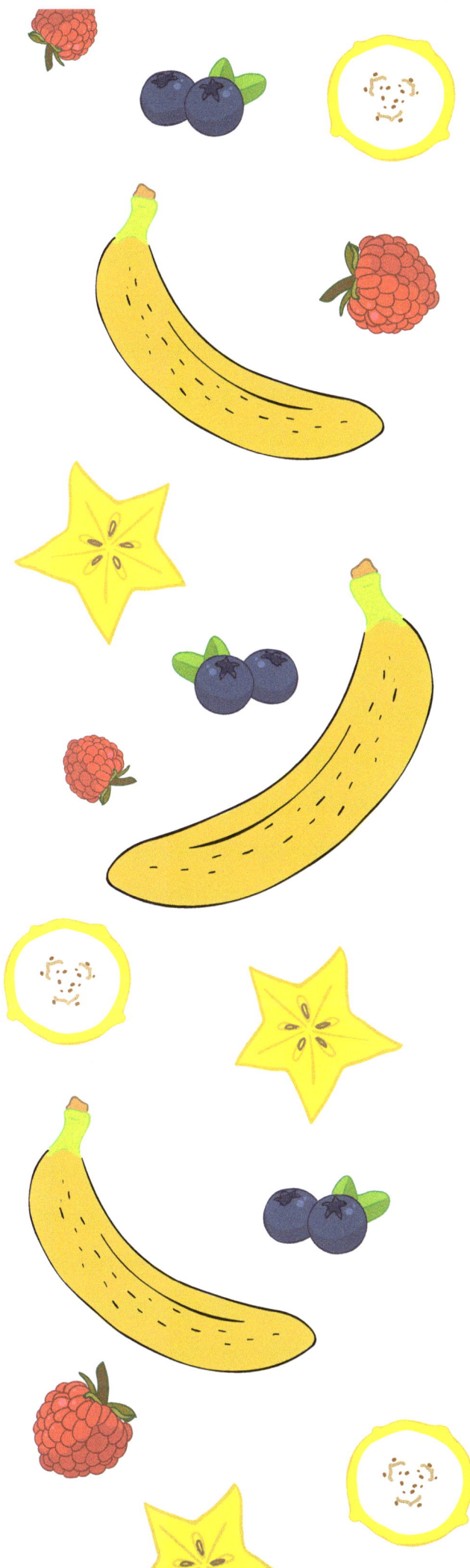

ACKNOWLEDGEMENTS

To my best friend and husband Michael: Words cannot adequately express my appreciation for you. Thank you for always believing in me. Without your love and endless support this book and series would not be possible.

To my daughters Shiloh and Elior: This book series is for you as we explore and discover the wonderful world of food. Shiloh, the way you engage with the world helps me to improve the way I help others. Thank you for your imagination and your adventurous palate. Elior, we can't wait until your adventures in taste-testing begin!

To my sister Brette: Thank you for editing and re-editing every morsel of this book x 2 and being my biggest cheerleader! My life would not be complete without you. Thank you for your friendship, love, and time.

To the extremely talented Mary Navarro: Thank you for transforming my vision into a reality and sharing my love and passion for inspiring children to live better by trying something new. I am so grateful for our ever-evolving work to provide children and families with the best tools possible to expand palates and make food fun.

To my family, friends, and the kiddos who helped make this dream come true: Thank you for your time and feedback. Your excitement, observations, and experiences help us to continuously improve our efforts and provide inspiration as we pursue our mission. It is a privilege to watch you Discover, Nourish, and Grow.

With gratitude and love,
Arielle Dani

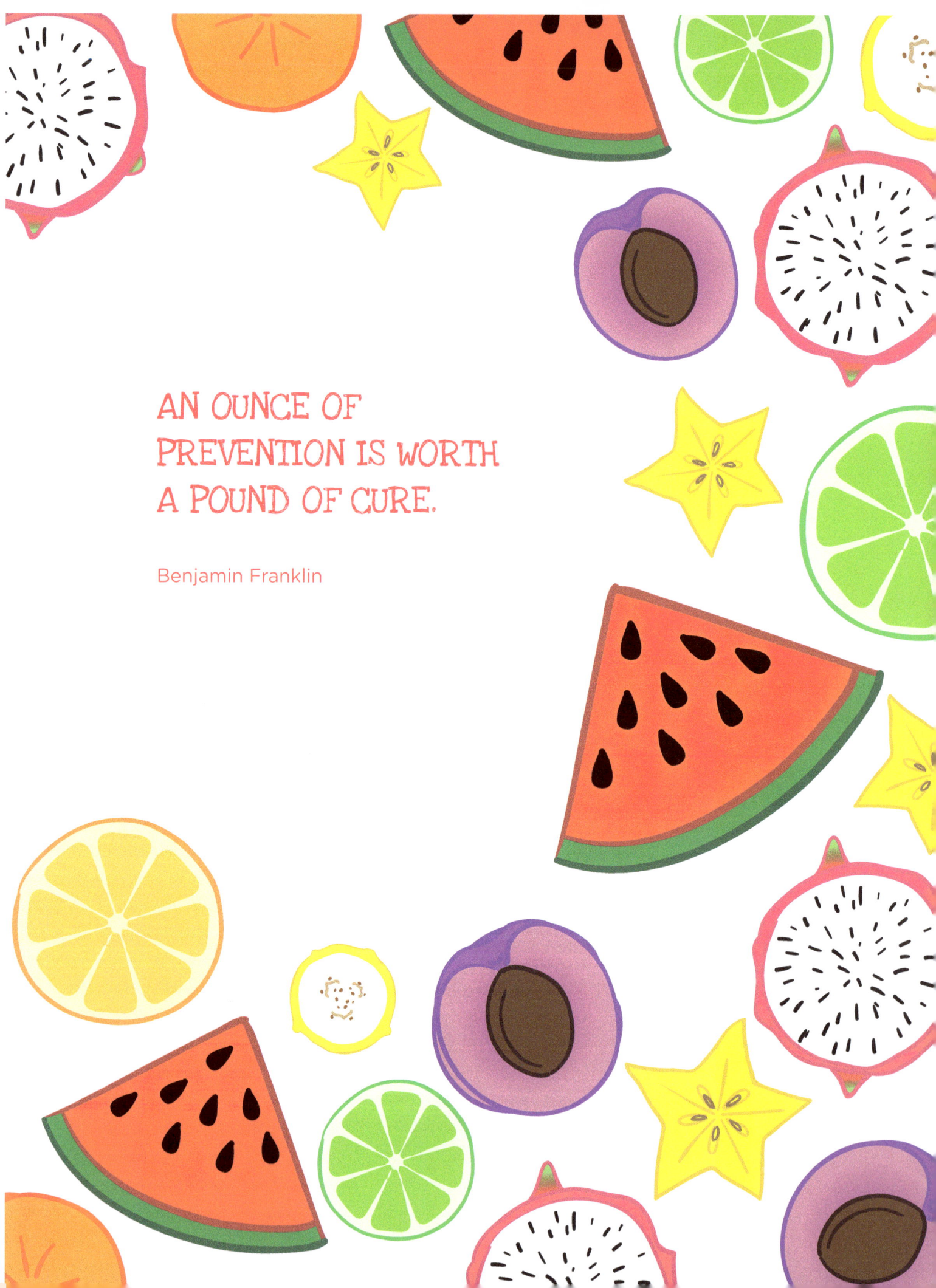

AN OUNCE OF PREVENTION IS WORTH A POUND OF CURE.

Benjamin Franklin

DEDICATION

To parents, grandparents, caregivers, and teachers:

Children's palates are based on senses and experiences. Early feeding, cultural background, taste-bud memory, visual presentation, knowledge, and preconception all influence taste and beliefs about food. This book series is intended to delight, inspire, and foster an interest in real food. A useful resource for children and adults alike, this book creates positive associations with mealtime.

Experiment with food. Conduct your own taste tests with new fruits and vegetables or old favorites prepared in different ways. Visit a farm. Pick local produce. Plan and grow a garden. Get kids involved in picking, storing, and cooking. Engage with kids, make food fun, and transform young palates.
Create memories – they will last a lifetime!

Now put your Food Explorer hats on and get ready for adventures in food.

Experience Delicious,
Discover – Nourish – Grow

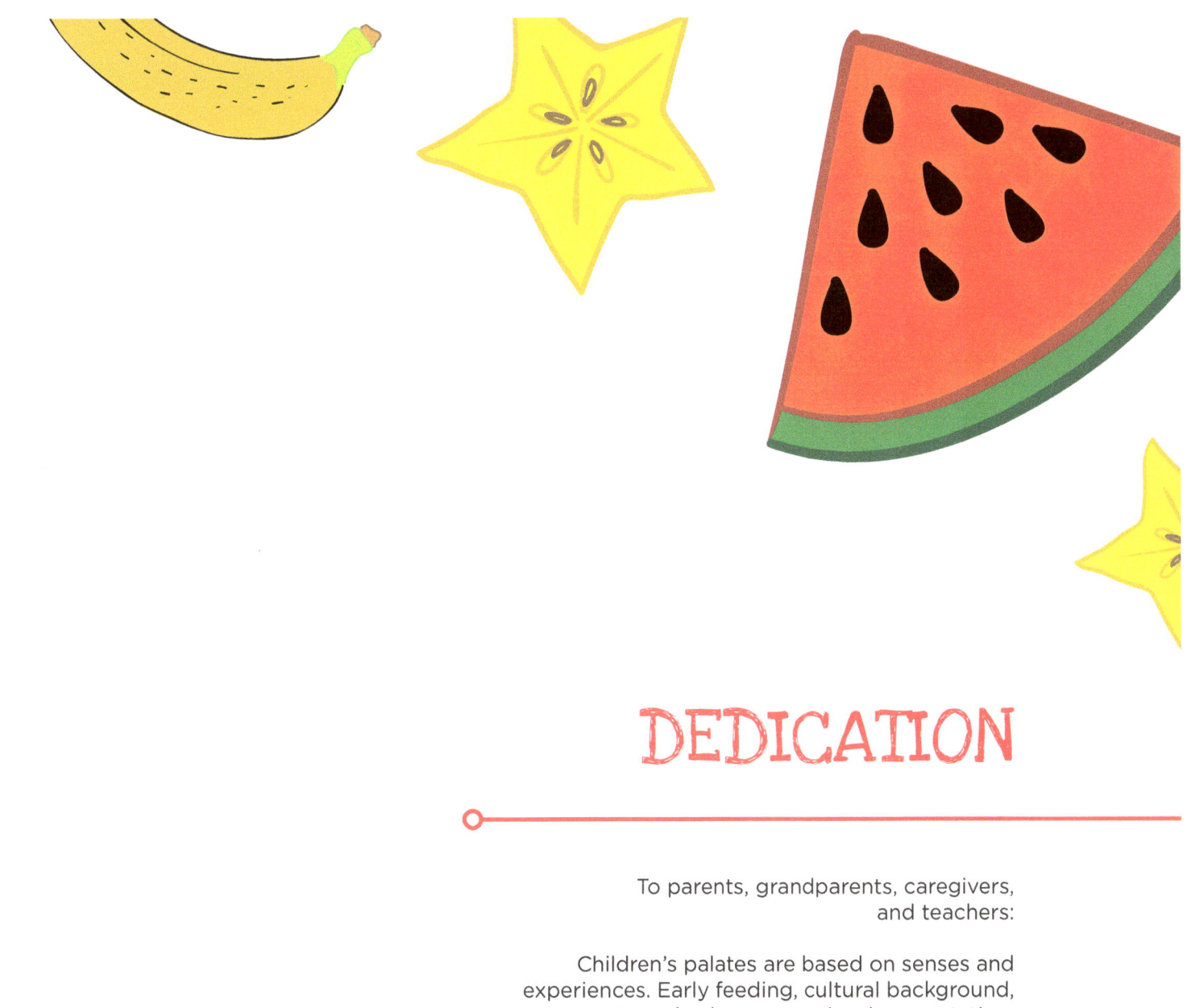

How To Read This Book

Review this page before reading the book for the best experience on your adventures with fruit. This book is designed to be easy to read so you can experiment and explore new foods!

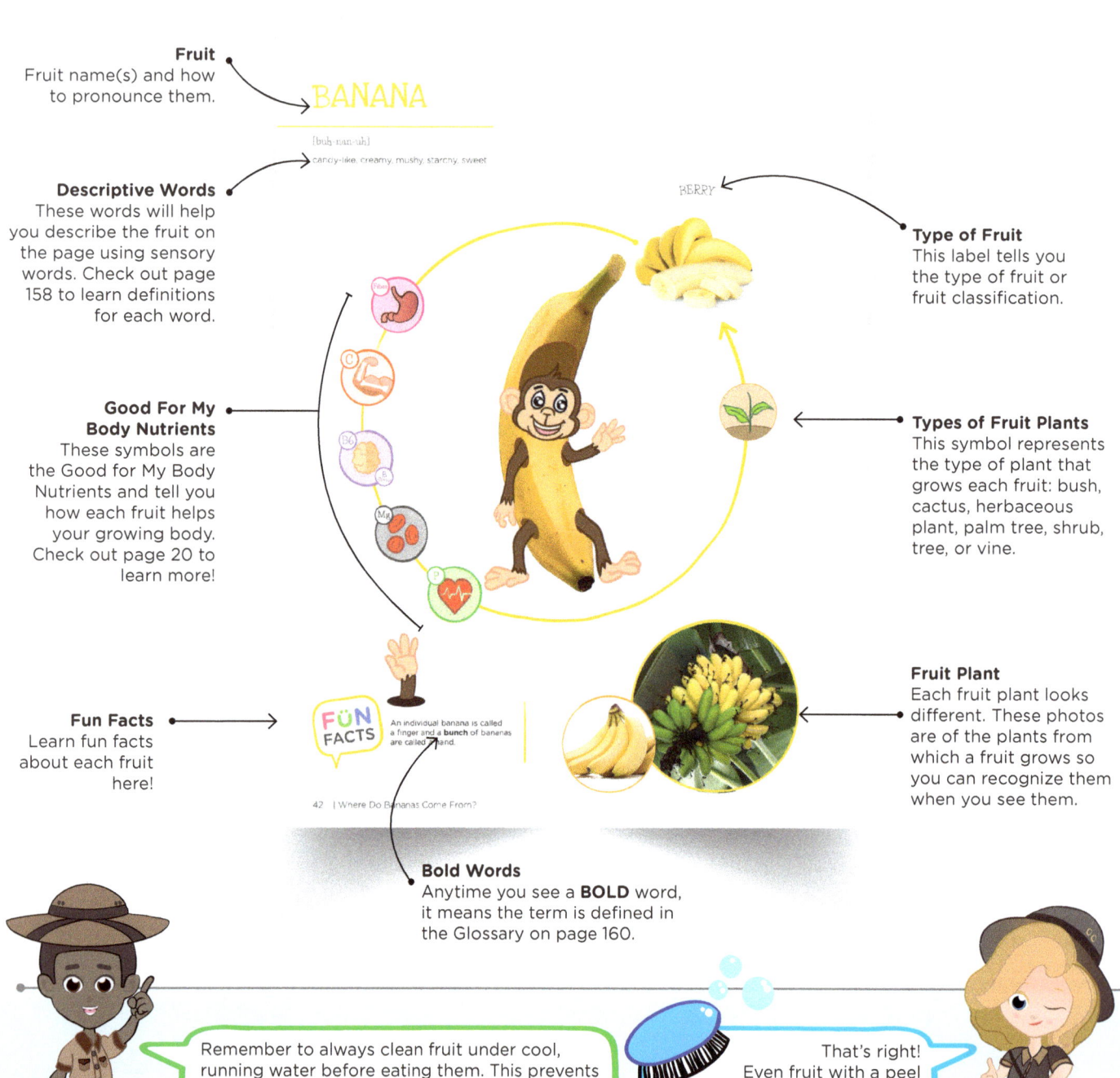

Fruit
Fruit name(s) and how to pronounce them.

Descriptive Words
These words will help you describe the fruit on the page using sensory words. Check out page 158 to learn definitions for each word.

Good For My Body Nutrients
These symbols are the Good for My Body Nutrients and tell you how each fruit helps your growing body. Check out page 20 to learn more!

Fun Facts
Learn fun facts about each fruit here!

Type of Fruit
This label tells you the type of fruit or fruit classification.

Types of Fruit Plants
This symbol represents the type of plant that grows each fruit: bush, cactus, herbaceous plant, palm tree, shrub, tree, or vine.

Fruit Plant
Each fruit plant looks different. These photos are of the plants from which a fruit grows so you can recognize them when you see them.

Bold Words
Anytime you see a **BOLD** word, it means the term is defined in the Glossary on page 160.

Remember to always clean fruit under cool, running water before eating them. This prevents harmful **bacteria** on the outside from getting on the inside. Harmful bacteria can come from your hands, knives, or other surfaces they come in contact with and make you sick!

That's right! Even fruit with a peel should be washed first. Try using a veggie scrubber under running water for fruit that has dirt or sand on the skin.

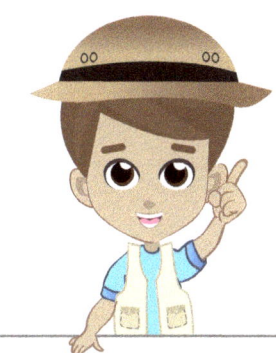

FRUITS VARIETIES

Many fruits have several **varieties** of the same type of fruit that we love to eat! The fruit varieties pages introduce you to some of the commonly consumed fruit varieties with interesting facts, how to recognize them, or details about **flavor** and **texture**.

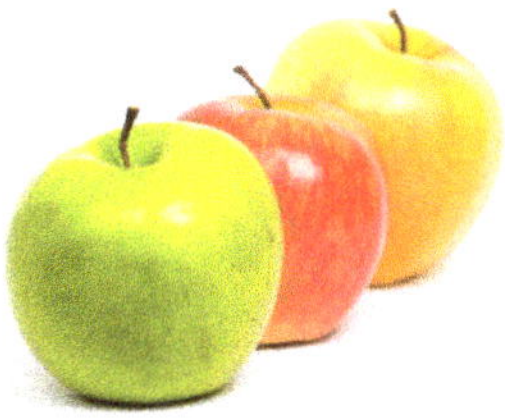

Pick
Learn how to PICK the perfectly delicious fruit here!

Peak Season
The lighter colored sections with small triangles tell you when a fruit is in peak season which means it is fresh, yummy, less expensive, and easier to find!

Store
Learn how to STORE your fruit and keep them fresh until you are ready to eat them.

Seasonality
A fruit may be in-season locally when the months are filled with color.

Fruit Preparation
These photos show you ways the fruit is often prepared.

Cooking Methods
These symbols highlight ways to cook or prepare each fruit and give you ideas for different ways to try them. Check out page 26 to learn more!

Fruit Tidbits
Learn extra information about each fruit from interesting facts to preparation methods.

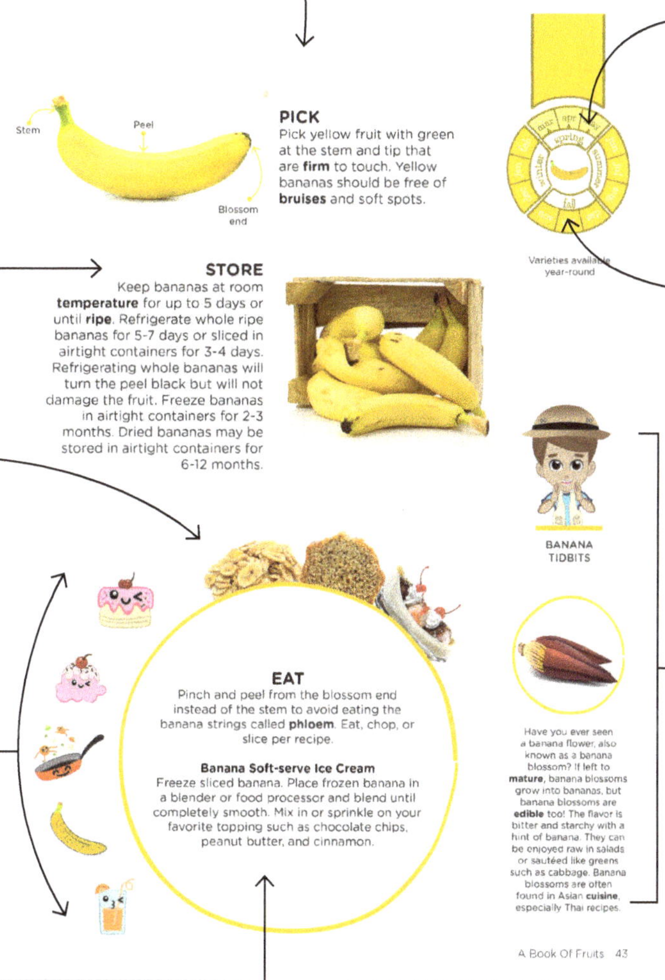
Stem
Peel
Blossom end
PICK
Pick yellow fruit with green at the stem and tip that are **firm** to touch. Yellow bananas should be free of **bruises** and soft spots.
mar
apr
spring
winter
summer
fall
Varieties available year-round
STORE
Keep bananas at room **temperature** for up to 5 days or until **ripe**. Refrigerate whole ripe bananas for 5-7 days or sliced in airtight containers for 3-4 days. Refrigerating whole bananas will turn the peel black but will not damage the fruit. Freeze bananas in airtight containers for 2-3 months. Dried bananas may be stored in airtight containers for 6-12 months.
BANANA TIDBITS
EAT
Pinch and peel from the blossom end instead of the stem to avoid eating the banana strings called **phloem**. Eat, chop, or slice per recipe.
Banana Soft-serve Ice Cream
Freeze sliced banana. Place frozen banana in a blender or food processor and blend until completely smooth. Mix in or sprinkle on your favorite topping such as chocolate chips, peanut butter, and cinnamon.
Have you ever seen a banana flower, also known as a banana blossom? If left to **mature**, banana blossoms grow into bananas, but banana blossoms are **edible** too! The flavor is bitter and starchy with a hint of banana. They can be enjoyed raw in salads or sautéed like greens such as cabbage. Banana blossoms are often found in Asian **cuisine**, especially Thai recipes.
A Book Of Fruits 43

Eat
Learn how to EAT each fruit from raw to cooked and ready for taste-testing. Try the simple recipe, then explore the flavors and textures using your 5 senses!

MY 5 SENSES

This book is all about fruit exploration! Learn how to use your 5 senses on page 22. Become a Food Explorer by picking a fruit to try and using your senses to experience it. Record your observations on the "My 5 Senses Worksheet" found on page 25 or print them from our website for FREE! (www.experiencedeliciousnow.com)

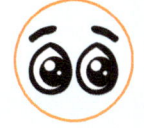

See
Feel
Smell
Taste
Hear

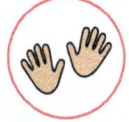

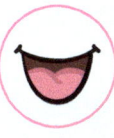

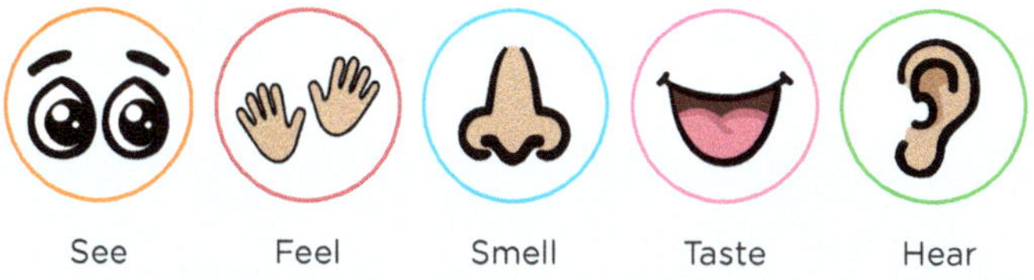

Table of Contents

What Are Fruit and How Do They Grow?	12-13
Types of Fruit Plants	14
Types of Fruit	15-17
How Do Seedless Fruit Grow?	18
When Do Fruit Grow?	19
Good for My Body Nutrients	20-21
Using Your 5 Senses	22-23
My 5 Senses Worksheet	24-25
Cooking Methods	26-27
Origin Map: North America	28
Origin Map: South America	29
Origin Map: Asia and Europe	30
Origin Map: Africa	31
Fruit	32-157
Descriptive Words	158-159
Glossary Words	160-163

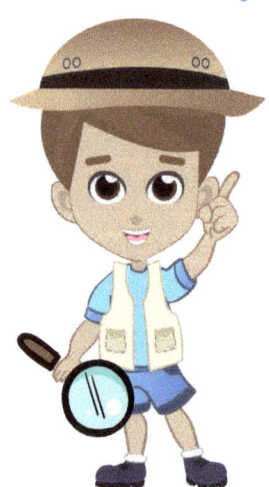

Welcome! We are the Food Explorers in search of delicious. Join us as we discover new tastes and textures on an adventure into the wonderful world of fruit.

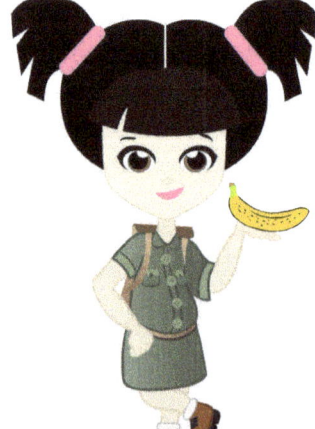

Over the following pages, we hope to enhance your experience with fun facts and interesting tidbits about our favorite fruit.

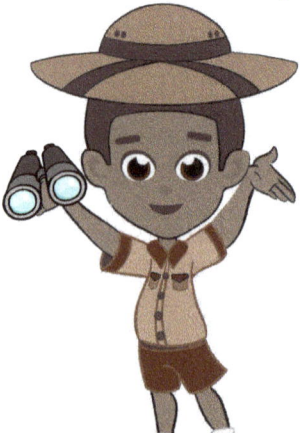

If you don't see your favorite fruit in the Table of Contents, it may be a variety of another similar fruit, for example, a nectarine can be found under Peach Varieties!

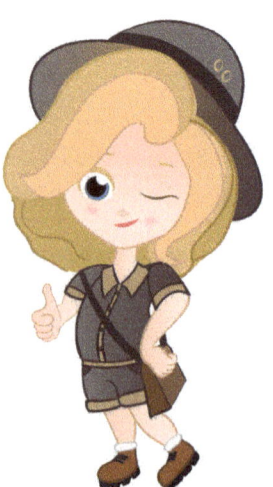

Let's dig in!

	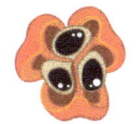			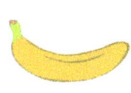			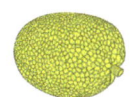
Acai p. 32	Akee p. 34	Apple Varieties p. 36	Apricot p. 40	Banana p. 42	Blackberry p. 44	Blueberry p. 46	Breadfruit p. 48
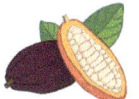	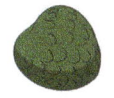			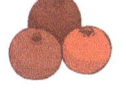		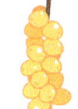	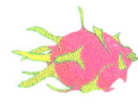
Cacao p. 50	Cherimoya p. 52	Cherry Varieties p. 54	Coconut p. 58	Cranberry p. 60	Currant p. 62	Date p. 64	Dragon Fruit p. 66
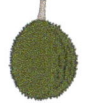	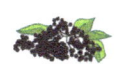			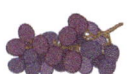	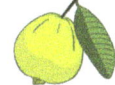	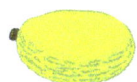	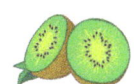
Durian p. 68	Elderberry p. 70	Fig p. 72	Goji Berry p. 74	Grape Varieties p. 76	Guava p. 80	Jackfruit p. 82	Kiwi p. 84
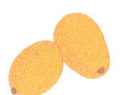	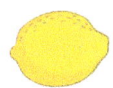	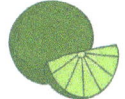	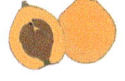				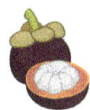
Kumquat p. 86	Lemon p. 88	Lime p. 90	Loquat p. 92	Lychee p. 94	Mamoncillo p. 96	Mango Varieties p. 98	Mangosteen p. 102
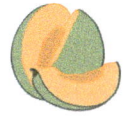	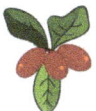	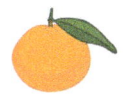	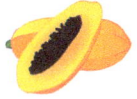	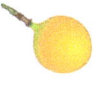	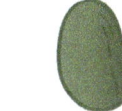	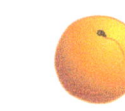	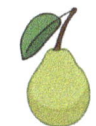
Melon Varieties p. 104	Miracle Berry p. 108	Orange Varieties p. 110	Papaya p. 116	Passion Fruit p. 118	Pawpaw p. 120	Peach Varieties p. 122	Pear Varieties p. 126
	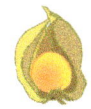			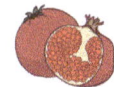		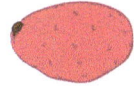	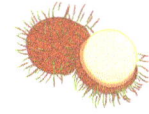
Persimmon p. 130	Physalis p. 132	Pineapple p. 134	Plum Varieties p. 136	Pomegranate p. 140	Pomelo p. 142	Prickly Pear p. 144	Rambutan p. 146
			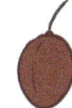				
Raspberry p. 148	Star Fruit p. 150	Strawberry Varieties p. 152	Tamarillo p. 156				

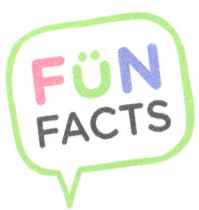

Horticulture is the science of growing fruits, vegetables, and flowers.

What are Fruit and How Do they Grow?

A fruit is the fully-grown and ready-to-eat part of a flower that is **edible** - meaning the part of the flower or plant that is safe to eat.

Most fruit have **seeds** that can grow into new plants.

Plants make their own food or **energy** through **photosynthesis**. They take water and **nutrients** from the soil, **carbon dioxide** from the air, and light from the sun, and **transform** it into **oxygen** and energy in order to grow.

Where Do Bananas Come From?

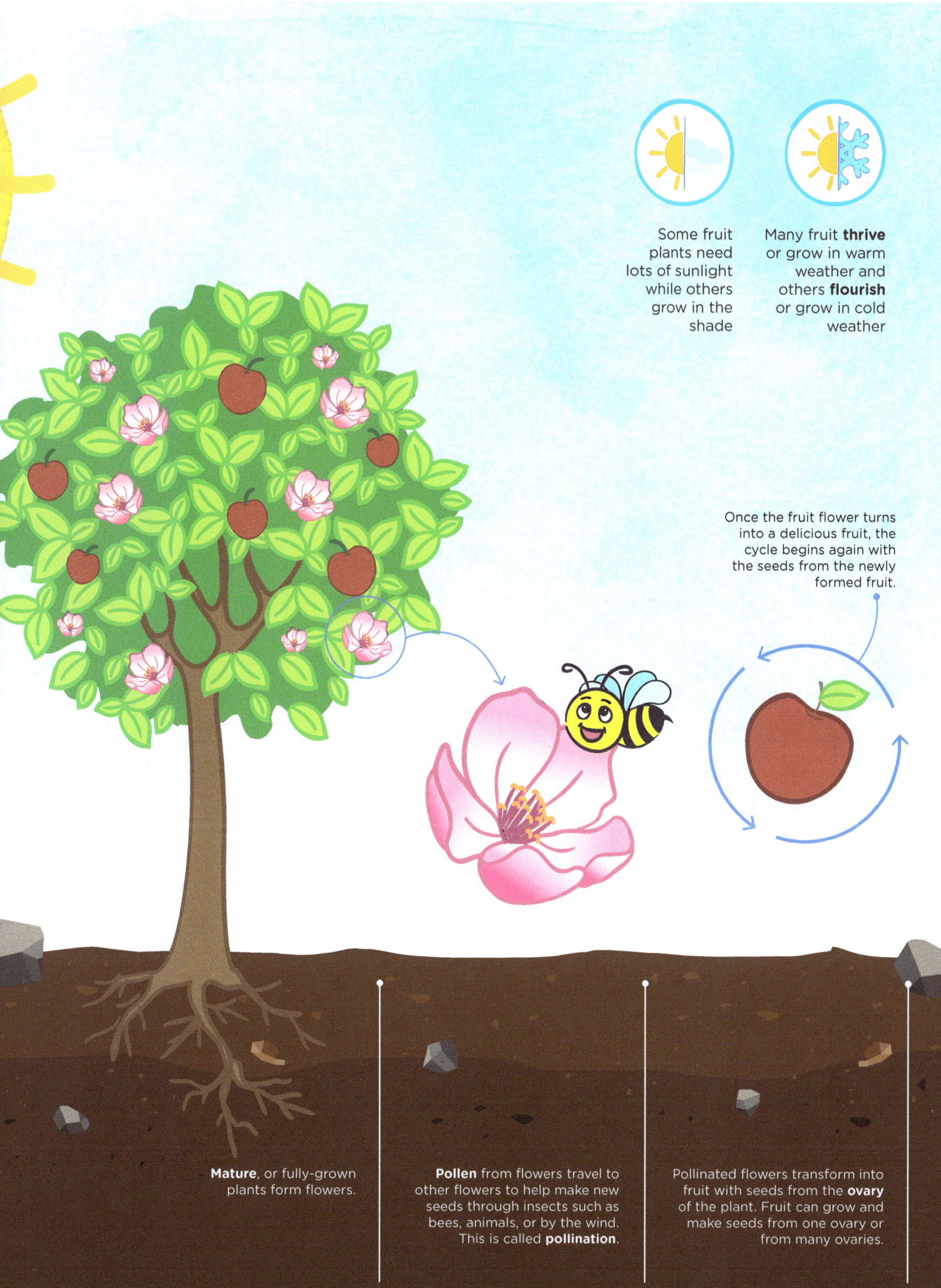

Types of Fruit Plants

Fruit grow from many different types of plants. Below are some examples:

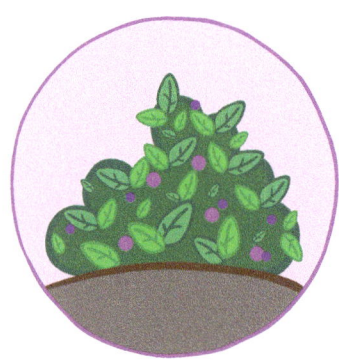

Bush [boo-sh]
small, connected, woody plants with branches and leaves that grow from or close to the ground

Cactus [kak-tuhs]
fleshy, leafless, plants with spiny stems and large flowers

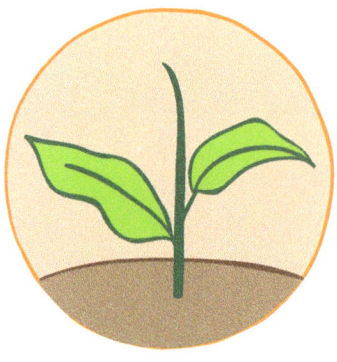

Herbaceous Plant [hur-bey-shuhs]
soft, stemmed plants that are not made of wood

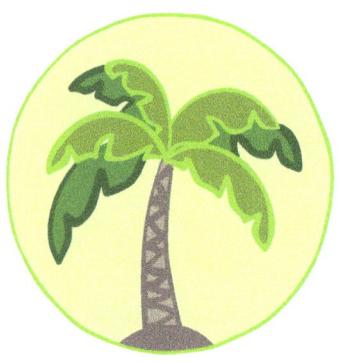

Palm Tree [pahm]
tall, branchless tree with a crown of large leaves

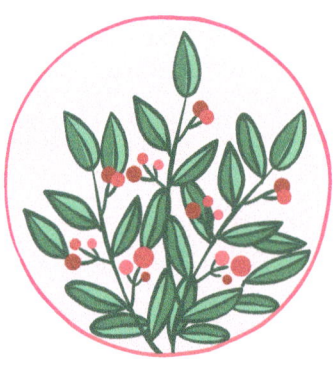

Shrub [shruhb]
small to medium woody plants with **thick** branches and leaves that grow from or close to the ground

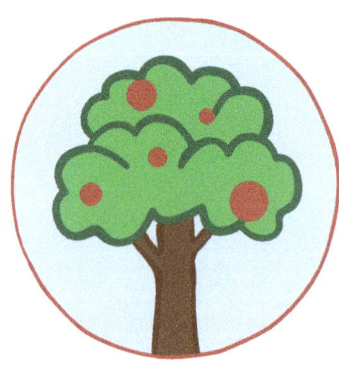

Tree [tree]
tall plant with a woody main stem or trunk and branches

Vine [vahyn]
long, thin-stemmed plants that trails and can grow along the ground or climb

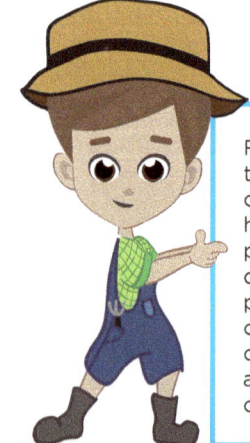

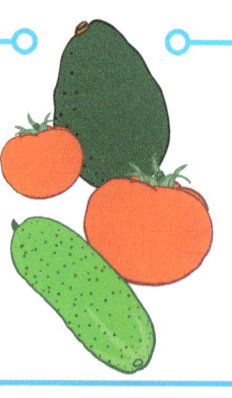

Fruits are **classified** based on how they grow. Some fruit are actually classified as vegetables because of how we eat them! A fruit is the **edible** part of a plant that we eat as a snack or for dessert, like an apple or apple pie. Other fruit such as avocados, cucumbers, and tomatoes are considered vegetables because they are often eaten as part of an appetizer or the main course of a meal.

Types of Fruit

Fruit are **diverse**. Fruit are **classified** based on how they grow and come in all different colors, shapes, and sizes. Some fruit can be eaten whole and other fruit may have tough outer skin, **seeds**, or **pits** that must be removed before you can enjoy them. The three basic fruit classifications, or types of fruit, are **simple fleshy fruit**, **aggregate fruit**, and **multiple fruit**.

Simple Fleshy Fruit
Grow from a SINGLE **ovary** in a SINGLE flower.

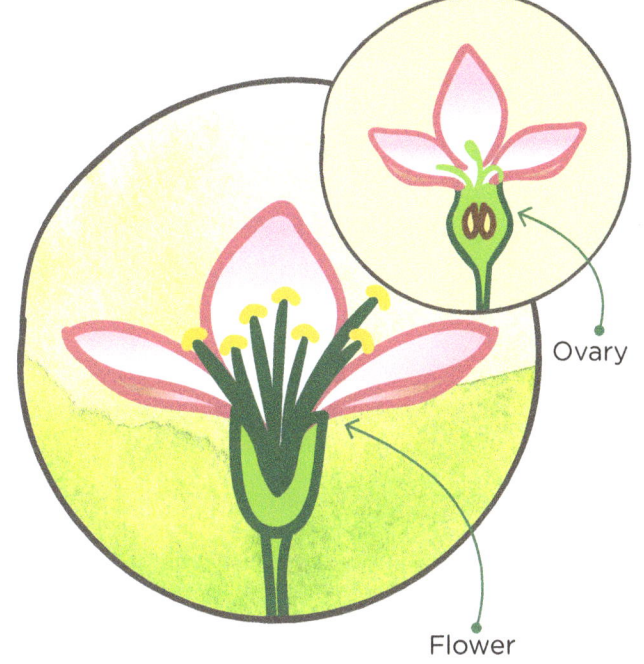

Aggregate Fruit
Grow from SEVERAL ovaries formed in a SINGLE flower.

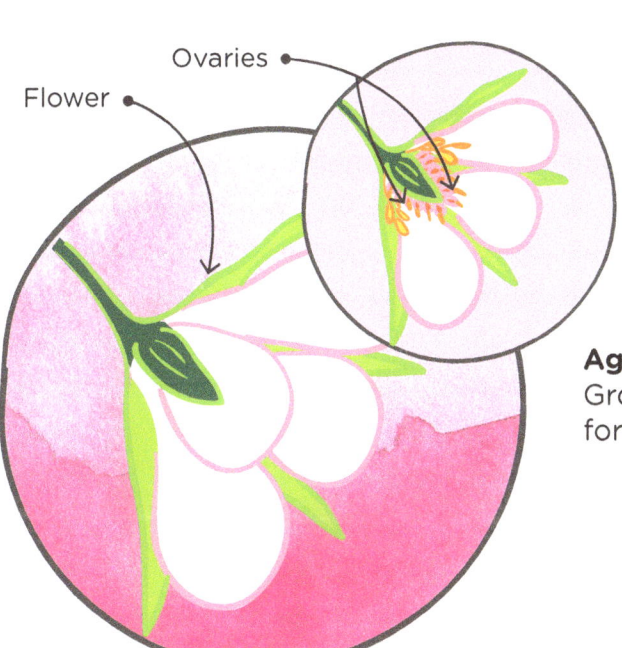

Multiple Fruit
Grow from SEVERAL ovaries formed from MULTIPLE flowers.

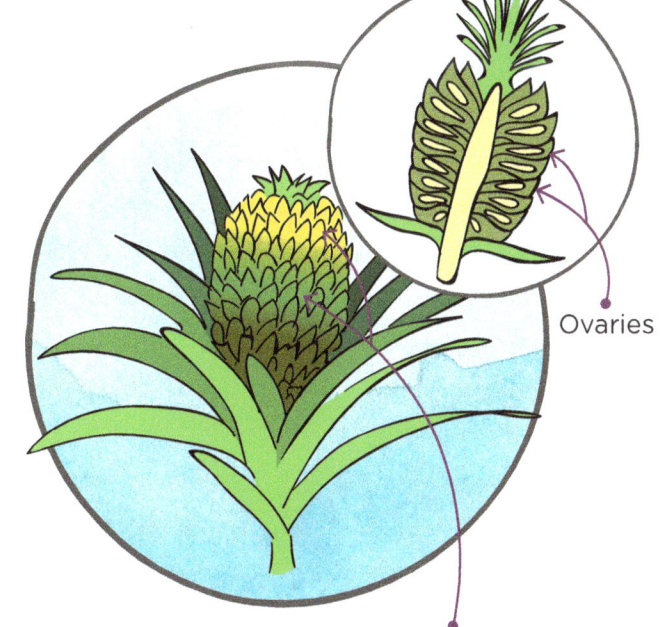

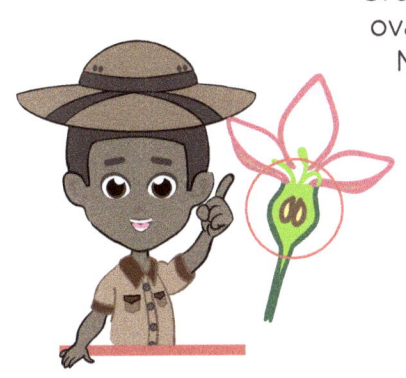

Ovaries are the part of the flower that make **seeds**.

A Book of Fruits

Types of Fruit

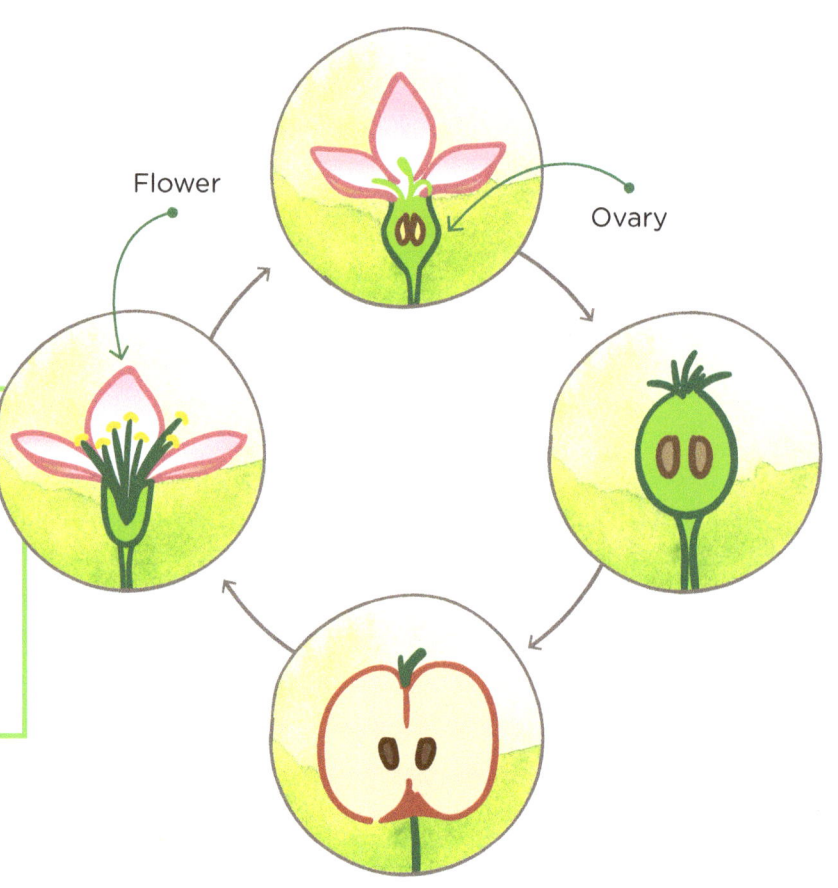

SIMPLE FLESHY FRUIT
Grow from a SINGLE **ovary** in a SINGLE flower. A flower with a single ovary forms a fruit. These fruits are grouped into categories based on how they grow.

Simple Fleshy Fruit Categories

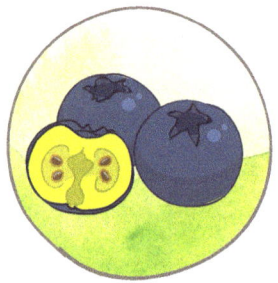

Berry [ber-ee]
fleshy soft-skinned fruit with several **seeds** such as grapes and blueberries

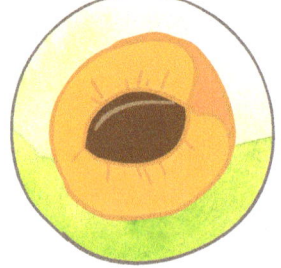

Drupe [droop]
fleshy fruit that surrounds a seed, also known as a **stone** or **pit**, such as plums and peaches

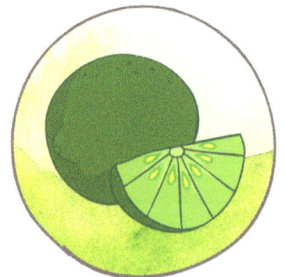

Hesperidium [hes-puh-rid-ee-uhm]
a special family of berries with a leathery outer skin or **rind** and divided fleshy interior such as oranges and lemons

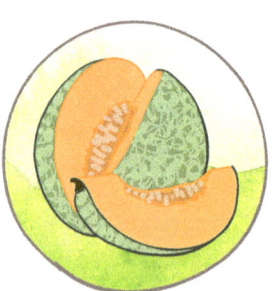

Pepo [pee-poh]
a family of berries with a hard-outer skin or rind such as cantaloupes and watermelons

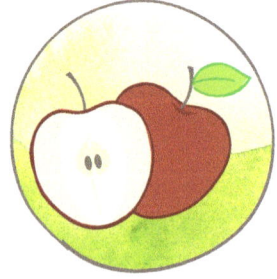

Pome [pohm]
fleshy fruit that surrounds a seeded core such as apples and pears

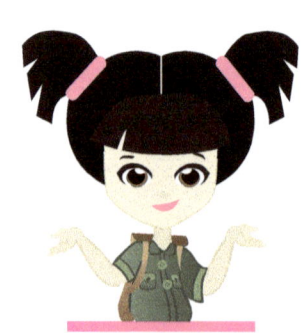

Fruit is a way that some plants spread their seeds and grow more fruit!

Types of Fruit

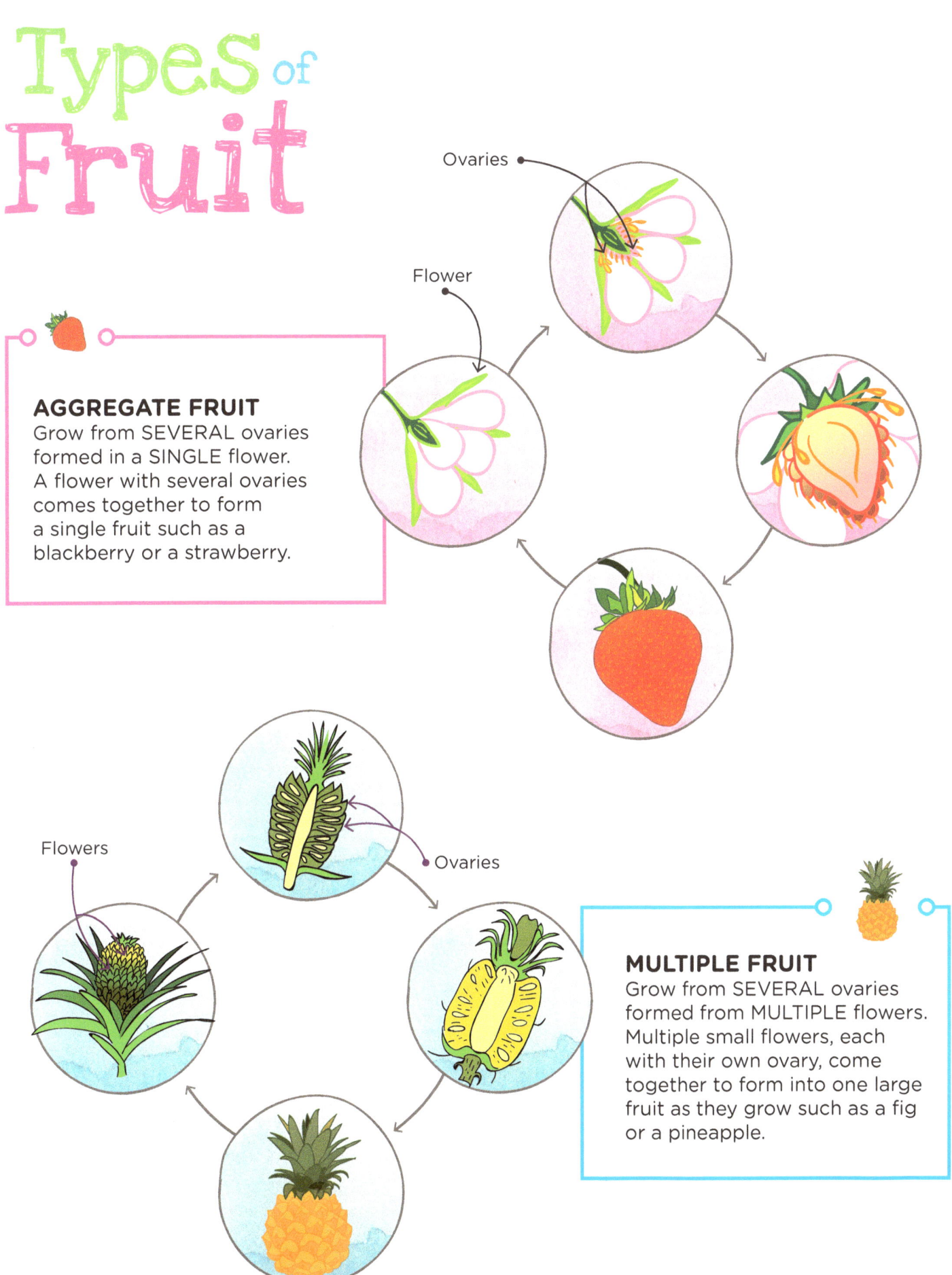

AGGREGATE FRUIT
Grow from SEVERAL ovaries formed in a SINGLE flower. A flower with several ovaries comes together to form a single fruit such as a blackberry or a strawberry.

MULTIPLE FRUIT
Grow from SEVERAL ovaries formed from MULTIPLE flowers. Multiple small flowers, each with their own ovary, come together to form into one large fruit as they grow such as a fig or a pineapple.

A Book of Fruits

How Do Seedless Fruit Grow?

Have you ever eaten a fruit that did not have any **seeds**? If plants grow from seeds, then how do seedless fruit grow more plants?

Seedless fruit varieties develop both naturally in the wild or can be **cultivated** by **farmers**. Farmers use a process called **parthenocarpy** to grow new fruit without seeds through **cuttings** of a root, stem, or leaf cut from a specific plant. Farmers can cultivate new fruit based on selecting desired qualities such as no seeds, an appealing **flavor**, or preferred **texture**.

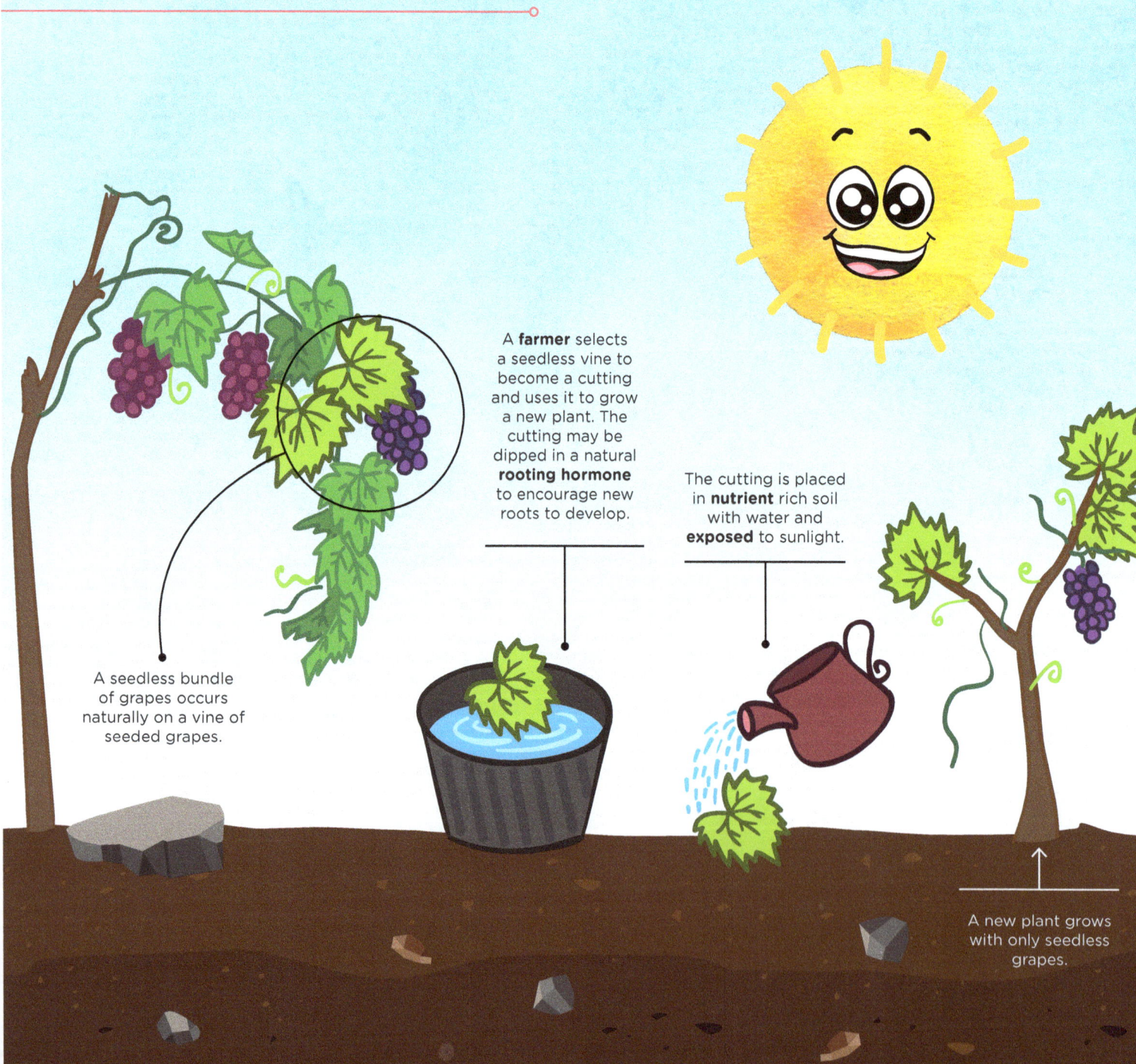

A seedless bundle of grapes occurs naturally on a vine of seeded grapes.

A **farmer** selects a seedless vine to become a cutting and uses it to grow a new plant. The cutting may be dipped in a natural **rooting hormone** to encourage new roots to develop.

The cutting is placed in **nutrient** rich soil with water and **exposed** to sunlight.

A new plant grows with only seedless grapes.

When Do Fruit Grow?

Fruits are **seasonal** which means they grow and are **harvested** based on the time of year and location. Varying **climates** mean that fruits and vegetables may only be available locally at certain times of year and can differ from place to place. Visit your local **farmer's** market to see what produce is in season near you!

When fruits are in season, they are fresh, yummy, less expensive, and easier to find!

Winter
December to February
Winter is the coldest season and sometimes brings snow

Spring
March to May
Spring is the rainy season when flowers start to blossom

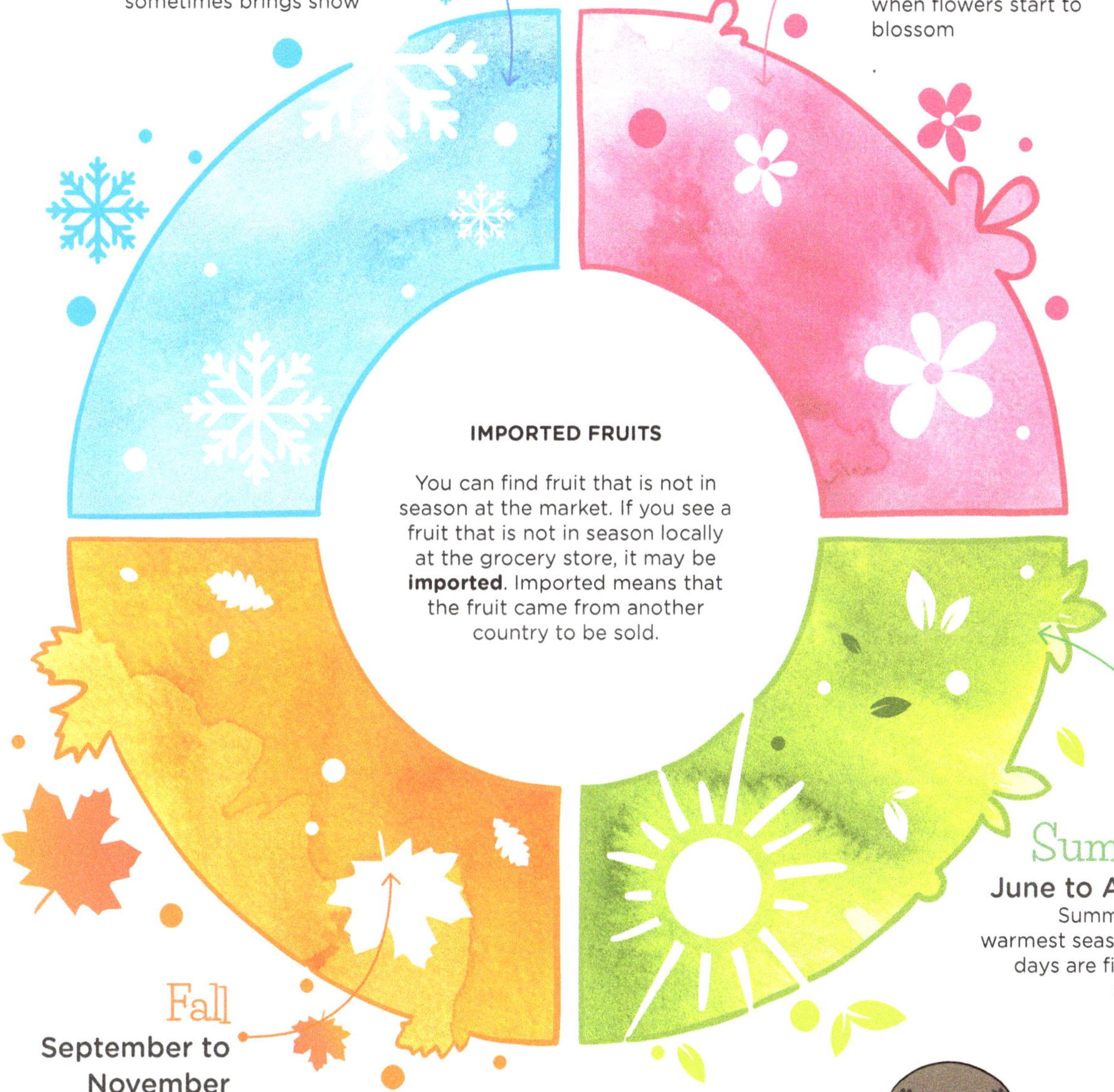

Summer
June to August
Summer is the warmest season when days are filled with sunshine

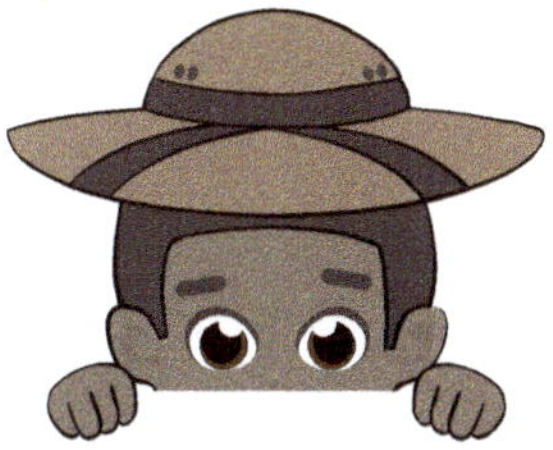

Fall
September to November
Fall brings cooler weather and leaves start to drop from trees

IMPORTED FRUITS
You can find fruit that is not in season at the market. If you see a fruit that is not in season locally at the grocery store, it may be **imported**. Imported means that the fruit came from another country to be sold.

Seasonality in this book is based on availability in North America.

A Book of Fruits 19

Good for my Body Nutrients

Fruit is important to keep our bodies healthy because they are filled with **nutrients**. Nutrients are the part of food that help our bodies function or work their best.

Each fruit contains many different nutrients such as **vitamins**, **minerals**, **antioxidants**, and **phytonutrients**. These nutrients work together in the body to help us grow healthy and strong, learn our best in school, play sports, and fight off sickness.

We call vitamins, minerals, and antioxidants Good for My Body Nutrients (GFMBN)!

When you see these **symbols** along with a fruit you will know how they help your growing body.

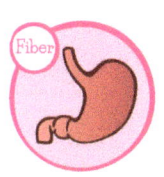
FIBER [fahy-ber]
helps keep your heart healthy, your insides clean by moving food through your **digestive system**, and makes your tummy feel full. **Digestion** is how your body gets **nutrients** and **energy** from the food you eat.

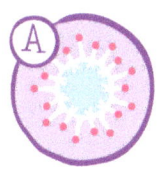
VITAMIN A
supports a healthy immune system, your body's defense to fight sickness. Vitamin A also helps with eyesight, especially at night, as well as with growth, development, and healthy skin.

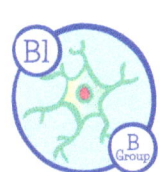
VITAMIN B1
(Thiamin) [thi-a-min]
supports your body's **nervous system**, the body's super highway that controls how your body works. Vitamin B1 also helps your body use energy from the food you eat.

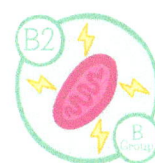
VITAMIN B2
(Riboflavin) [ri-bo-flay-vin]
helps your body use energy from the food you eat so your body works at its best. Vitamin B2 also assists other vitamins to do their jobs in your body which helps keep you healthy and active!

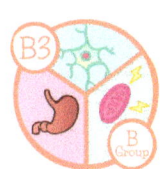
VITAMIN B3
(Niacin) [ni-a-cin]
supports many functions in the body from assisting with digestive health, to supporting your body's nervous system, and using energy from the food you eat. Vitamin B3 also helps with growth and healthy skin.

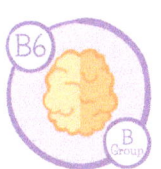
VITAMIN B6
(Pyridoxine) [pyr-i-dox-ine]
supports brain function and helps your body make red blood cells that carry **oxygen** throughout your body. Vitamin B6 also helps your body use energy from the food you eat and supports a healthy immune system.

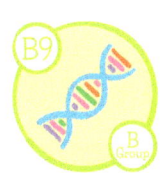
VITAMIN B9
(Folate) [foll-ate]
helps make **DNA**, the instruction manual for your body. Vitamin B9 also helps your body make red blood **cells** that carry oxygen throughout your body so you can run and play.

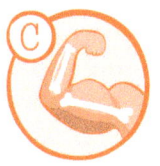
VITAMIN C
promotes strong muscles and bones so you can be active and play your favorite sports. Vitamin C also supports healthy skin, teeth, brain cells, and helps heal cuts when you get a scrape.

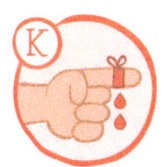
VITAMIN K
helps blood to **clot** or stop bleeding when you get cuts and scrapes.

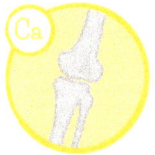
CALCIUM [kal-see-uhm]
is a **mineral** that helps build strong bones and teeth, keeps your heart beating strong, and supports your body's nervous system.

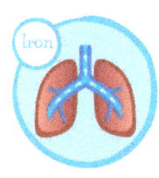
IRON [ahy-ern]
is a mineral that works like a big yellow school bus transporting oxygen from your lungs to your whole body and keeps you moving.

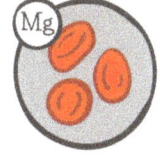
MAGNESIUM [mag-nes-c-um]
is a mineral used by every cell in your body. Magnesium helps turn the food we eat into energy, and supports healthy bones, muscles, and nerves.

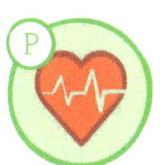
POTASSIUM [po-tas-c-um]
is a mineral that helps your heart and muscles function. Potassium aids in maintaining the balance of water and **electrolytes** in your body so you can feel good and play sports longer!

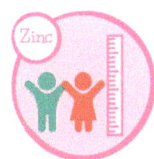
ZINC [zingk]
is a mineral important for growing up healthy. Zinc helps your **immune system** fight off sickness, and heals cuts and scrapes. Zinc also supports your sense of smell for tasting new foods!

Good for My Body Nutrients (GFMBN) are based on data from a 1 cup serving using the United States Department of Agriculture (USDA) nutrient database, or accessible research studies. GFMBN are defined as a "good source" based on the Recommended Dietary Allowances (RDAs) providing at least 10% of the percent Daily Value (% DV) of the Reference Daily Intakes (RDIs) with Daily Reference Values (DRVs) established by the Food and Drug Administration (FDA).

Using Your 5 Senses

Bananas, you've probably eaten a least a few, but have you explored them?

Do you like bananas? What do you like about them? How do you like to eat them? Do you eat bananas on top of breakfast cereal or baked into bread?

Exploring foods with our 5 senses is fun and can help us discover and engage with what we eat. Learning and using descriptive words is a tool that helps us identify unique qualities about foods and explain what we like or dislike about something.

When you sit down for a meal or snack take a moment to think about how it looks, how it smells, how it sounds, how it feels in your mouth, and how it tastes using your 5 senses.

It's like your very own experiment every time you eat!

5 Senses

Can you describe a banana? Each preparation method can change the experience. We can use our 5 senses to discover things we never knew we liked about a food!

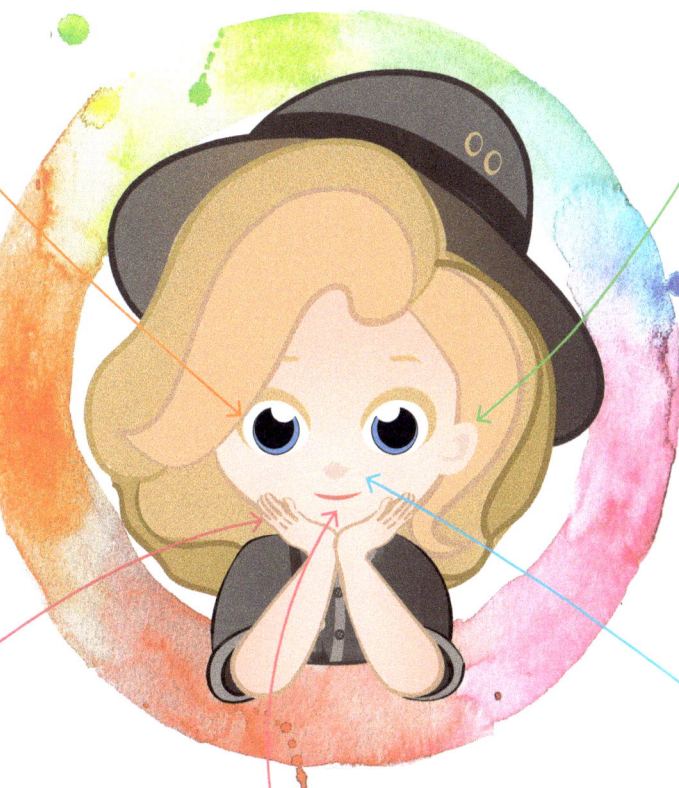

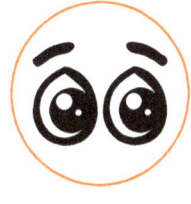

See

Let's take a closer look at the banana. What colors and **textures** do you SEE? It is green, yellow, yellow with brown spots, or black? Do bananas remind you of anything?

Hear

What sound do you HEAR when you run your fingers over raw peeled banana? Is it silent or does it make a sticky sound? Now take a bite. Did you HEAR anything? Keep chewing. Are there any sounds? Is each bite a sticky nibble or a quiet chew?

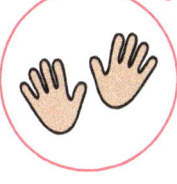

Feel

How does a banana skin FEEL in your hands? Is the texture soft, smooth, or both? What about when you peel the skin back? What does the texture FEEL like in your hands or when you take a bite? Is it **firm**, sticky, or mushy? Is each bite soft and tender? Try this with a raw banana and when baked into banana bread!

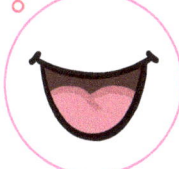

Taste

How does a banana TASTE? What is the **flavor**? Can you describe it? Is it sweet or starchy? Does it have a flavor at all? Does it TASTE different when it is raw than when it is baked into something? Which do you like better and why?

Smell

Have you ever sniffed a banana? That might sound silly, but SMELLING food is a big part of tasting! Hold a piece of banana up to your nose and take a good whiff. What does a banana SMELL like? Does it SMELL floral, sweet, or candy-like? Does it have a scent at all?

A Book of Fruits

My 5 Senses

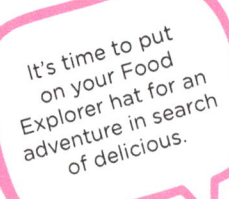

It's time to put on your Food Explorer hat for an adventure in search of delicious.

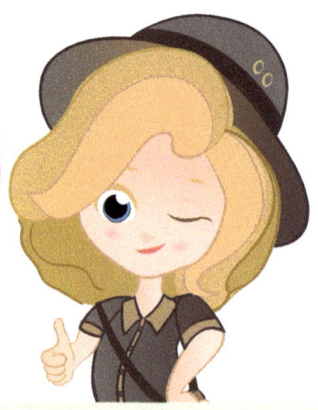

Pick a fruit and use your senses to experience it!

Notice the colors and shapes of the fruit. Feel the fruit in your fingers and listen for any sounds. Lift the fruit to your nose and give it a smell. Now take a bite. How does it taste? What does the **texture** feel like in your mouth? Does it make funny sounds when you chew it? How was it **prepared**? Was it raw, juiced, or baked?

Download the "My 5 Senses Worksheet" for FREE on our website.

www.experiencedeliciousnow.com

Fill out the worksheet for each fruit and the different way you experience them. Write down as many descriptive words as you can! Use the Descriptive Words table on pages 158-159 to help you!

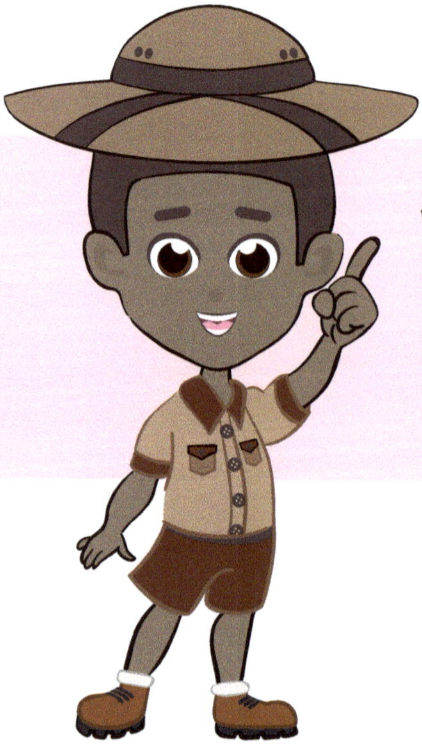

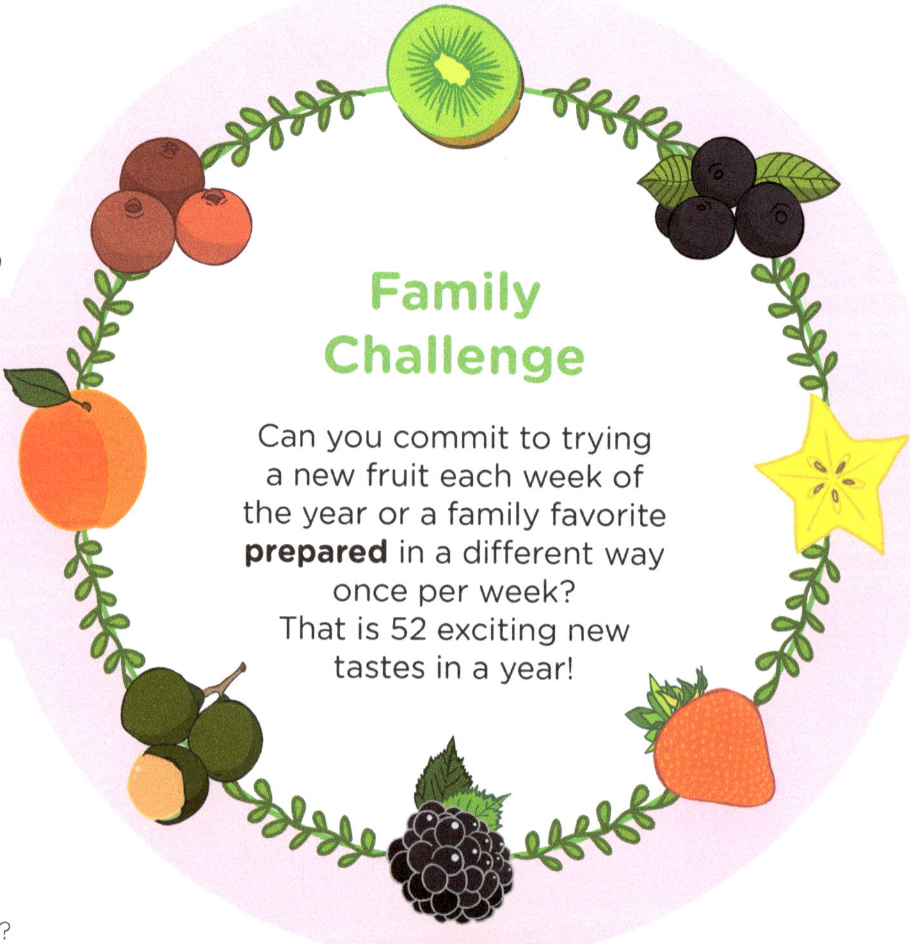

Family Challenge

Can you commit to trying a new fruit each week of the year or a family favorite **prepared** in a different way once per week? That is 52 exciting new tastes in a year!

5 Senses

Can you describe a banana? Each preparation method can change the experience. We can use our 5 senses to discover things we never knew we liked about a food!

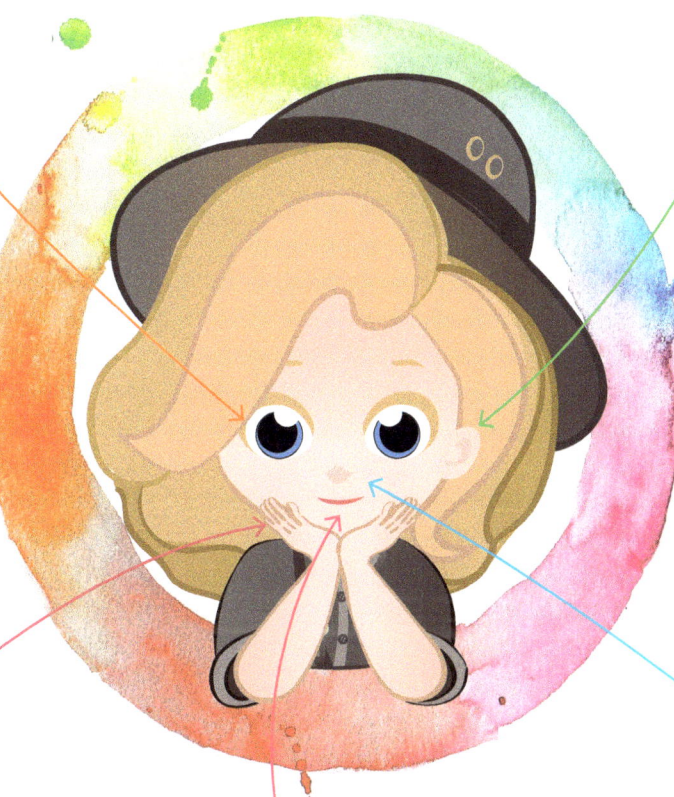

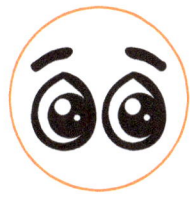

See

Let's take a closer look at the banana. What colors and **textures** do you SEE? It is green, yellow, yellow with brown spots, or black? Do bananas remind you of anything?

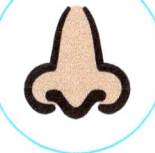

Hear

What sound do you HEAR when you run your fingers over raw peeled banana? Is it silent or does it make a sticky sound? Now take a bite. Did you HEAR anything? Keep chewing. Are there any sounds? Is each bite a sticky nibble or a quiet chew?

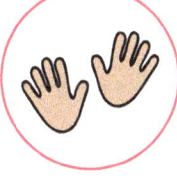

Feel

How does a banana skin FEEL in your hands? Is the texture soft, smooth, or both? What about when you peel the skin back? What does the texture FEEL like in your hands or when you take a bite? Is it **firm**, sticky, or mushy? Is each bite soft and tender? Try this with a raw banana and when baked into banana bread!

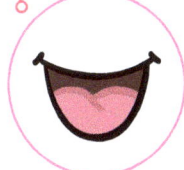

Taste

How does a banana TASTE? What is the **flavor**? Can you describe it? Is it sweet or starchy? Does it have a flavor at all? Does it TASTE different when it is raw than when it is baked into something? Which do you like better and why?

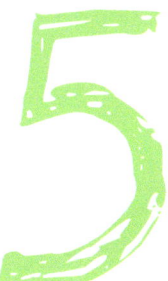

Smell

Have you ever sniffed a banana? That might sound silly, but SMELLING food is a big part of tasting! Hold a piece of banana up to your nose and take a good whiff. What does a banana SMELL like? Does it SMELL floral, sweet, or candy-like? Does it have a scent at all?

A Book of Fruits

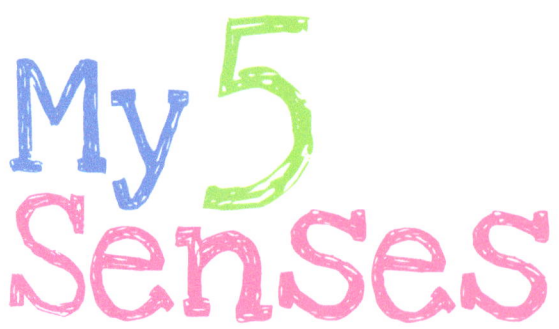

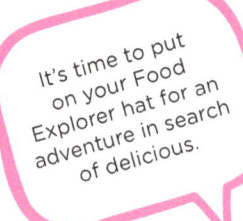

It's time to put on your Food Explorer hat for an adventure in search of delicious.

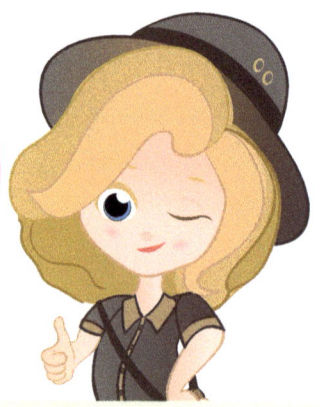

Pick a fruit and use your senses to experience it!

Notice the colors and shapes of the fruit. Feel the fruit in your fingers and listen for any sounds. Lift the fruit to your nose and give it a smell. Now take a bite. How does it taste? What does the **texture** feel like in your mouth? Does it make funny sounds when you chew it? How was it **prepared**? Was it raw, juiced, or baked?

Download the "My 5 Senses Worksheet" for FREE on our website.

www.experiencedeliciousnow.com

Fill out the worksheet for each fruit and the different way you experience them. Write down as many descriptive words as you can! Use the Descriptive Words table on pages 158-159 to help you!

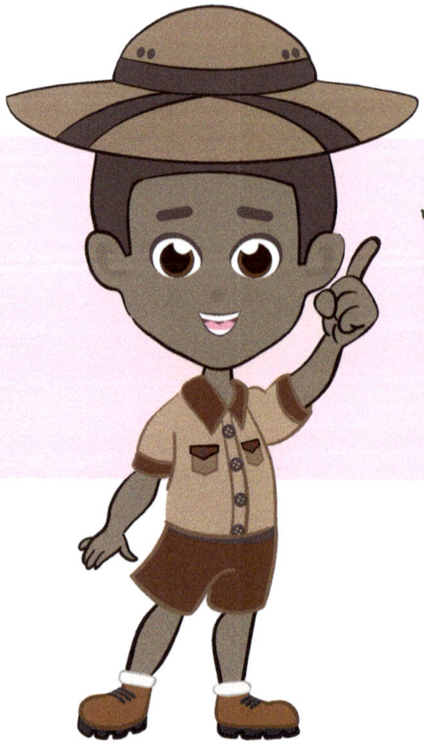

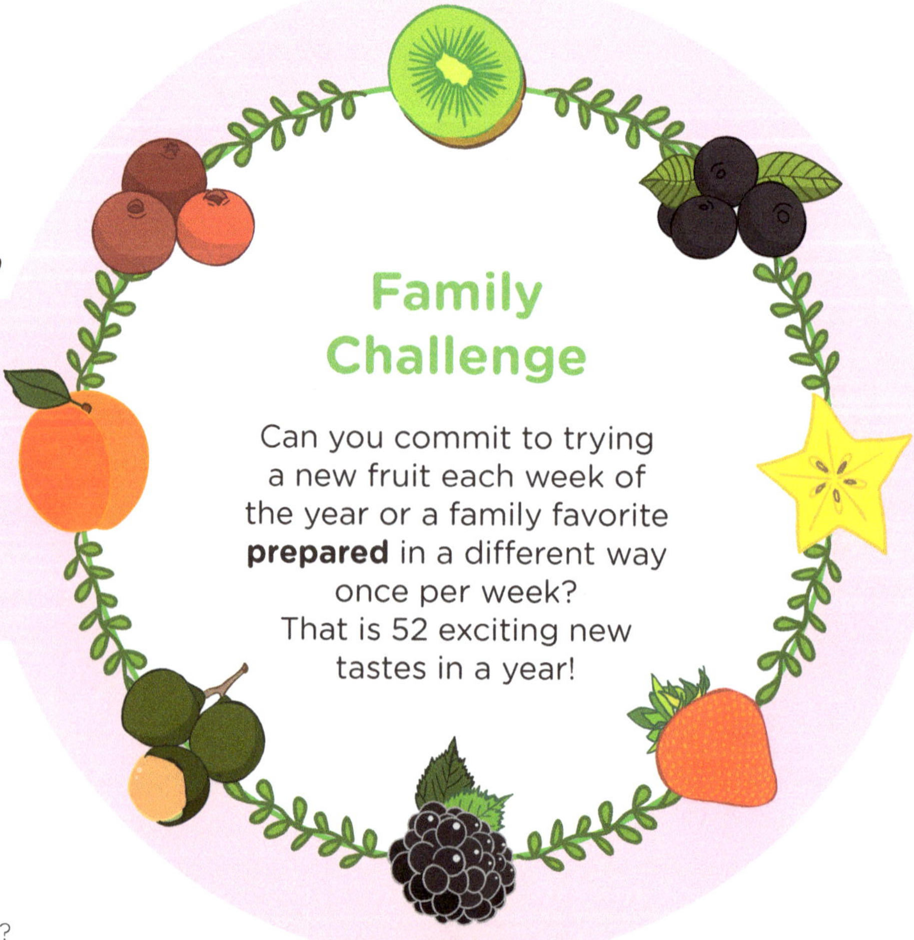

Family Challenge

Can you commit to trying a new fruit each week of the year or a family favorite **prepared** in a different way once per week? That is 52 exciting new tastes in a year!

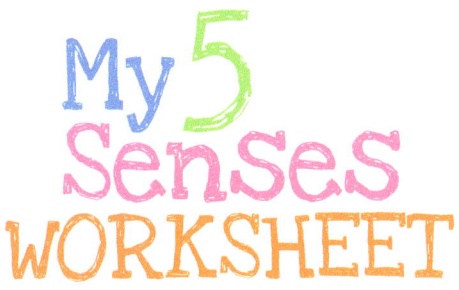
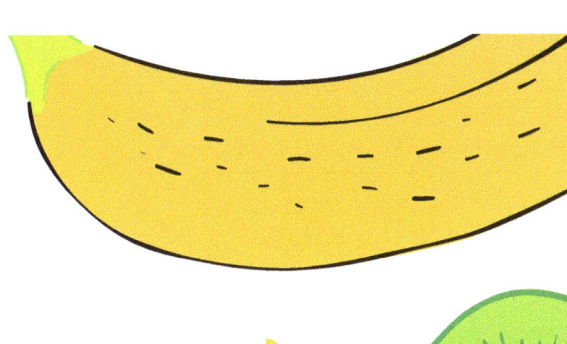

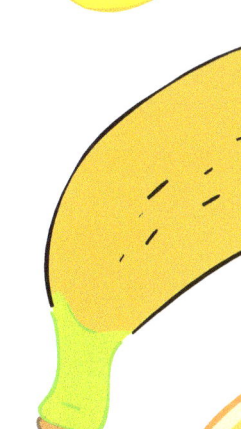

Fruit Name _____

Preparation Method _____

Did you like this fruit?

  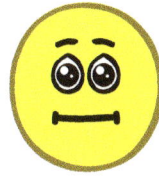   

Cooking Methods

There are so many wonderful and delicious ways to **prepare** fruits! In this book you will see **symbols** that give you ideas for how to try a new fruit. Below are a few explanations of common cooking methods to get you started.

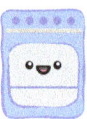
Bake or Roast
Cook with dry heat, typically in an oven.

Dried
A food that water or juice has been removed through sun drying, dry heat, or **dehydrators**.

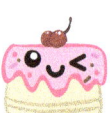
Baked Goods
Cooked food usually made from some type of flour or grain with dry heat. Baking typically refers to foods such as breads, cakes, cookies, muffins, pastries, and pies.

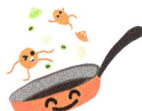
Fry, Sauté, Stir-fry
Cooking food in oil or fat is known as frying. To sauté, heat food in a small amount of fat (e.g., butter, oil) in a pan or wok on top of a stove or heat source. Preparing stir-fry is similar to sautéing food; however, stir-frying is typically at a higher **temperature** and the food is stirred when being cooked.

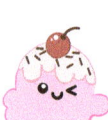
Dessert
Sweet foods such as cakes, cookies, ice cream, pies, and pudding. Desserts are typically served at the end of a meal.

Garnish
A food that is meant to be eaten as a topping or as an addition to other foods. Garnishes add **flavor**, **texture**, or decoration.

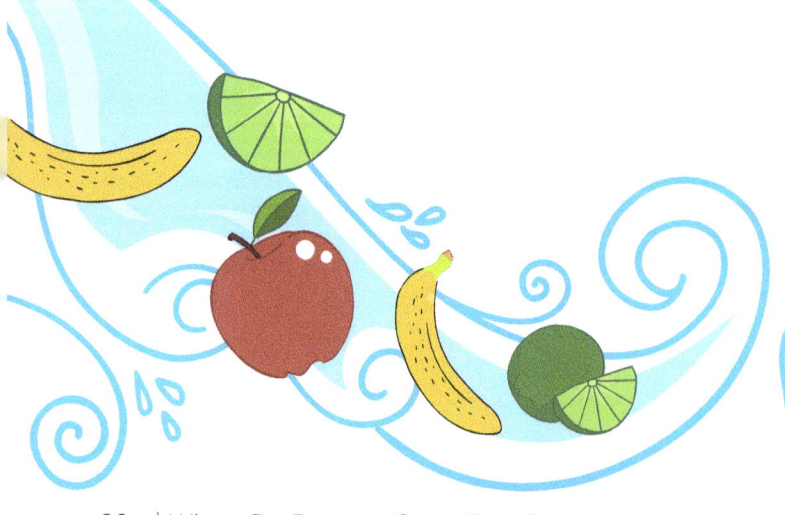

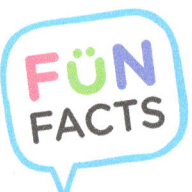
The flesh on some fruits such as apples and bananas turn brown when **exposed** to **oxygen** or air. To prevent browning, brush or dip fruit slices in lemon, lime, pineapple, or orange juice. The **vitamin** C in these juices helps protect fruit from the air.

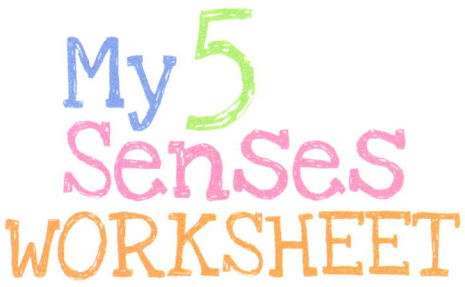
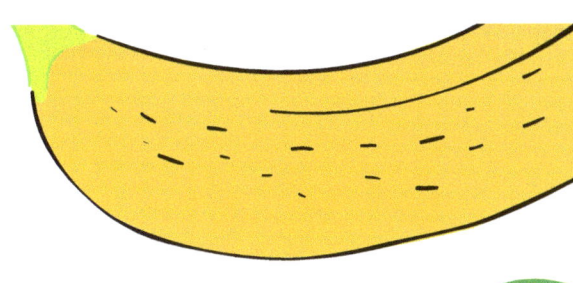

Fruit Name _____

Preparation Method _____

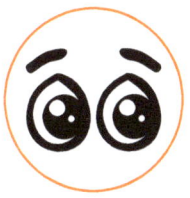
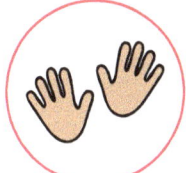
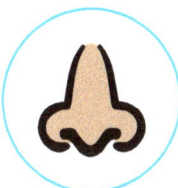
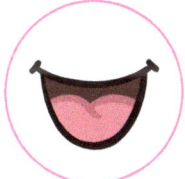
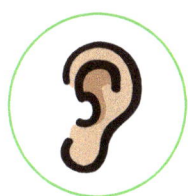

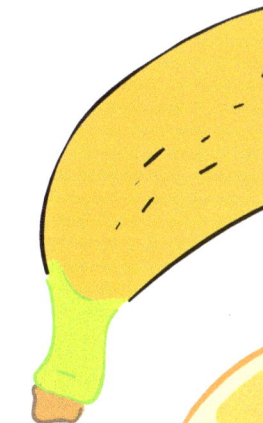

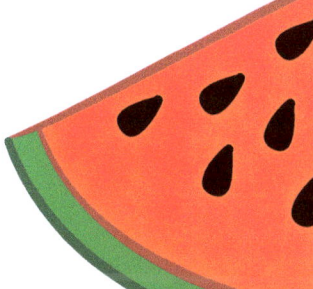

Did you like this fruit?

  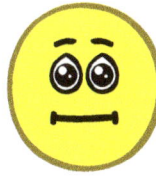   

Cooking Methods

There are so many wonderful and delicious ways to **prepare** fruits! In this book you will see **symbols** that give you ideas for how to try a new fruit. Below are a few explanations of common cooking methods to get you started.

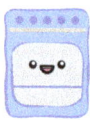

Bake or Roast
Cook with dry heat, typically in an oven.

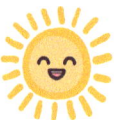

Dried
A food that water or juice has been removed through sun drying, dry heat, or **dehydrators**.

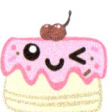

Baked Goods
Cooked food usually made from some type of flour or grain with dry heat. Baking typically refers to foods such as breads, cakes, cookies, muffins, pastries, and pies.

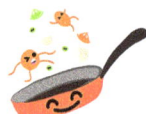

Fry, Sauté, Stir-fry
Cooking food in oil or fat is known as frying. To sauté, heat food in a small amount of fat (e.g., butter, oil) in a pan or wok on top of a stove or heat source. Preparing stir-fry is similar to sautéing food; however, stir-frying is typically at a higher **temperature** and the food is stirred when being cooked.

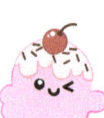

Dessert
Sweet foods such as cakes, cookies, ice cream, pies, and pudding. Desserts are typically served at the end of a meal.

Garnish
A food that is meant to be eaten as a topping or as an addition to other foods. Garnishes add **flavor**, **texture**, or decoration.

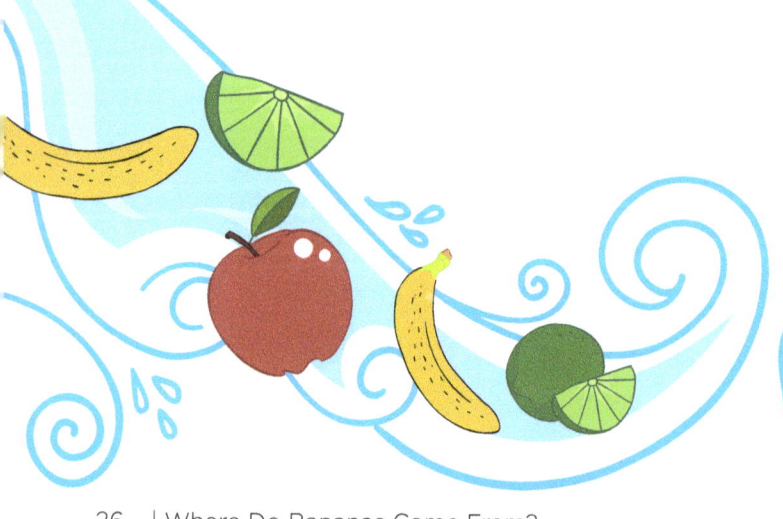

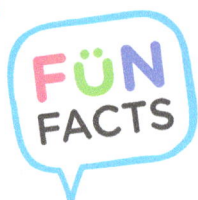

The flesh on some fruits such as apples and bananas turn brown when **exposed** to **oxygen** or air. To prevent browning, brush or dip fruit slices in lemon, lime, pineapple, or orange juice. The **vitamin** C in these juices helps protect fruit from the air.

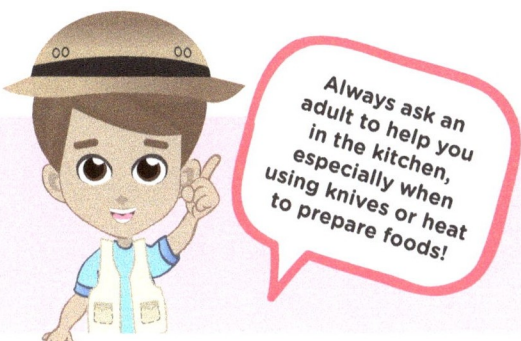

Always ask an adult to help you in the kitchen, especially when using knives or heat to prepare foods!

Temperature is a measurement that indicates how hot or cold something is and can be measured using a thermometer in degrees **Fahrenheit** or degrees **Celsius**. Fahrenheit is labeled as degrees F in this book.

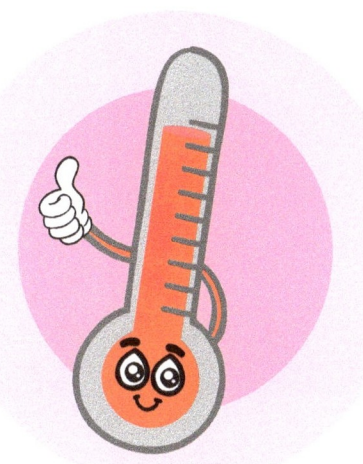

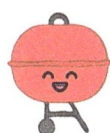
Grill or Barbeque
Cook foods with direct, dry heat from fire on a grated surface with thin, parallel, metal bars.

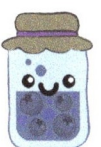
Pickle or Ferment
Food storage and preparation methods that may include placing food in vinegar, **brine**, or **helpful bacteria**, also known as **probiotics**.

Jam, Jelly, Marmalade, Sauce, or Syrup
Foods **prepared** to be eaten as a topping or as an addition to other foods. They are available in many consistencies and textures including liquid, semi-liquid, **thick**, and chunky.

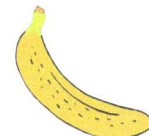
Raw or Fresh
Raw food is when something is eaten in its natural, uncooked form.

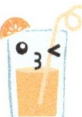
Juice or Smoothie
A preparation method of fruits and vegetables that **transforms** them into a liquid ready to drink. Juicing removes the liquid from a food and smoothies blend food into a liquid.

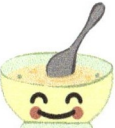
Soup or Stew
A preparation method when liquids are blended, boiled, or simmered with ingredients such as meats, beans, fruits, and vegetables. Stews typically have less liquid than soups and are a thicker texture.

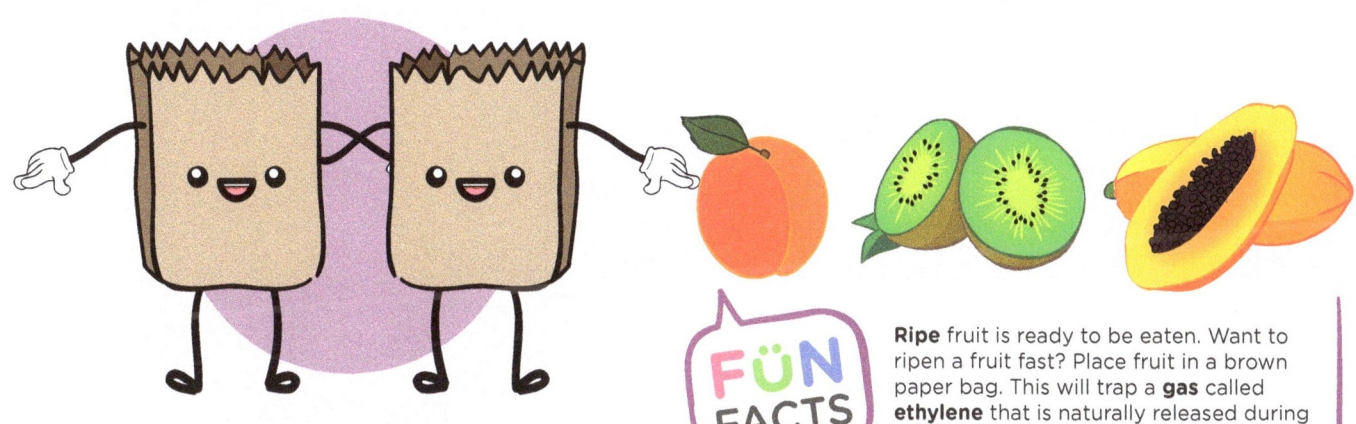

FUN FACTS

Ripe fruit is ready to be eaten. Want to ripen a fruit fast? Place fruit in a brown paper bag. This will trap a **gas** called **ethylene** that is naturally released during ripening and helps to soften fruit.

A Book of Fruits

North America

Have you ever wondered where people first discovered the fruits you eat? These maps of the world will show you where early Food Explorers are thought to have originally tasted the fruits in this book!

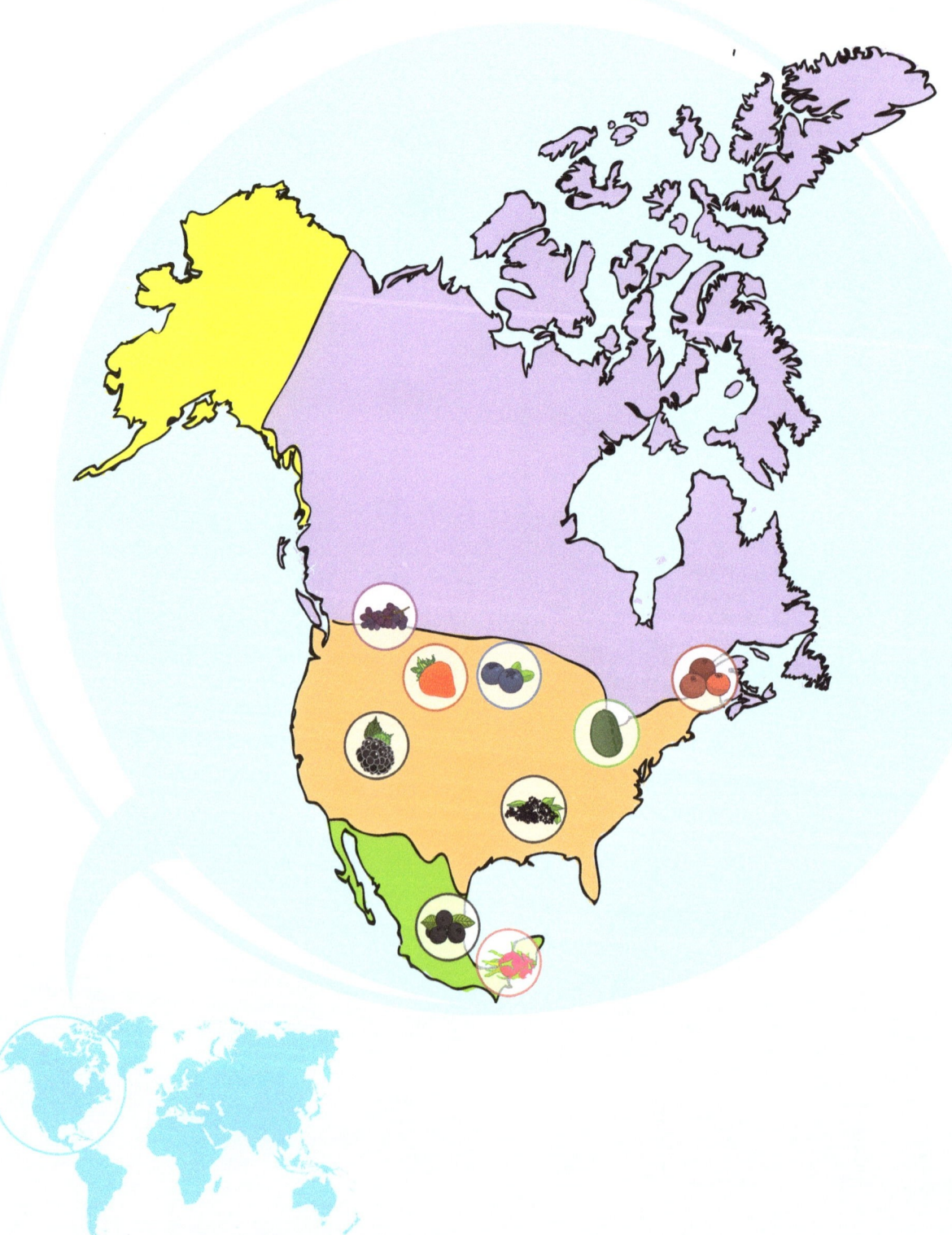

South America

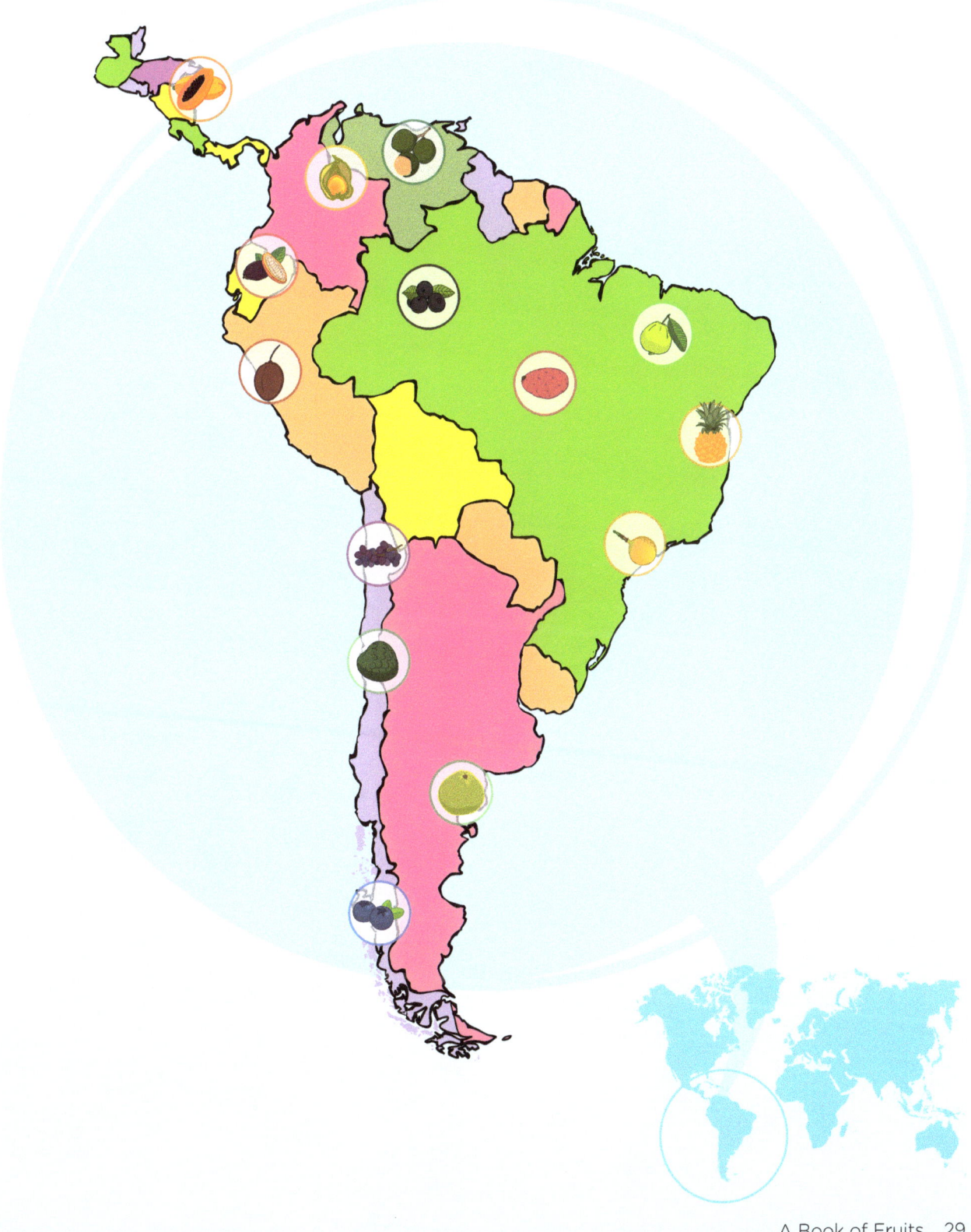

Asia and Europe

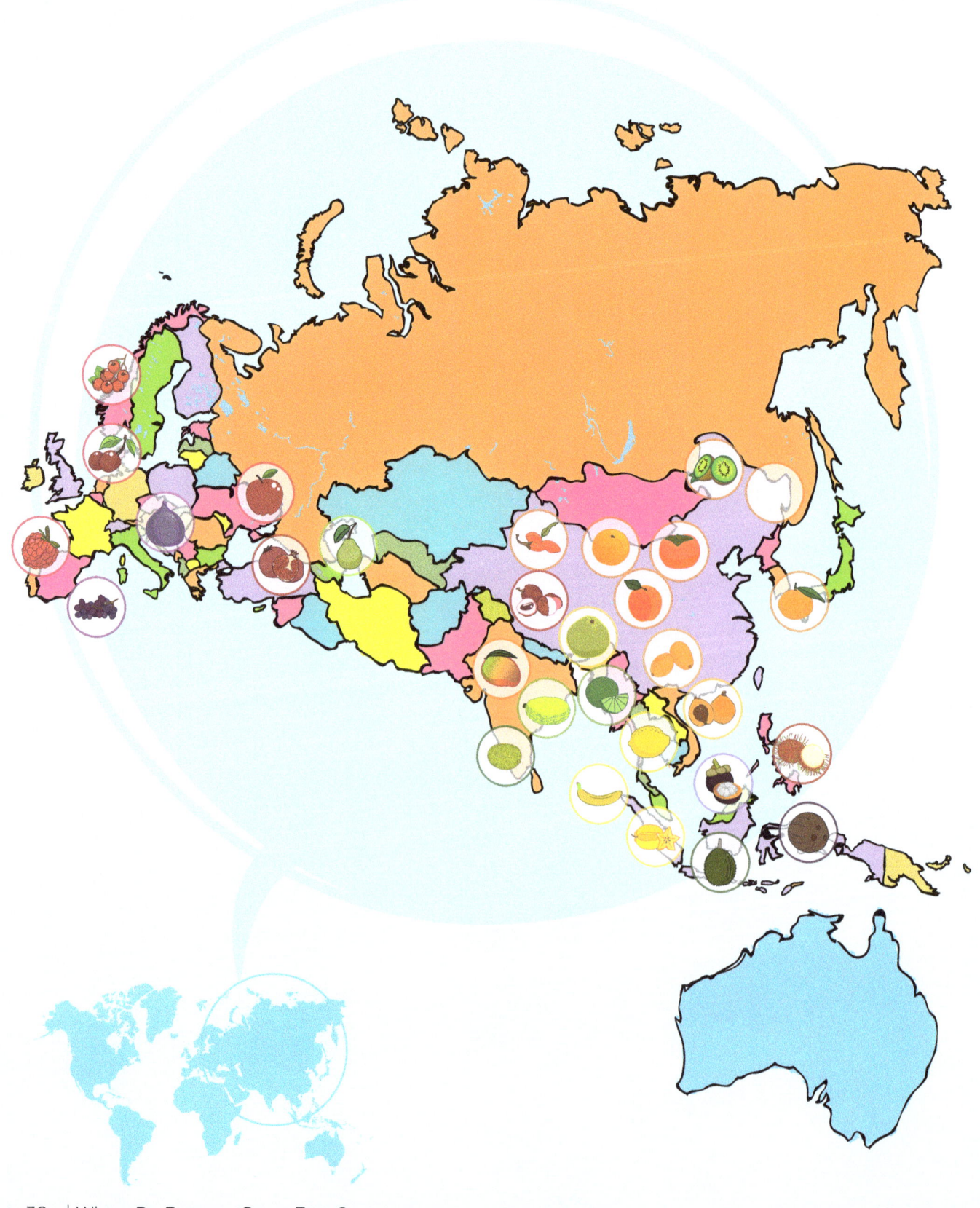

Africa

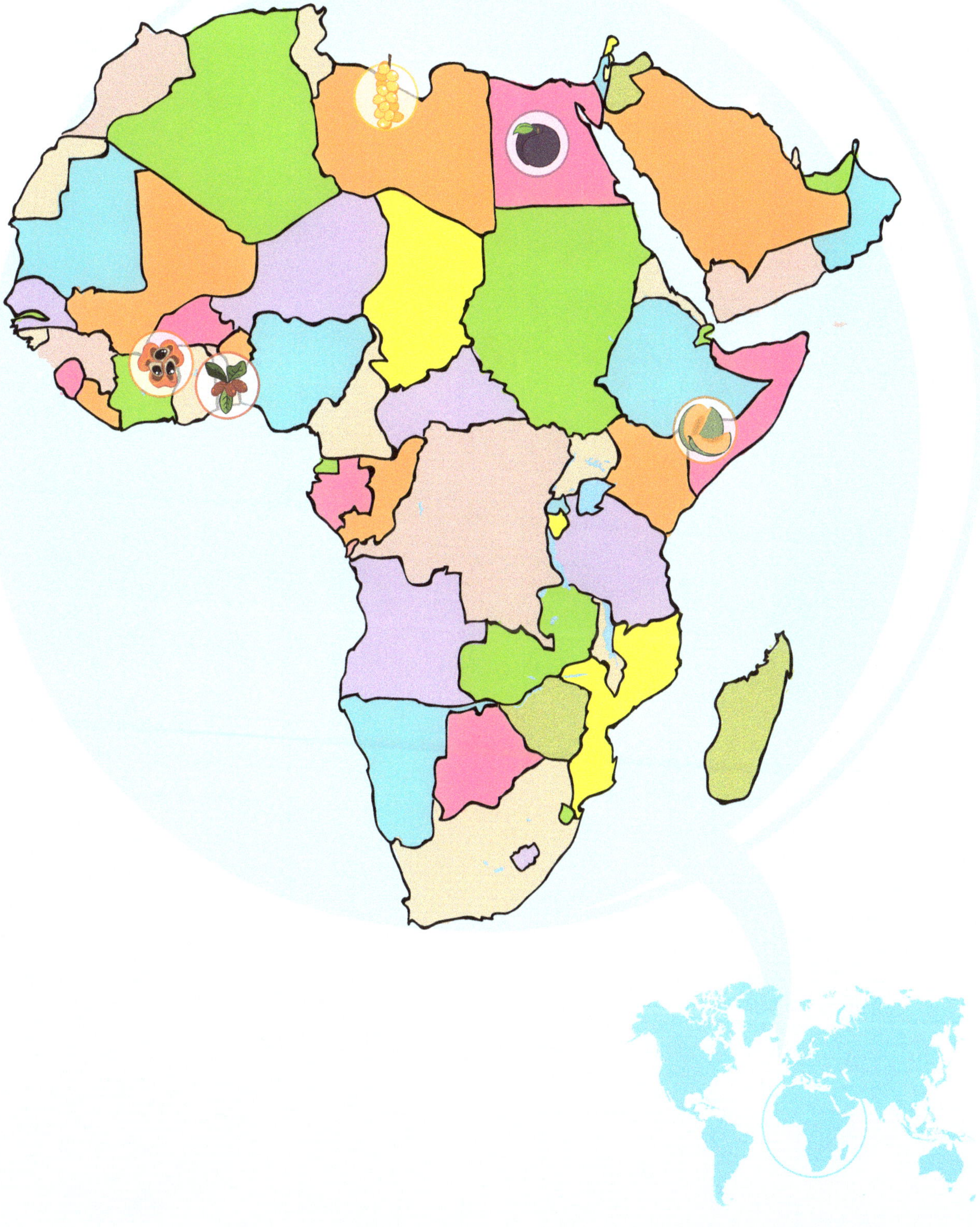

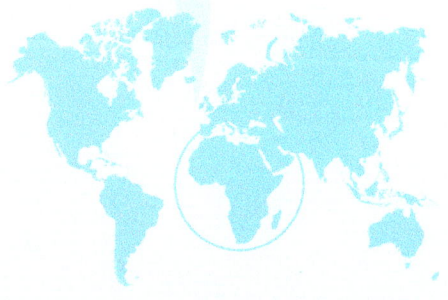

A Book of Fruits 31

ACAI

[ah-sahy-ee]

bitter, refreshing, rich, tart, tropical

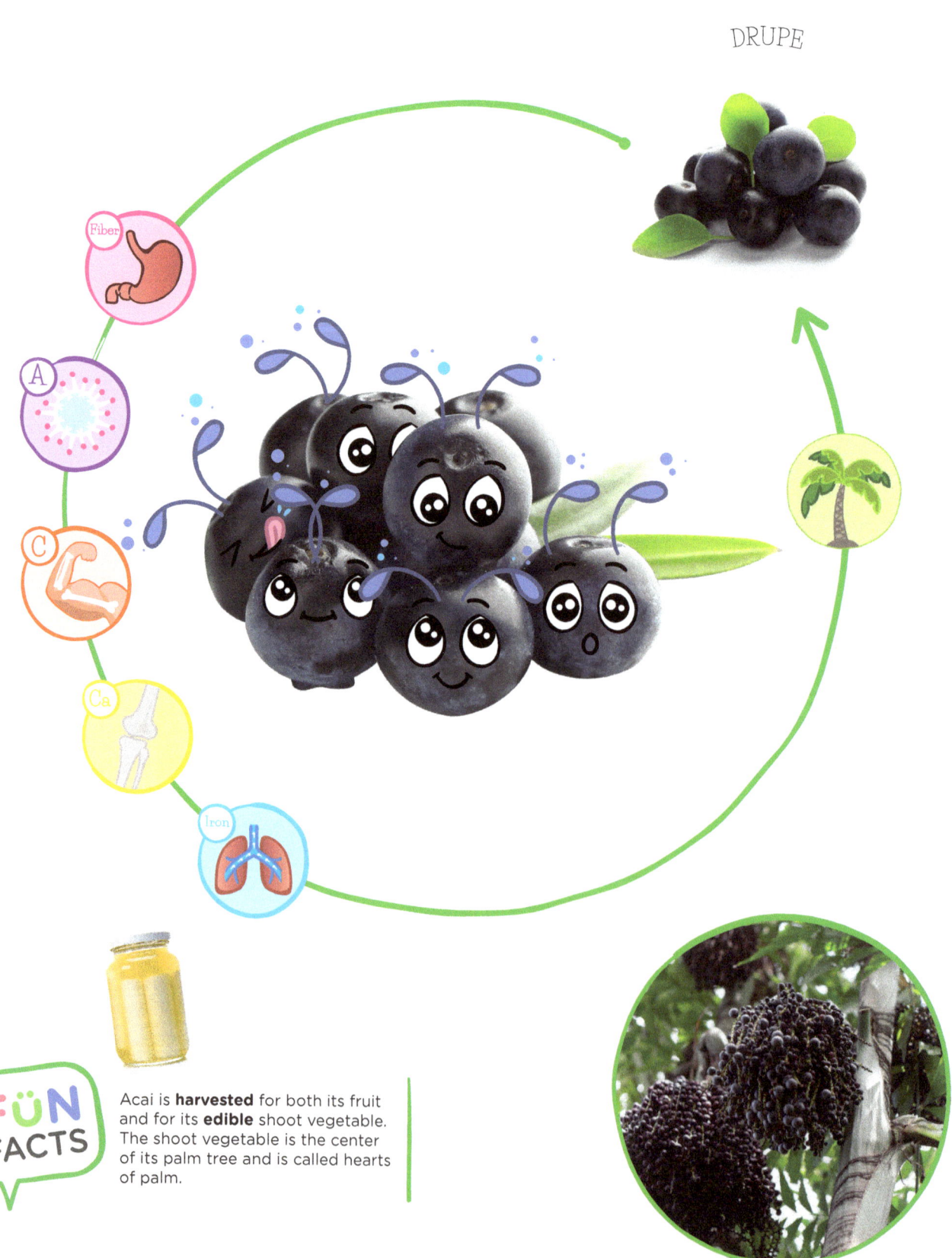

FUN FACTS: Acai is **harvested** for both its fruit and for its **edible** shoot vegetable. The shoot vegetable is the center of its palm tree and is called hearts of palm.

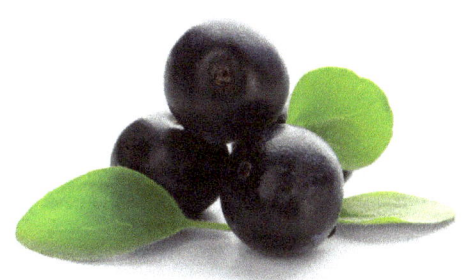

PICK
Acai is typically sold as a dried powder, frozen **puree**, added to juice, or in **prepared** food products outside of the countries where they grow because they **spoil** very quickly.

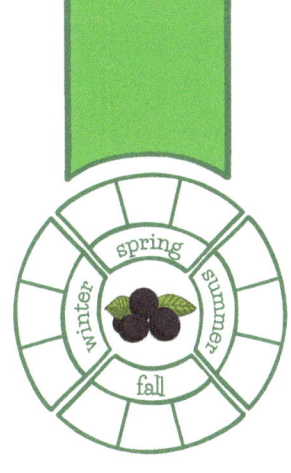

Available imported year-round

STORE
Store per packaging.

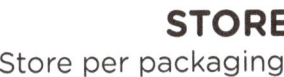

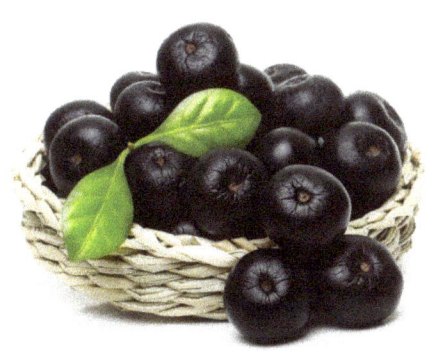
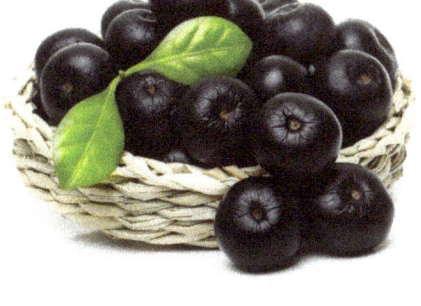

EAT
Acai is typically sold as a dried powder or frozen **puree**.

Acai Smoothie Bowl
Combine 1 cup frozen berries, 1 frozen banana, 4 tablespoons rolled oatmeal, 2 teaspoons acai powder, and 6 ounces coconut milk in a blender and mix until smooth. The **texture** should be **thick** like ice cream. Sprinkle your favorite toppings on the smoothie bowl such as chopped nuts, sliced fruit, chia, flaxseeds, and dried coconut.

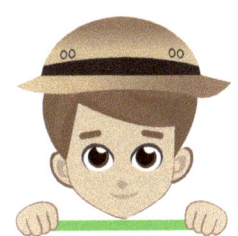

ACAI TIDBITS

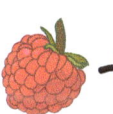 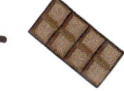

The **flavor** of acai is often compared to a cross between a blackberry or raspberry and a piece of dark chocolate.

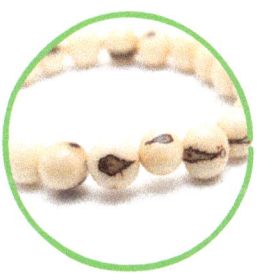

The seed makes up about 80% of the fruit and is often made into jewelry.

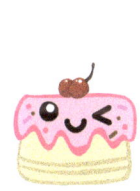
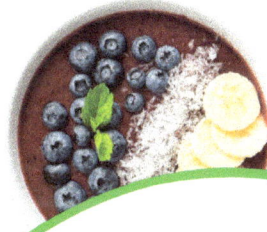
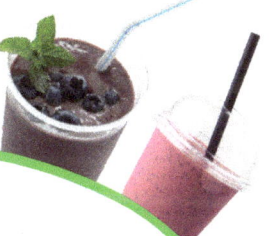
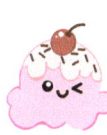
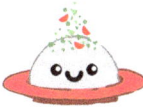

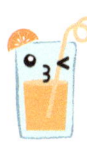

A Book of Fruits

ACKEE
AKEE

[uh-kee] | [ak-ee]

buttery, creamy, mild, nutty, spongy

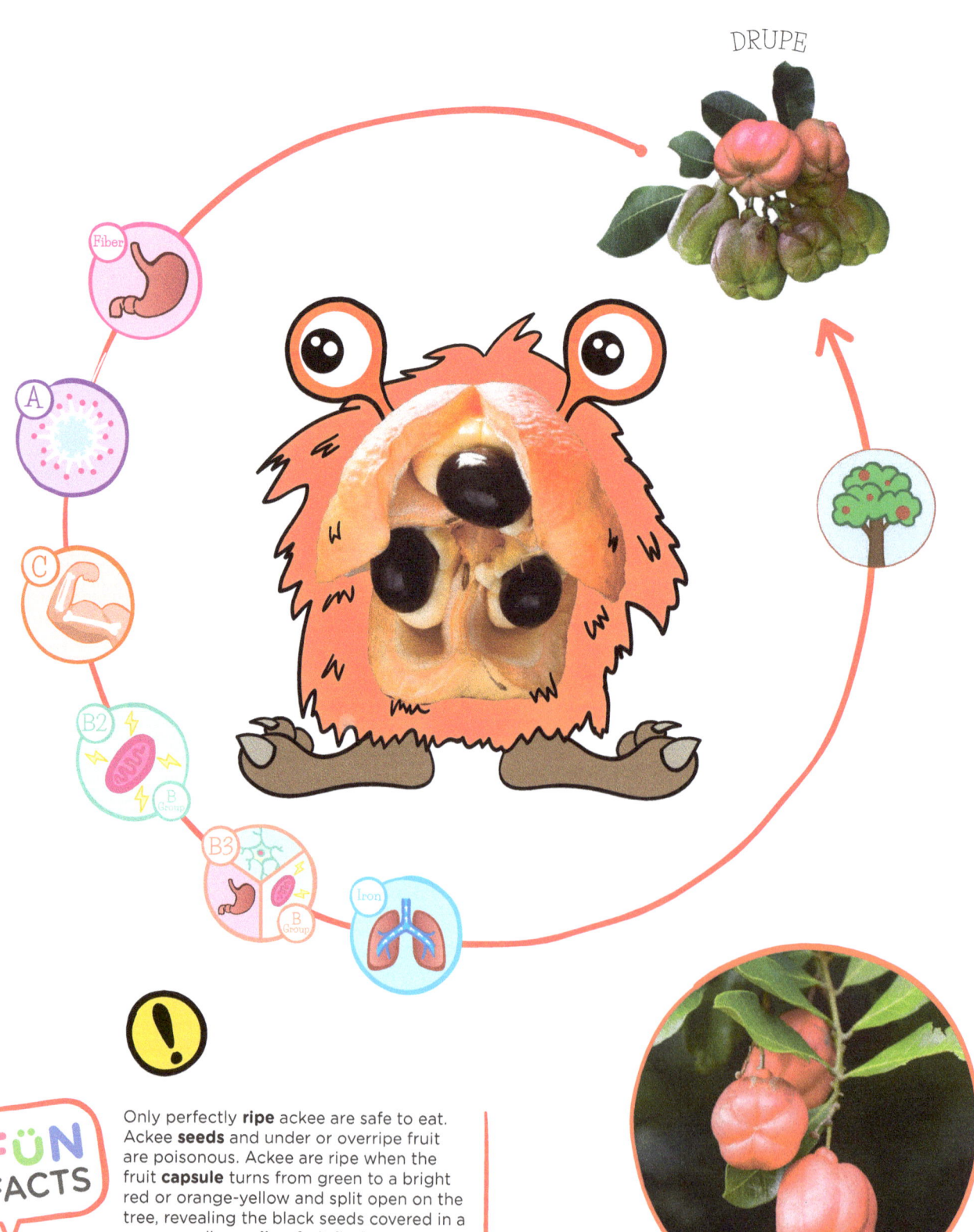

DRUPE

Fun Facts: Only perfectly **ripe** ackee are safe to eat. Ackee **seeds** and under or overripe fruit are poisonous. Ackee are ripe when the fruit **capsule** turns from green to a bright red or orange-yellow and split open on the tree, revealing the black seeds covered in a creamy yellow **aril** or fruit flesh.

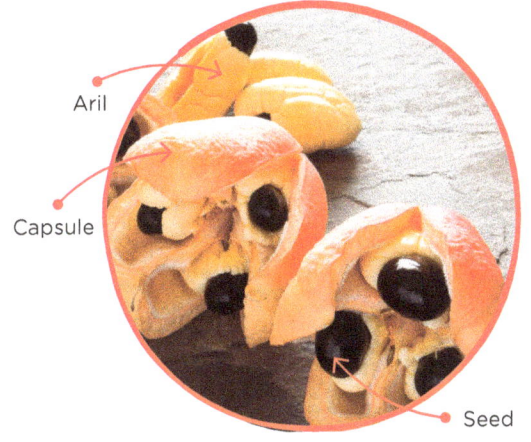

PICK
Ackee is only sold canned or frozen in the United States by certified companies that ensure the fruit is safe to eat. Underripe and overripe fruit is **poisonous** and **spoils** very quickly.

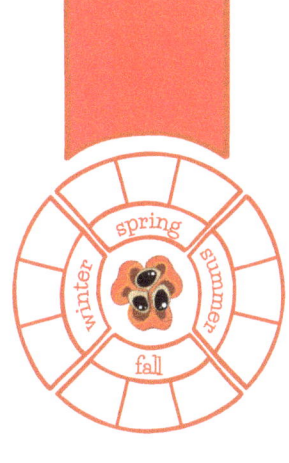

Available imported year-round

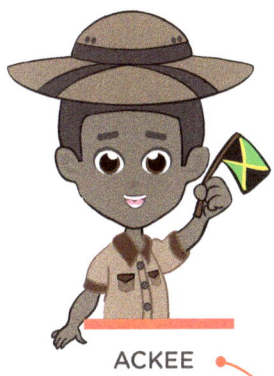

STORE
Store per packaging.

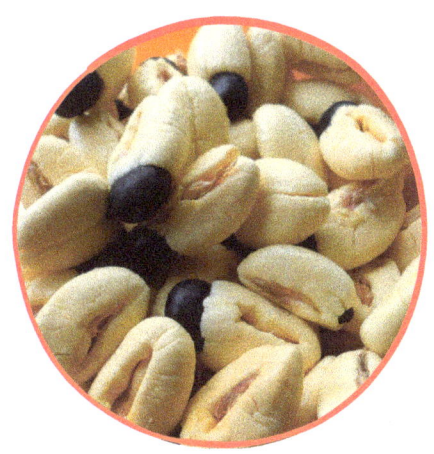

EAT
Ackee is only sold canned or frozen in the United States. Boil frozen and canned ackee in salted water for 5 minutes and use per recipe.

Sautéed Ackee
Chop and sauté 1 medium-sized onion and 1/2 cup diced red pepper over medium-high heat in coconut oil until onions are **translucent**. Stir in 2 cloves minced garlic, 1 medium chopped tomato, 1/2 teaspoon thyme. Drain and rinse canned ackee, stir into a pan with the other ingredients, mix gently and simmer for 5 minutes, then salt and pepper to taste. For an added kick, try adding a chopped habanero pepper.

ACKEE TIDBITS
Ackee is the national fruit of Jamaica and is served in the national dish, "Ackee and Saltfish." Jamaicans say ackee is perfectly ripe when the fruit yawns or smiles which means that it opens naturally on the tree before it is **harvested**.

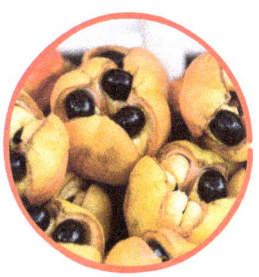

Ackee fruit is technically not a **drupe**, but a fleshy aril from a **dehiscent** capsule. This means that the fruit splits open when they are ripe.

A Book of Fruits 35

APPLE

[ap-uhl]

crunchy, juicy, sweet, tart, waxy

POME

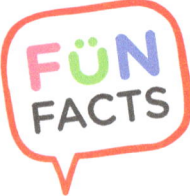

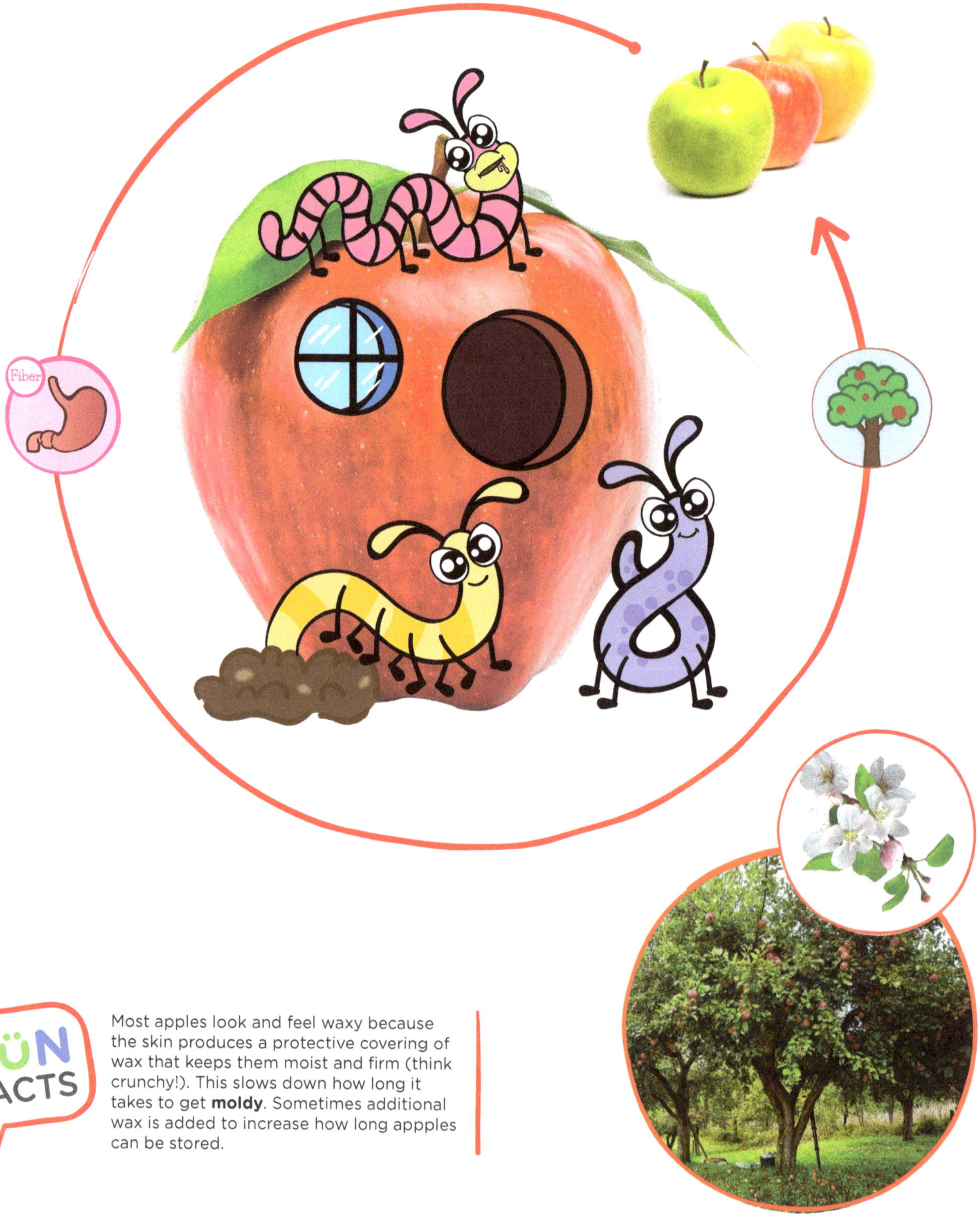

Fun Facts: Most apples look and feel waxy because the skin produces a protective covering of wax that keeps them moist and firm (think crunchy!). This slows down how long it takes to get **moldy**. Sometimes additional wax is added to increase how long appples can be stored.

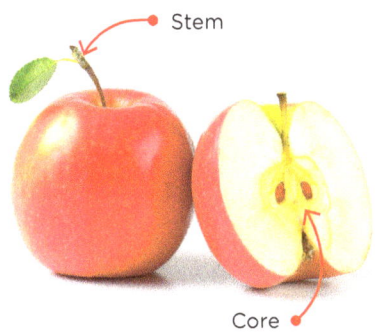

PICK
Pick deep-colored, **firm**, smooth fruit with fresh green stems attached. Apple varieties should be free of **bruises** and soft spots. Colors differ depending on **variety**.

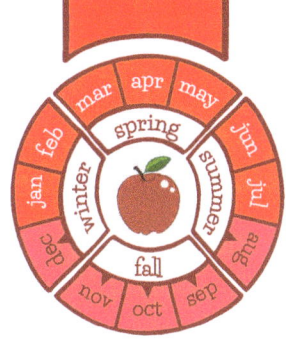

Varieties available year-round; Imported year-round

Peak Season
August–December

STORE
Keep apples at room **temperature** for up to 7 days. Refrigerate whole apples in a plastic bag for 1-2 months or sliced in airtight containers for 3-4 days. Freeze apples in airtight containers for 10-12 months. Dried apples may be stored in airtight containers for 6-12 months. Keep away from foods with strong odors.

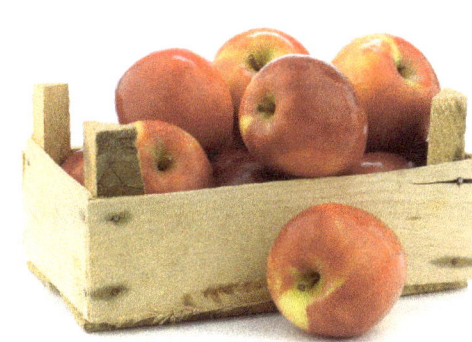

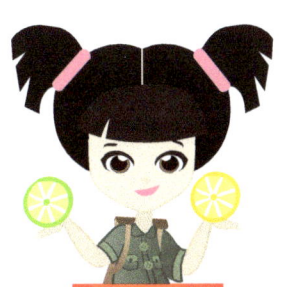

APPLE TIDBITS
Apples turn brown when sliced. Brush or dip slices in lemon, lime, pineapple, or orange juice to prevent browning.

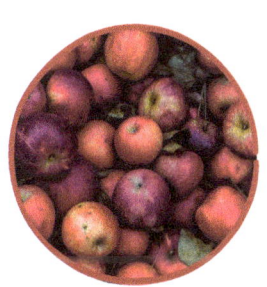

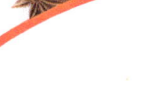

EAT
Clean the skin and remove the core. Eat, chop, or slice per recipe.

Microwave Baked Apple
Place cored apple in a microwave safe dish. Fill the center core area with 1 tablespoon dried fruit such as raisins or chopped dates and 1 tablespoon nuts such as walnuts or pecans. Sprinkle with 1 teaspoon brown sugar and 1/4 teaspoon cinnamon. Cover dish with lid or tightly wrapped plastic and microwave on high for 4-5 minutes. Apples are ready when the skin is soft to touch. Allow the apple to cool before eating.

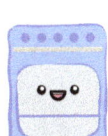

There are over 7,500 varieties of apples grown through the world and 100 varieties grown commercially in the United States. They range in size from a little larger than a cherry to as big as a grapefruit. How many have you tried?

A Book of Fruits

APPLE VARIETIES

BRAEBURN [BRAY-BURN]

A two-toned, red and yellow-green apple with red striping. This crisp, tangy, sweet-tart variety has hints of spices such as nutmeg and cinnamon. Braeburn apples are considered an all-purpose apple. They are great fresh, baked, or roasted. Try roasting this **variety** with root vegetables for a sweet and savory dish.

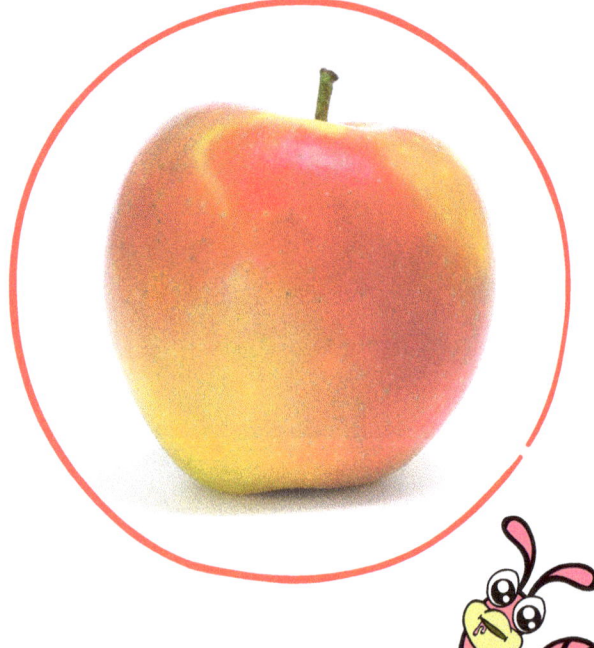

FUJI [FOO-JEE]

A light red apple with a yellow blush. This dense, juicy, crisp variety is mild and sweet with hints of both honey and citrus. Fuji apples are great roasted, baked, sautéed, and boiled into sauce. Try adding slices to a quiche before baking.

GOLDEN DELICIOUS [GOHL-DUHN DIH-LISH-UHS]

First discovered in West Virginia, this green to golden-yellow variety is **firm** and crisp with a sweet-tart, honeyed **flavor**. Golden Delicious apples are great fresh, baked, dried, juiced, or made into butters and sauces. Try making apple butter out of this variety.

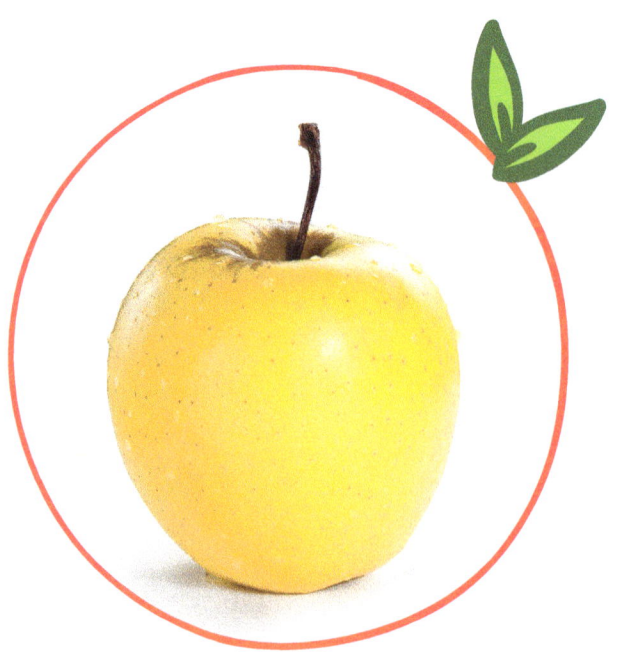

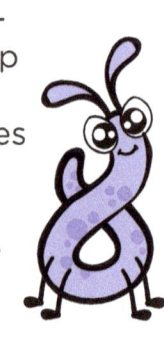

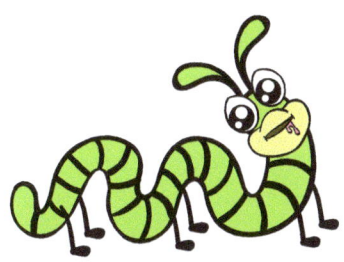

GRANNY SMITH [GRAN-EE SMITH]

In 1868, Maria Ann (Granny) Smith found a **seedling** growing on her property in Australia where she would toss crabapples. The seedling produced a never before seen, hard, light green apple with dotted white skin and a juicy, tart flavor. Granny Smith apples are great fresh and used in baking.

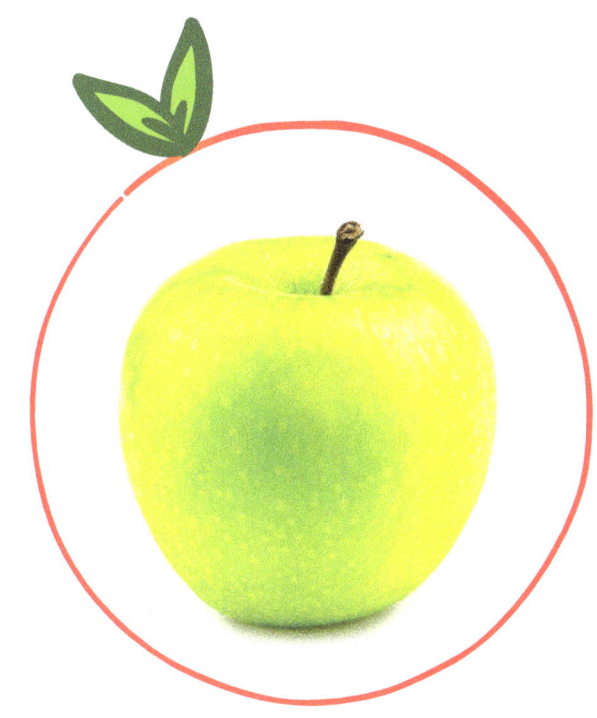

PINK LADY [PINGK LEY-DEE]

A yellow apple with a pink to reddish-pink blush. The Pink Lady™ variety has a distinct, sweet-tart flavor, dry crunch, and an effervescent or fizz-like burst of flavor. Try them fresh in salads, apple sauce, pies, tarts, and pancakes.

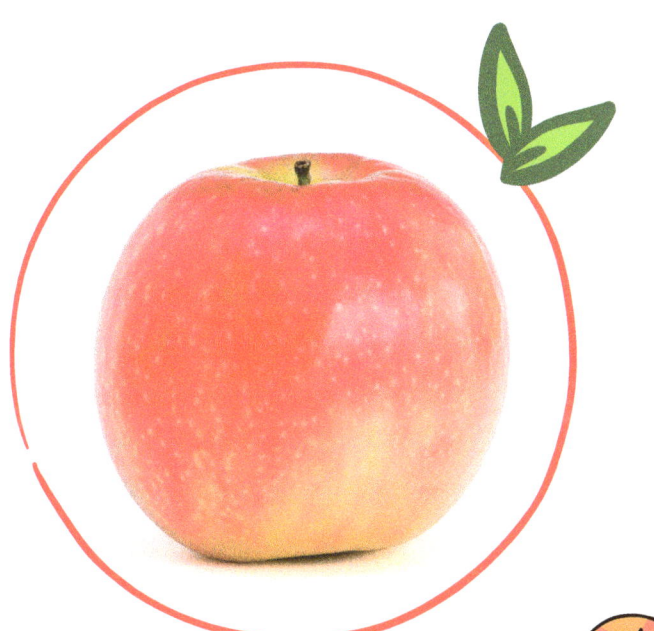

RED DELICIOUS [RED DIH-LISH-UHS]

A bright red apple with a sweet, crisp, flavor and slightly floral aroma. The Red Delicious variety are best used when they are fresh because their flesh does not maintain their firm **texture** when cooked. Try adding them to fruit salad or on a fruit and cheese platter.

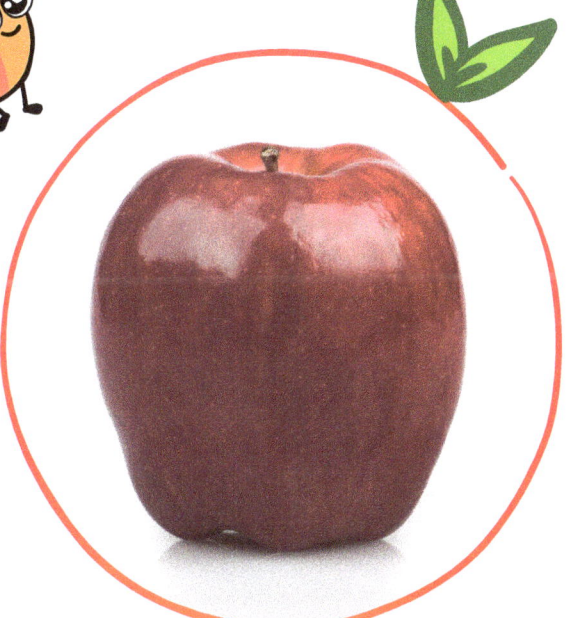

A Book of Fruits 39

APRICOT

[ap-ri-kot]

honeyed, musky, sweet, tart, velvety

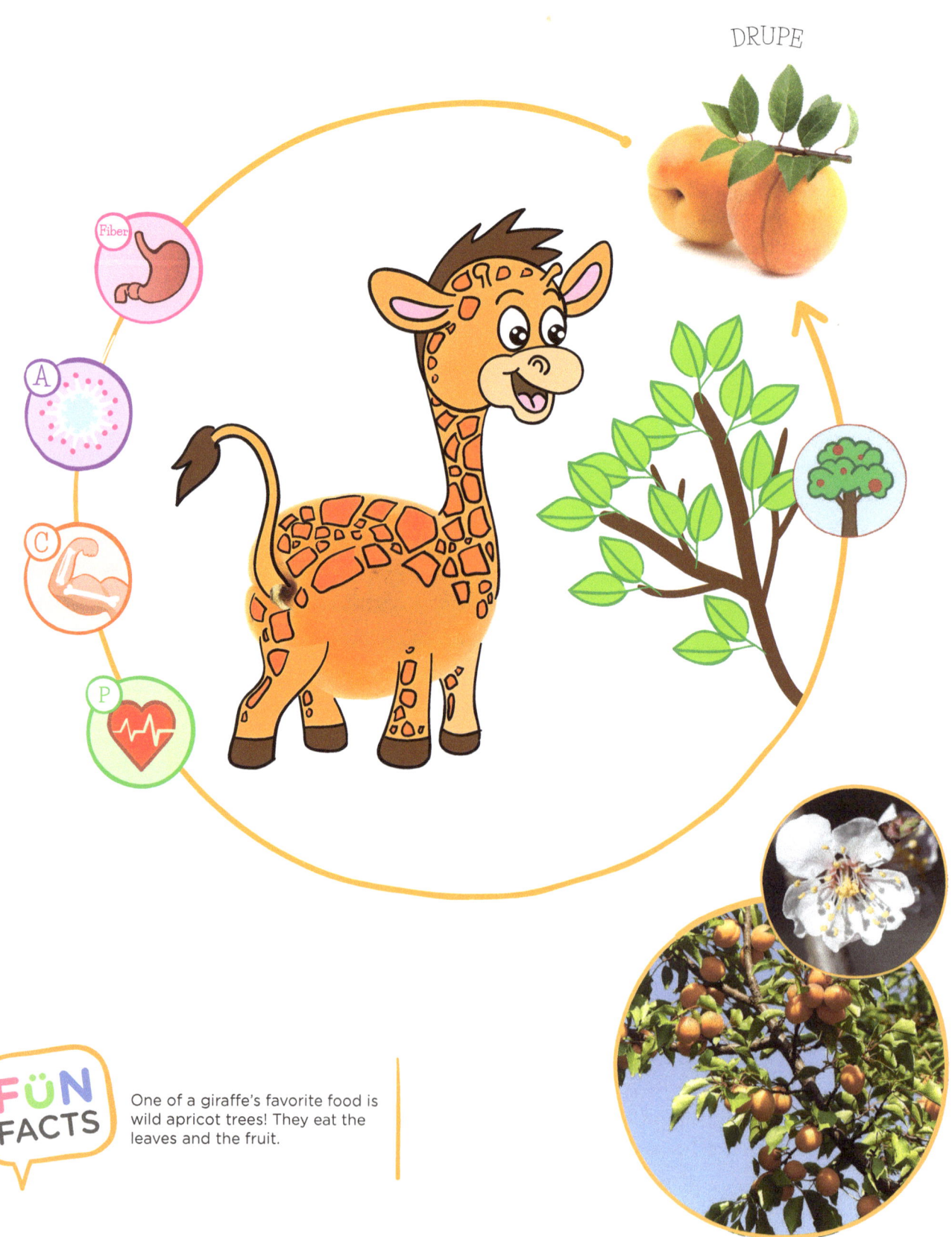

DRUPE

FUN FACTS One of a giraffe's favorite food is wild apricot trees! They eat the leaves and the fruit.

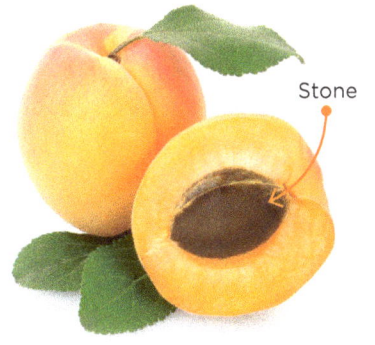

PICK
Pick orange-yellow to orange fruit with a red blush that are soft to touch. Apricots should free of **bruises** and mushy spots.

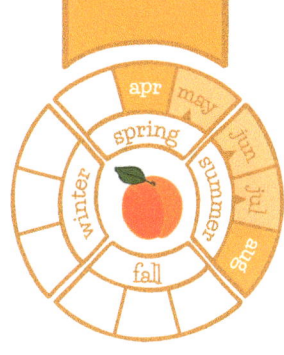

Available April to August

Peak Season
May-July

STORE
Keep apricots at room **temperature** for up to 3 days or until **ripe**. Refrigerate whole apricots in a plastic bag for 4-5 days or sliced in airtight containers for 3-4 days. Freeze apricots in airtight containers for 10-12 months. Dried apricots may be stored in airtight containers for 6-12 months.

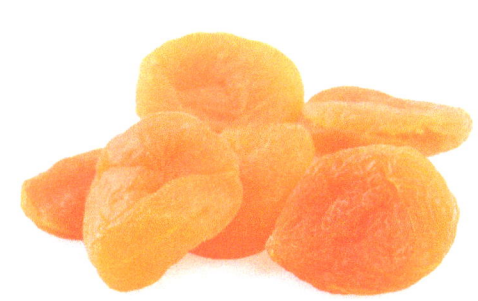

APRICOT TIDBITS

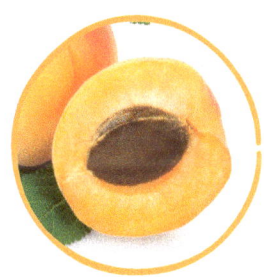

Apricots have a single seed in the center that is in a hard, stony shell, called a stone. This is why apricots are sometimes called a stone fruit.

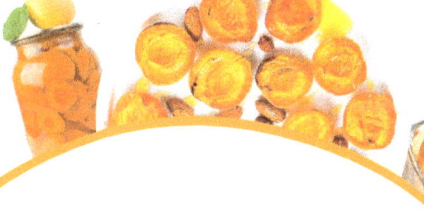
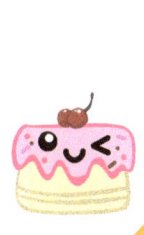
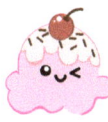
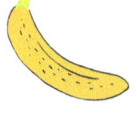
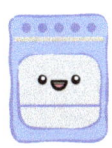

EAT
Clean the skin, slice or break in half with fingers, and remove the **stone** from the center. Eat, chop, or slice per recipe.

Apricot Mascarpone Toast
Spread 1 tablespoon of mascarpone cheese on a **thick** piece of toasted, seeded bread, sprinkle with 1/8 teaspoon cardamom, top with 1 de-stoned and sliced apricot, and **drizzle** honey over the top.

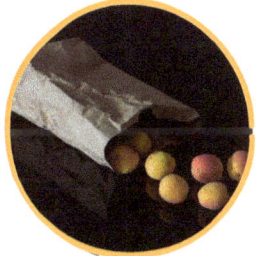

Place unripe apricots in a paper bag to ripen more quickly. Apricots are best enjoyed at room temperature.

A Book of Fruits 41

BANANA

[buh-nan-uh]

candy-like, creamy, mushy, starchy, sweet

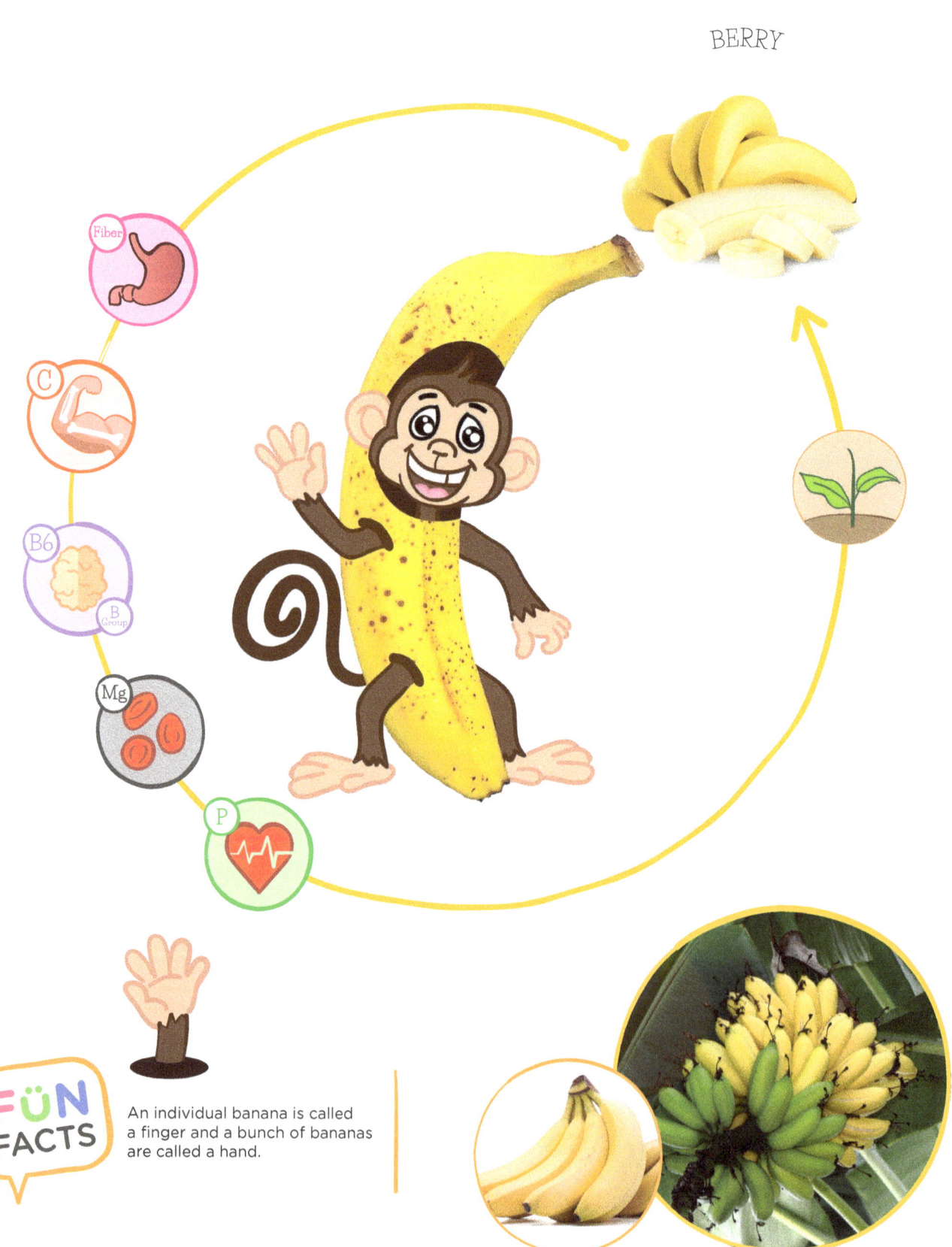

BERRY

FUN FACTS An individual banana is called a finger and a bunch of bananas are called a hand.

42 | Where Do Bananas Come From?

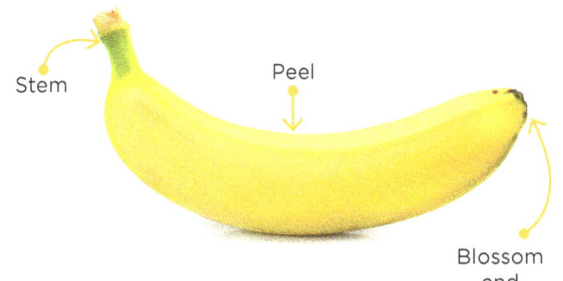
Stem • Peel • Blossom end

PICK
Pick yellow fruit with green at the stem and tip that are **firm** to touch. Yellow bananas should be free of **bruises** and soft spots.

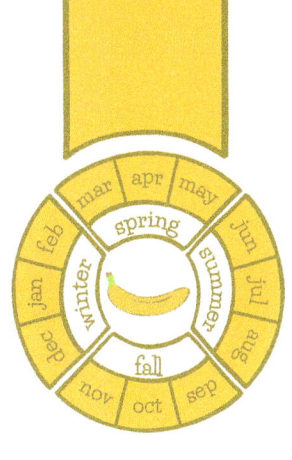
Varieties available year-round

STORE
Keep bananas at room **temperature** for up to 5 days or until **ripe**. Refrigerate whole ripe bananas for 5-7 days or sliced in airtight containers for 3-4 days. Refrigerating whole bananas will turn the peel black but will not damage the fruit. Freeze bananas in airtight containers for 2-3 months. Dried bananas may be stored in airtight containers for 6-12 months.

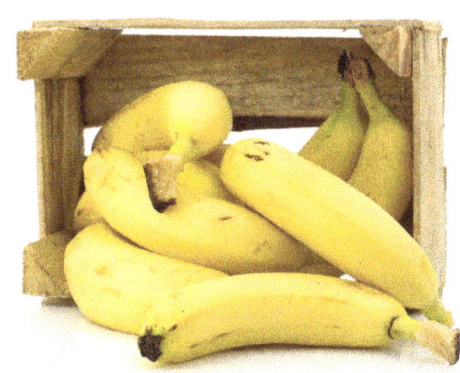

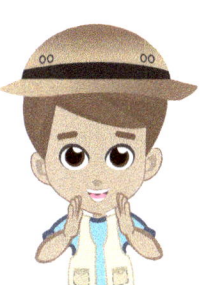

BANANA TIDBITS

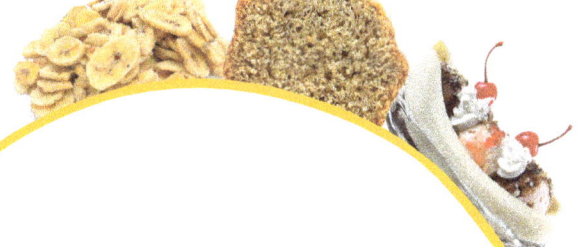

EAT
Pinch and peel from the blossom end instead of the stem to avoid eating the banana strings called **phloem**. Eat, chop, or slice per recipe.

Banana Soft-serve Ice Cream
Freeze sliced banana. Place frozen banana in a blender or food processor and blend until completely smooth. Mix in or sprinkle on your favorite topping such as chocolate chips, peanut butter, and cinnamon.

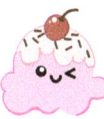
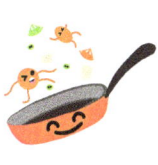
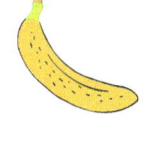
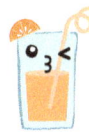

Have you ever seen a banana flower, also known as a banana blossom? If left to **mature**, banana blossoms grow into bananas, but banana blossoms are **edible** too! The **flavor** is bitter and starchy with a hint of banana. They can be enjoyed raw in salads or sautéed like greens such as cabbage. Banana blossoms are often found in Asian **cuisine**, especially Thai recipes.

BLACKBERRY

[blak-ber-ee]

earthy, grainy, juicy, sweet, tart

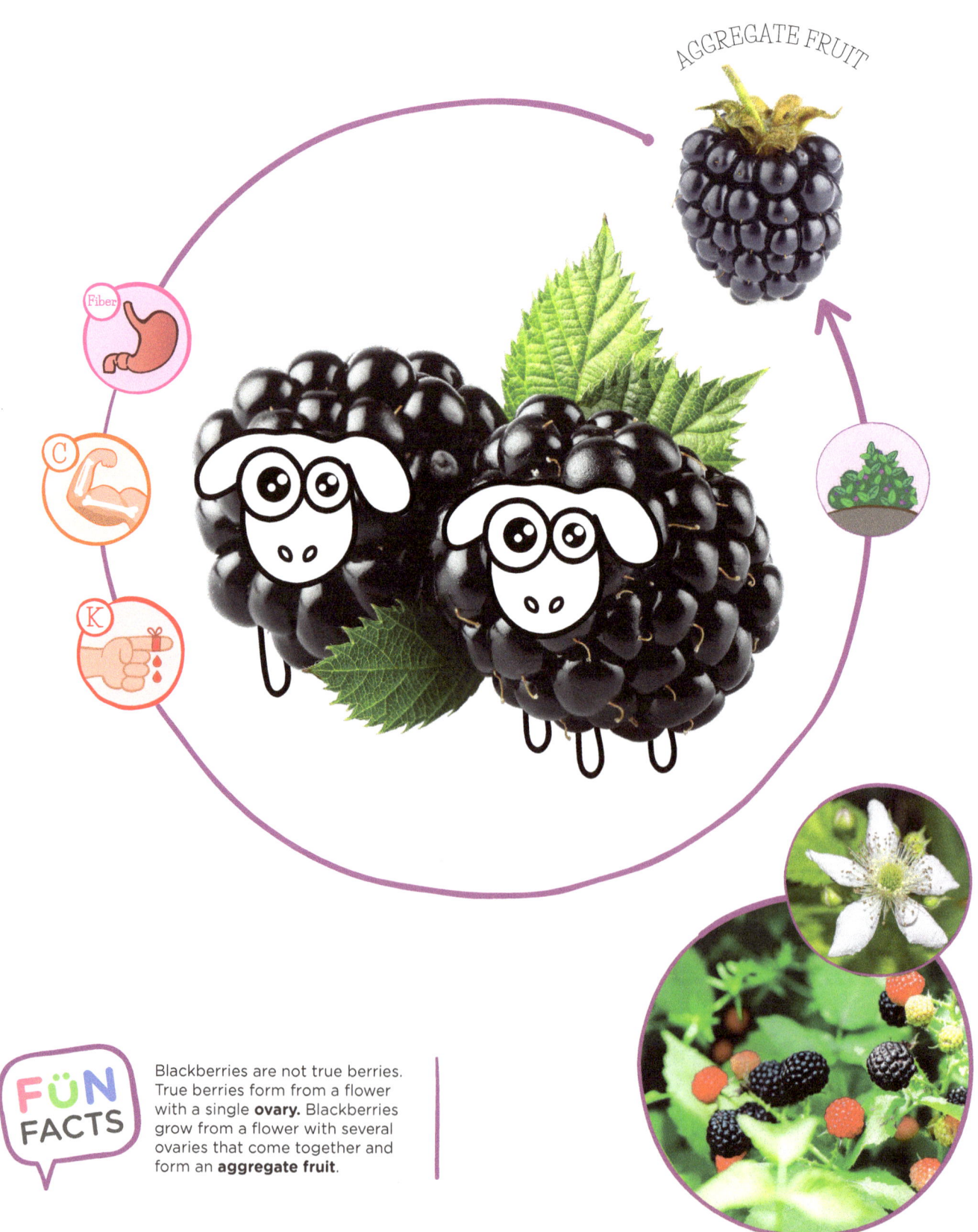

AGGREGATE FRUIT

FUN FACTS: Blackberries are not true berries. True berries form from a flower with a single **ovary.** Blackberries grow from a flower with several ovaries that come together and form an **aggregate fruit**.

Where Do Bananas Come From?

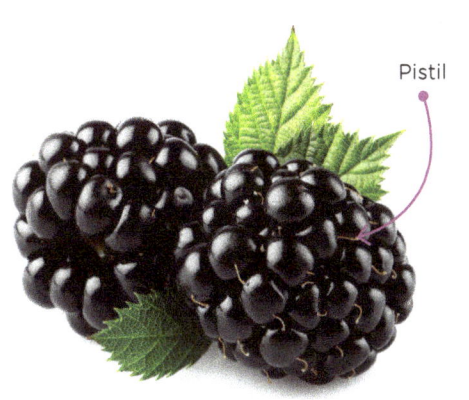
Pistil

PICK
Pick dark, shiny, **plump** fruit. Check the bottom of the package to make sure there is not any juice or **mold** and that blackberries are not crushed.

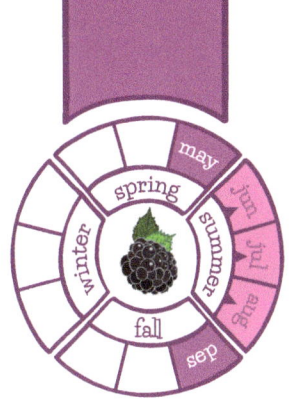

Available May to September; Imported year-round

Peak Season
June-August

STORE
Keep blackberries at room **temperature** and eat them the day they are picked or purchased. Refrigerate blackberries in their plastic container or place the berries loosely in a shallow container covered with plastic wrap for 2-3 days. Freeze blackberries in airtight containers for 10-12 months. Before storing blackberries, throw away any crushed or **moldy** fruit.

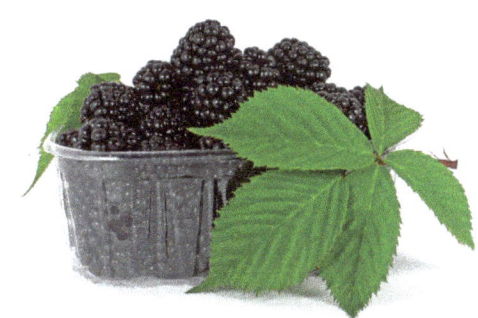

BLACKBERRY TIDBITS

EAT
Clean just before eating or using.

Blackberry Pie
Pre-heat oven to 425 degrees F. Combine 3 ½ cups blackberries with 1/3 cup white sugar, and 1/2 cup all-purpose flour. Pour mixture into an unbaked pie crust, spread 1/2 cup blackberries on top of the mixture and squeeze 1/2 a lemon over the top. Cover with second unbaked pie crust and pinch the top and bottom crust edges together, then slice vents in the top. Brush the top crust with 1 tablespoon milk and sprinkle with 1 tablespoon white sugar. Bake for 15 minutes then reduce the temperature of the oven to 375 degrees F and bake an additional 20-25 minutes until the filling is bubbling and the crust is golden brown.

Blackberries are related to roses and, like roses, grow on thorny brambles or bushes. Be careful when **foraging** for blackberries to prevent cuts and scratches.

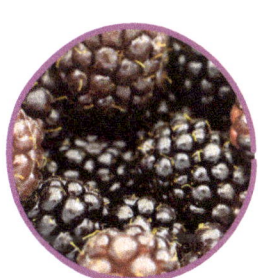

The name blackberry sometimes refers to a group of bush berries that are **hybrids** of the blackberry. This includes boysenberries, marionberries, and loganberries.

A Book of Fruits 45

BLUEBERRY

[bloo-ber-ee]

gritty, plump, sour, sweet, tart

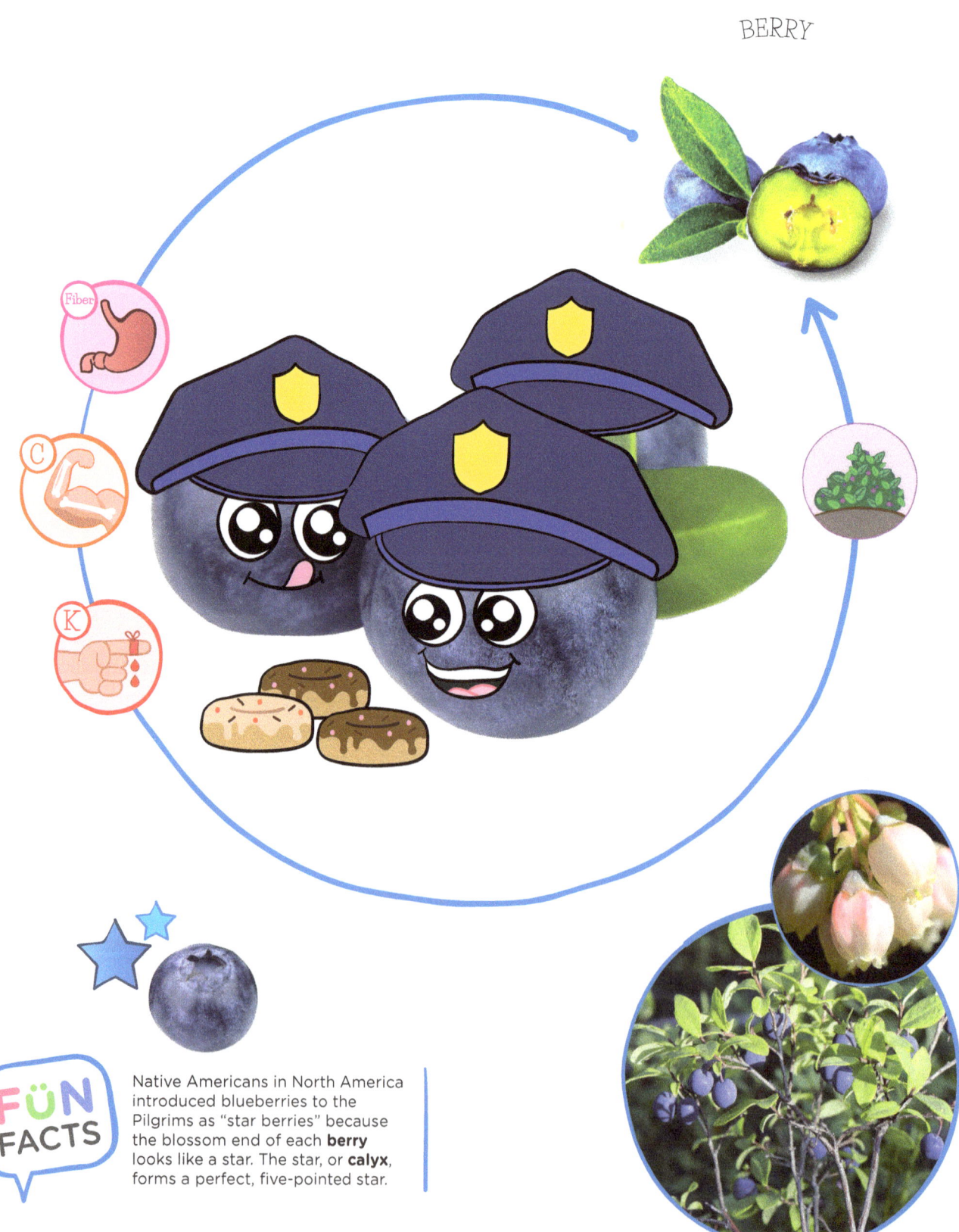

FUN FACTS: Native Americans in North America introduced blueberries to the Pilgrims as "star berries" because the blossom end of each **berry** looks like a star. The star, or **calyx**, forms a perfect, five-pointed star.

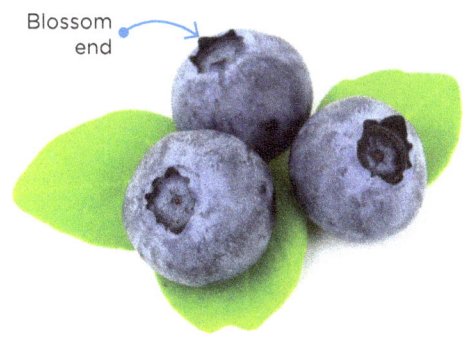
Blossom end

PICK
Pick purple-blue to blue-black, **plump**, **firm**, smooth, and dry fruit. Blueberry skin should have a powdery **bloom**, a natural, protective, waxy coating. Check the bottom of the package to make sure there is not any juice or **mold** and that blueberries are not crushed.

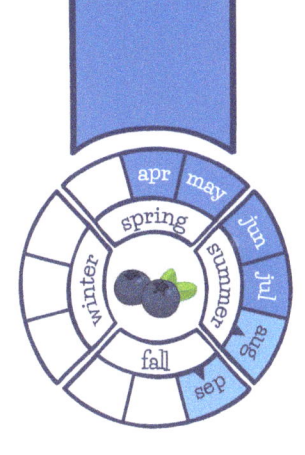

Available April to September; Imported year-round

Peak Season
August-September

STORE
Keep blueberries at room **temperature** and eat them the day they are picked or purchased. Refrigerate blueberries in their plastic container or place the berries loosely in a shallow container covered with plastic wrap for 1-2 weeks. Freeze blueberries in airtight containers for 10-12 months. Dried blueberries may be stored in airtight containers for 6-12 months. Before storing blueberries, throw away any crushed or moldy fruit.

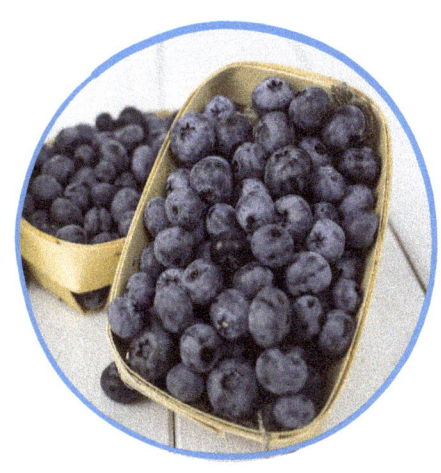

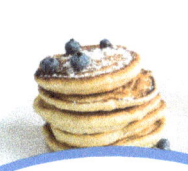

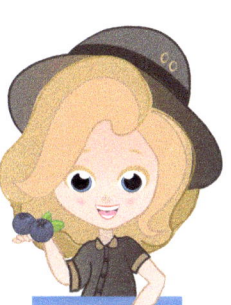

BLUEBERRY TIDBITS

EAT
Clean just before eating or using.

Blueberry Chutney
Combine 1 1/2 cinnamon sticks, 1/2 teaspoon whole cloves, and 1/2 teaspoon allspice berries in a small cheese cloth and tie closed. In a saucepan, heat 6 ounces red wine vinegar, spice bag, and simmer over medium heat for 5 minutes. Stir in 4 cups fresh blueberries, simmer for 5 minutes, and then cover the saucepan. Remove saucepan from the heat and allow mixture to sit at room temperature for 8-12 hours. Strain mixture, separating the berries and spice bag from the liquid. Return the liquid to the saucepan, add 1/2 cup white sugar, 1/2 cup brown sugar, and bring to a boil until **thickened**, about 4 minutes, to make syrup. Spoon berries into a glass jar and cover with syrup. Refrigerate chutney for up to 1 month.

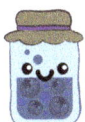
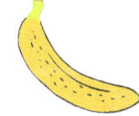

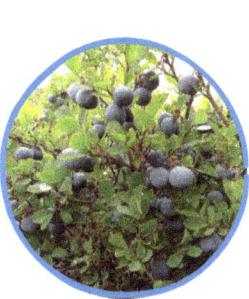

Cultivated blueberries are planted and grow on high bushes that are 4 to 7 feet tall. The berries are large in size and have a sweet and mild **flavor**. Wild blueberries grow naturally on low bushes that are less than 2 feet high. The berries are smaller in size, and have a more intense sweet and tangy flavor.

A Book of Fruits 47

BREADFRUIT

[bred-froot]
aromatic, bland, custard-like, fleshy, mealy, musty, starchy, sticky, sweet, tacky

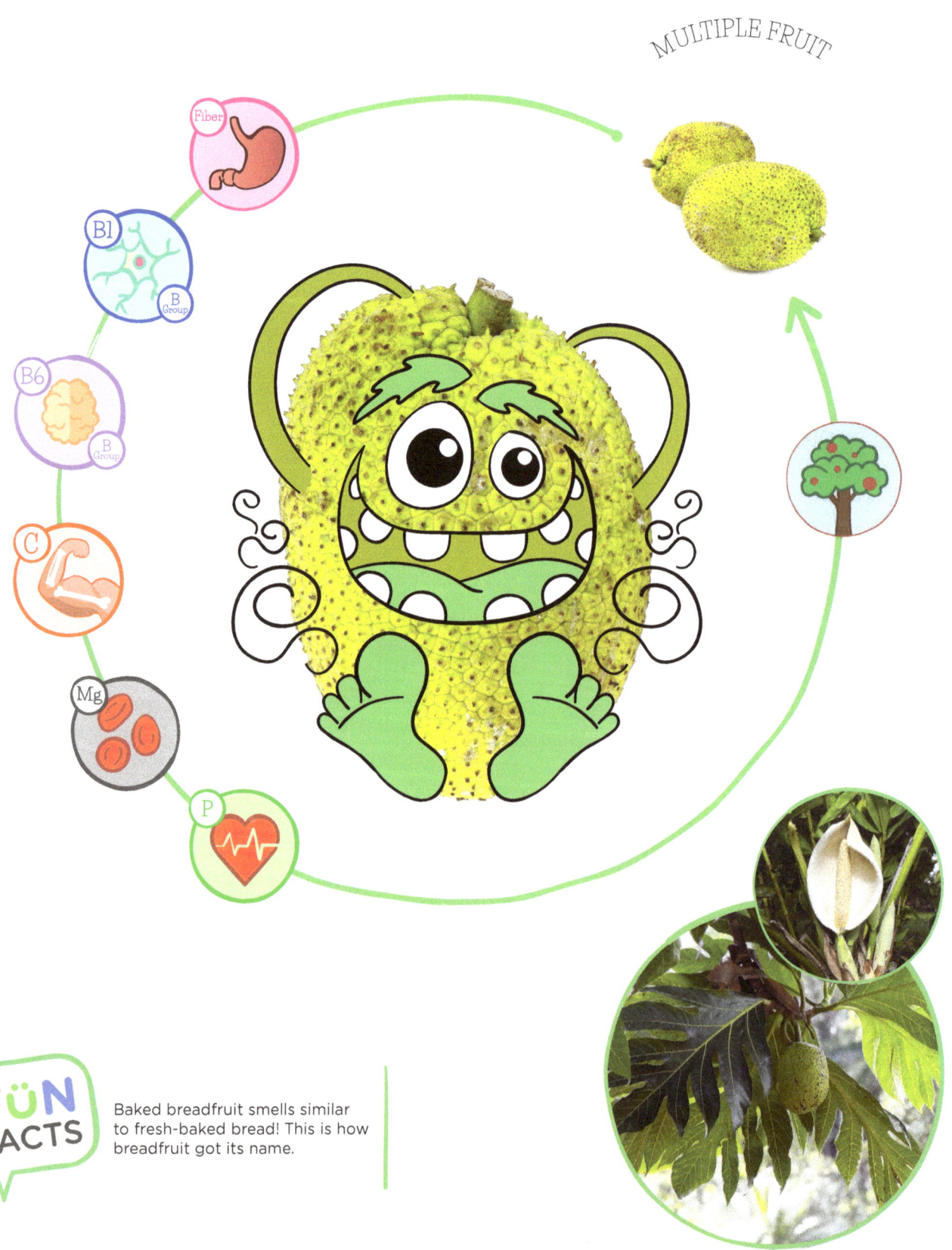

MULTIPLE FRUIT

FUN FACTS: Baked breadfruit smells similar to fresh-baked bread! This is how breadfruit got its name.

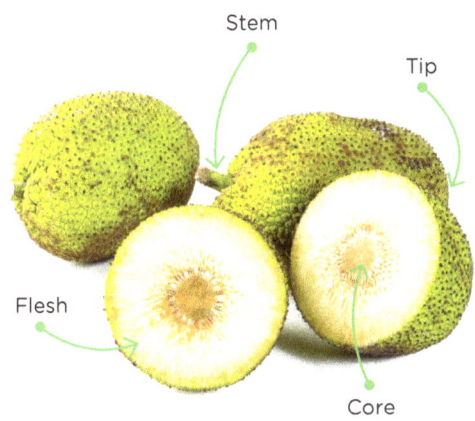

Stem, Tip, Flesh, Core

PICK
Pick underripe, greenish-yellow fruit with small brown cracks between the bumpy skin. Underripe fruit should be **firm** and smooth. Pick **ripe**, yellow-green to yellow-brown fruit with a sweet, aromatic, perfumed aroma. Ripe breadfruits should be smooth, soft to touch, and free of **bruises** and mushy spots.

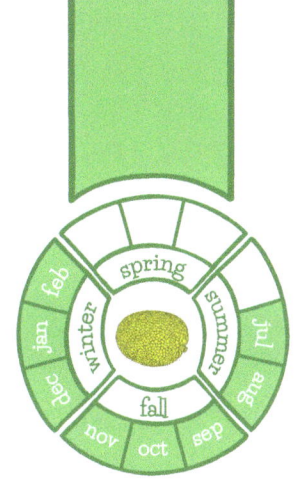

Available July to February; Imported year-round

STORE
Keep ripe breadfruits at room **temperature** and **prepare** them the day they are purchased or keep them under water for up to 3 days. Refrigerate ripe breadfruits for up to 10 days and underripe fruit for up to 15 days. Breadfruits can also be stored or preserved by drying them in the sun, freezing the **flesh**, or burying the fruit in the ground to **ferment**.

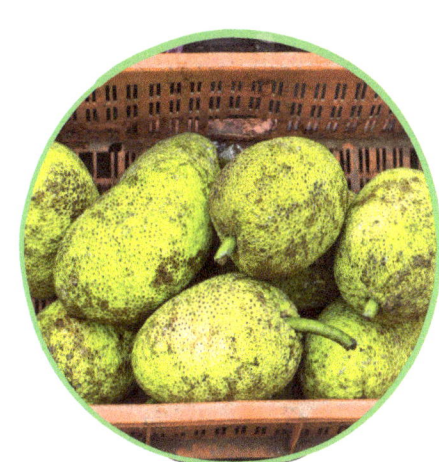

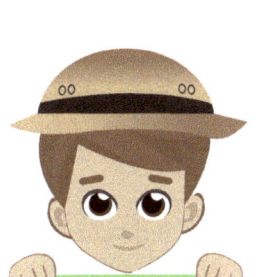

BREADFRUIT TIDBITS

Breadfruit is enjoyed differently depending on whether it is underripe or ripe. Underripe fruit is eaten like a vegetable and used for potato-like dishes. Ripe fruit is eaten as a fruit and used for sweet treats.

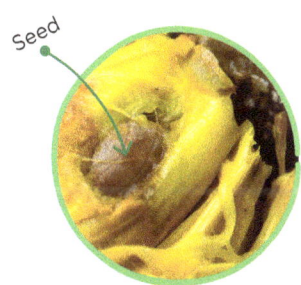

Seed

Breadfruit seeds are **edible** and can be eaten after boiling, steaming, or roasting. They have a mild, nutty **flavor** that is a little sweet.

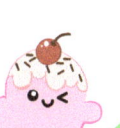
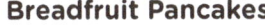
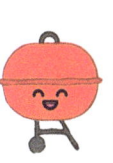
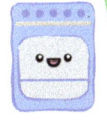

EAT
Clean the skin and chop or slice per recipe.

Breadfruit Pancakes

Hold a small ripe breadfruit, about 1 1/2 pounds, in one hand and pull the stem straight out with the other hand or slice in half stem to tip and remove the core. Scoop the soft flesh in to a blender. To make batter, add 2 eggs, 1/3 cup coconut milk, 1 teaspoon baking powder, 1 teaspoon cinnamon, 1/2 teaspoon vanilla extract, and 1/4 teaspoon nutmeg to blender and combine until smooth. Heat a lightly oiled griddle or frying pan over medium-low heat with coconut oil. Pour or scoop the batter onto the griddle using 1/4 cup for each pancake. Cook covered until edges are dry or about 3 minutes and then flip. Cook the other side about 2 minutes until pancake is browned on both sides.

A Book of Fruits 49

CACAO
COCOA

[kuh-kah-oh] | [koh-koh]

acidic, astringent, bitter, floral, nutty

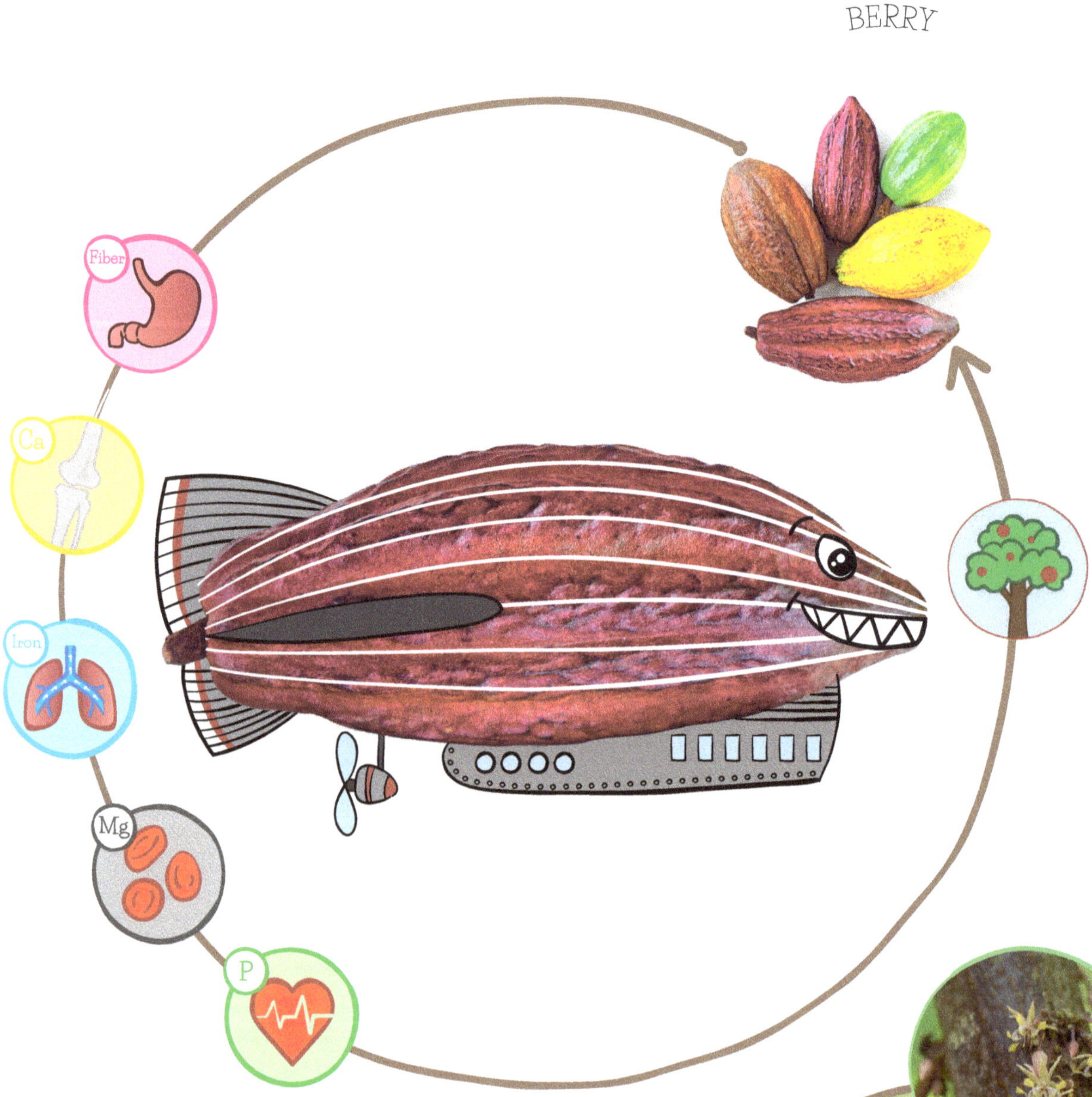

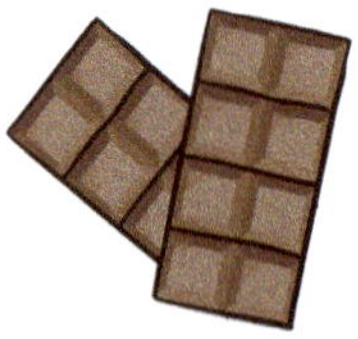

BERRY

FUN FACTS

Cacao **seeds** or beans are the source of chocolate! Each tree produces approximately 30 berry-like pods a year containing 30-50 cacao beans. It takes about 500 beans to make 1 pound of chocolate. This means that each tree can produce about 2 pounds of chocolate a year.

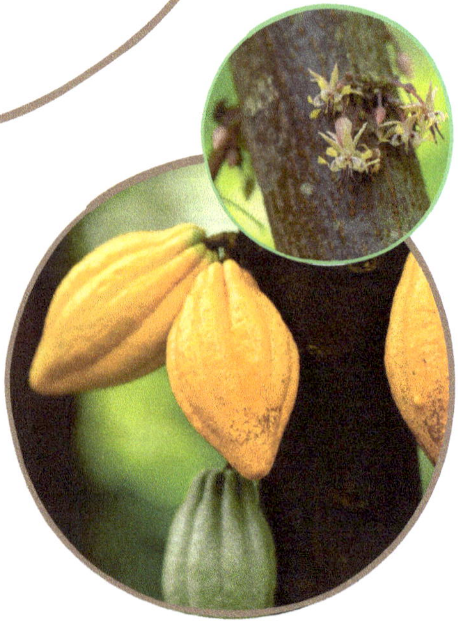

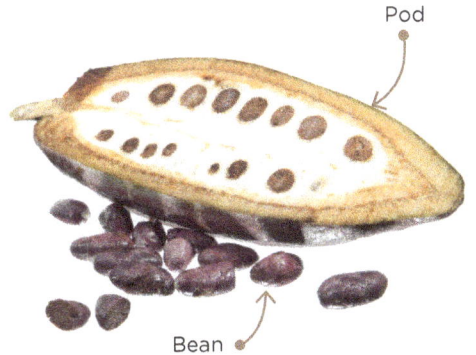
Pod · Bean

PICK
Raw cacao beans are prepackaged and sold as dried powder or "nibs" within the United States after the beans have been removed from the pods, **processed**, and graded for quality.

Available imported year-round

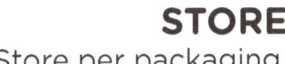

STORE
Store per packaging.

Nibs

CACAO TIDBITS

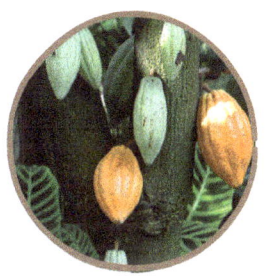

Cacao is a **cauliflory** plant. This means that the pods grow from the trunk of the tree rather than on the overhanging branches. The location of the pods close to the ground allows animals that cannot climb or fly to pollinate and spread seeds.

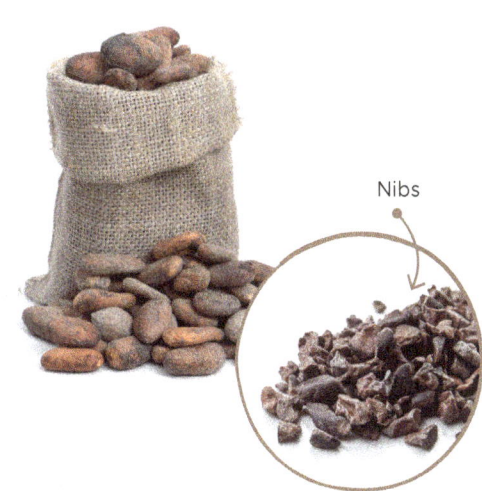

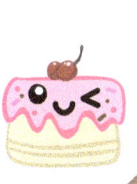

EAT
Raw cacao is typically sold as a dried powder or "nibs."

Raw Cacao Peanut Butter Balls
Combine 1 cup rolled oatmeal, 1/4 cup peanut butter, 1/4 cup honey, 2 tablespoons raw cacao powder, and 1/8 teaspoon salt in a food processor and blend until well mixed. Form 1 inch balls with your hands. Refrigerate for up to 1 week. Makes about 12 balls.

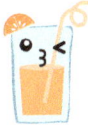

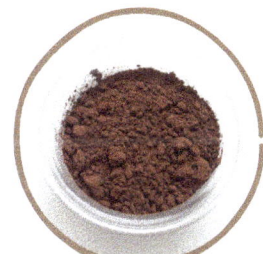

The tree and the beans are called cacao. The powder made from the seeds that is turned into chocolate is called cocoa.

A Book of Fruits

CHERIMOYA
CUSTARD APPLE

[cher-uh-moi-uh] | [kuhs-terd ap-uhl]

ambrosial, creamy, custard-like, juicy, sweet

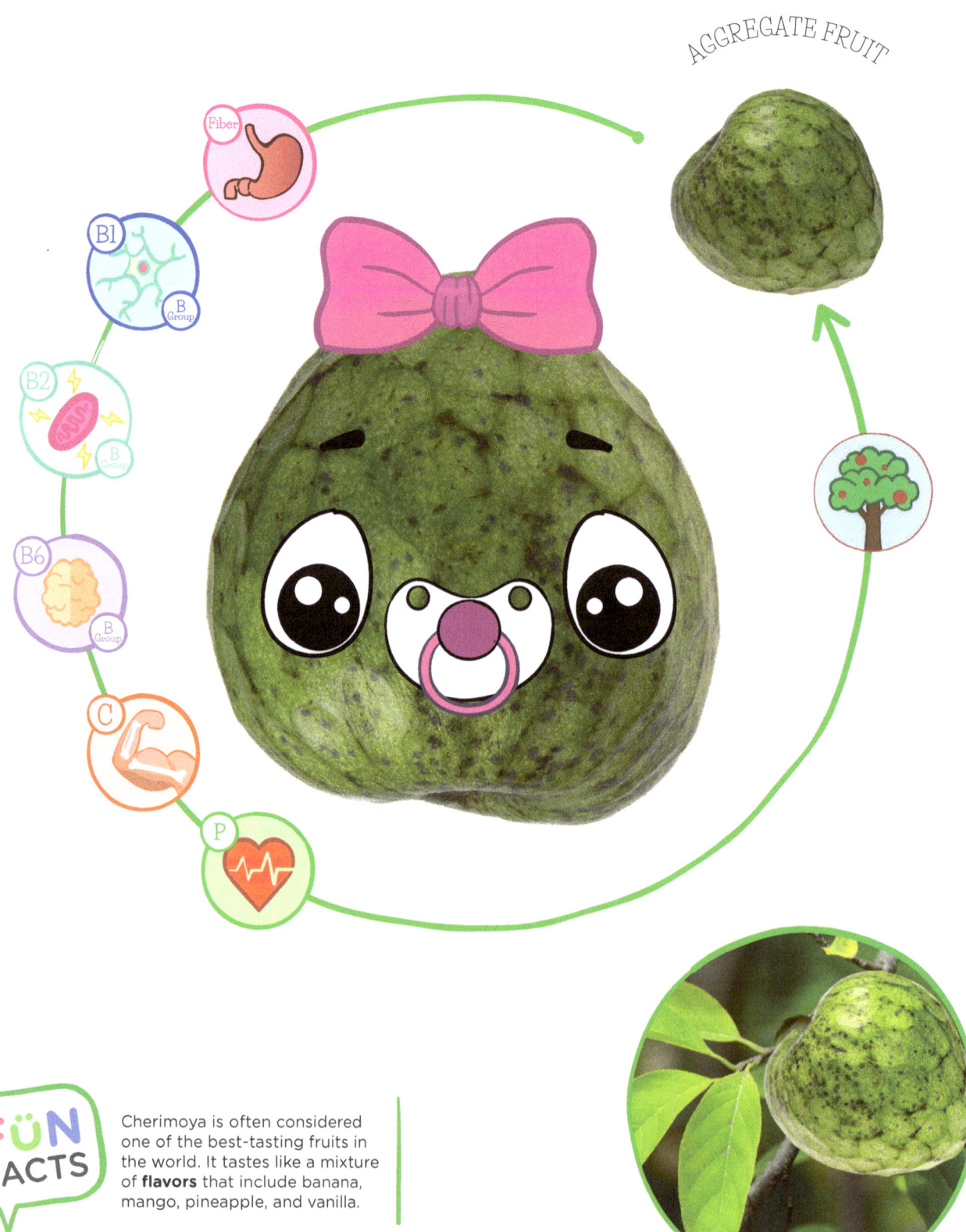

AGGREGATE FRUIT

FUN FACTS: Cherimoya is often considered one of the best-tasting fruits in the world. It tastes like a mixture of **flavors** that include banana, mango, pineapple, and vanilla.

52 | Where Do Bananas Come From?

PICK
Pick pale green or creamy yellow fruit that are soft to touch. Overripe fruit is dark brown. Cherimoyas should be free of mushy spots and **mold**.

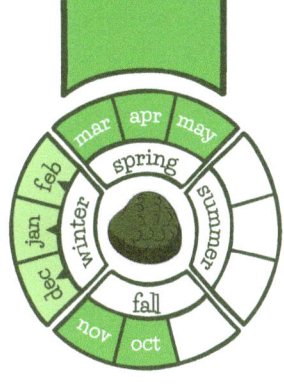

Available October to May

Peak Season
December-February

STORE
Keep cherimoyas at room **temperature** for up to 5 days or until **ripe**. Refrigerate whole cherimoyas 2-4 days or sliced in airtight containers for 1-2 days. Freeze cherimoyas in airtight containers for 10-12 months.

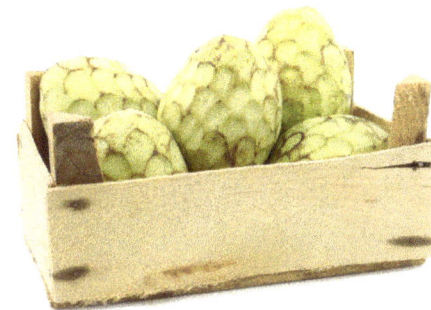

CHERIMOYA TIDBITS

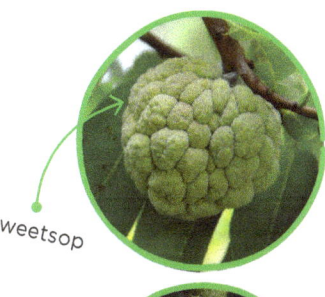

Sweetsop

EAT
Clean the skin, slice in half from stem to tip, spoon out the **flesh**, and remove the **seeds**.

Cherimoya Frozen Yogurt
Puree 2 pounds deseeded cherimoya (about 2 cherimoyas), 1/2 cup coconut **flavored** yogurt, and 1 tablespoon lime juice. Pour puree into ice cube trays and freeze. Place cubes in a food processor and blend until light and fluffy. Scoop frozen yogurt into bowls and top with lime **zest**.

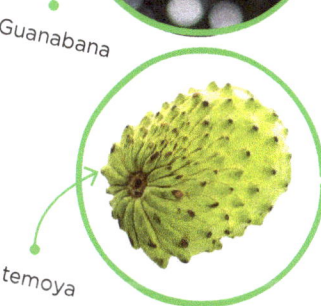

Guanabana

Atemoya

Fruits that look similar to cherimoya with dark green skin, heart-shaped, and have small black seeds are the sweetsop, guanabana and atemoya. The atemoya is a **hybrid** between the cherimoya and the sweetsop.

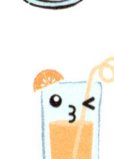

A Book of Fruits 53

CHERRY

[cher-ee]

candy-like, juicy, sour, sweet, tart

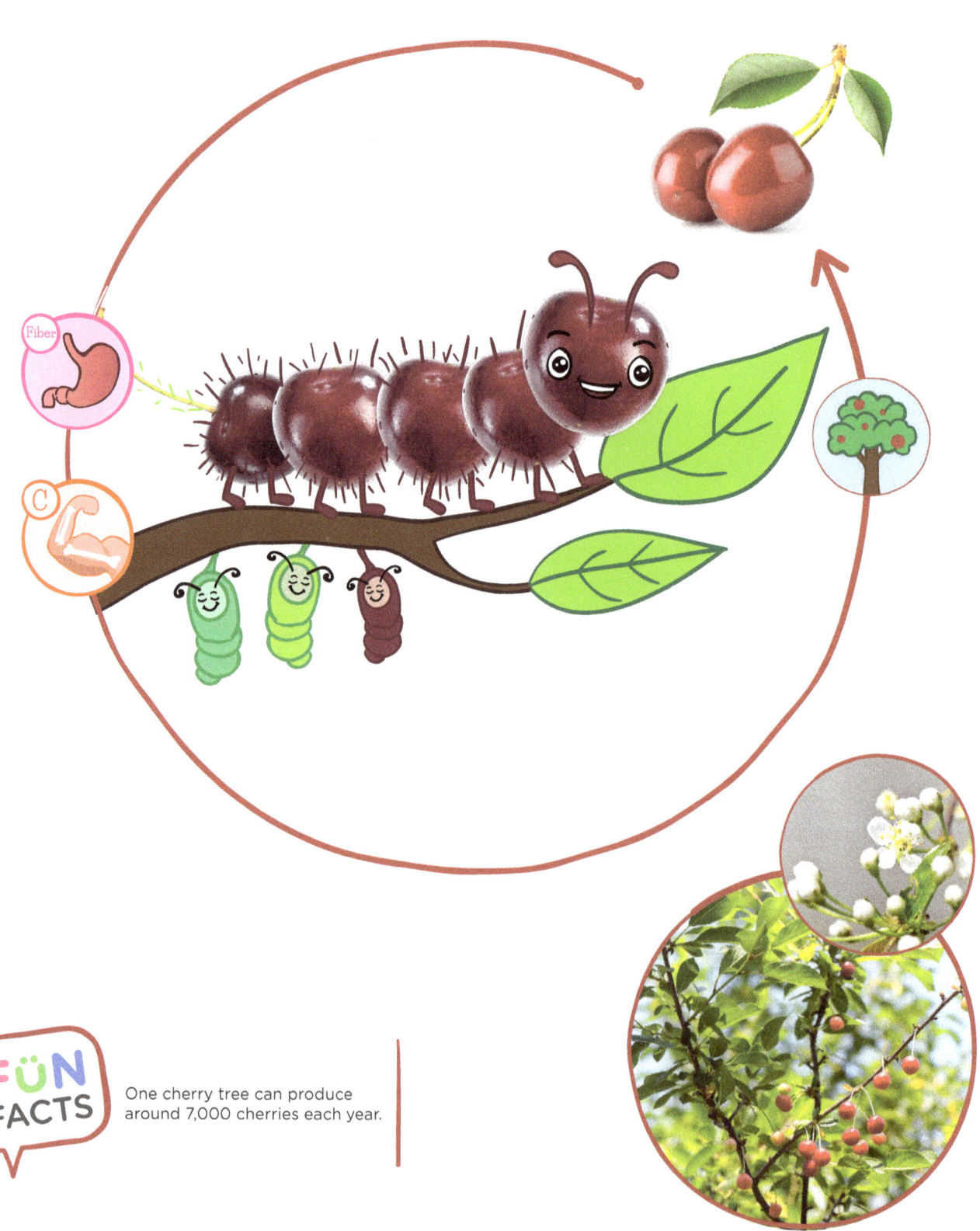

DRUPE

FUN FACTS One cherry tree can produce around 7,000 cherries each year.

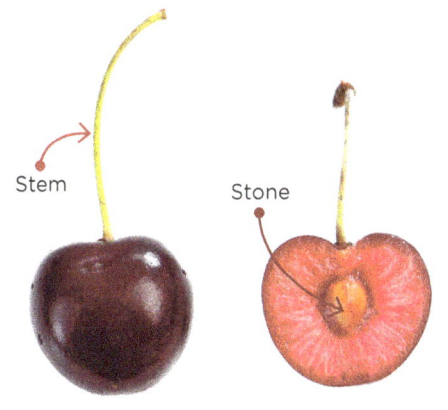

PICK
Pick shiny, **firm**, fruit with fresh green stems attached. Cherry varieties should be free of **bruises** and soft spots. Colors differ depending on **variety**.

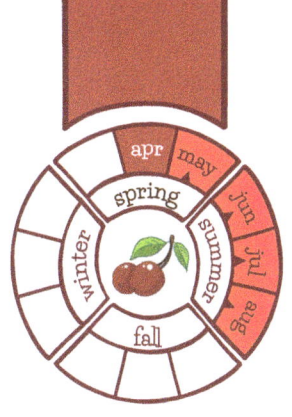

Available April to August; Imported year-round

Peak Season
May-August

STORE
Keep cherries at room **temperature** and eat them the day they are picked or purchased. Refrigerate cherries in a plastic bag for 4-10 days. Freeze cherries in airtight containers for 10-12 months. Dried cherries may be stored in airtight containers for 6-12 months. Before storing cherries, throw away any crushed or **moldy** fruit. Keep away from foods with strong odors.

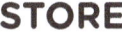
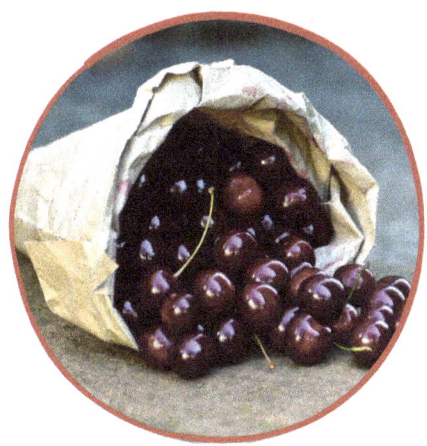
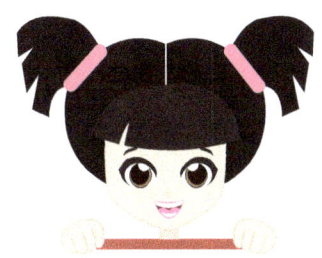

CHERRY TIDBITS

Hanami, also known as the cherry blossom festival, is a Japanese tradition of welcoming spring. During Hanami people gather and celebrate the beauty of nature.

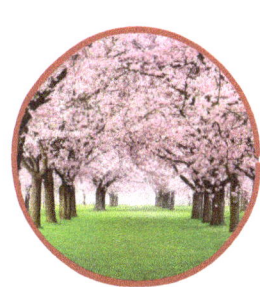

EAT
Clean just before eating or using. Bite, slice in half, or use a cherry pitter to remove the **stone** from the center. Eat, chop, or slice per recipe.

Fermented Sour Cherries
Clean 1/2 pound of sour cherries and remove the stones. Combine cherries in a bowl with 1 cup white sugar, stir, and set aside for 2 hours. Stir again, then place a plate over the mixture with a can or jar on top to make sure the cherries are **submerged** in their juices. Stir the cherries once a day for 2 weeks allowing them to **ferment** in the bowl. Each time making sure the cherries are submerged in their own juices. After 2 weeks transfer cherries and juice to a clean glass jar and store in the refrigerator for up to 1 month. Serve with oatmeal, over cheese, pancakes, or add as a garnish to drinks.

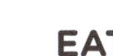
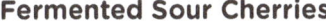
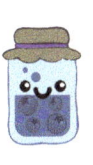

There are two main types of cherries: sweet cherries and sour or tart cherries. Sweet cherries are typically large and taste great fresh, added to salads, or eaten in desserts. Tart cherries are smaller and often **processed** for baking, jellies, and juices.

A Book of Fruits

CHERRY VARIETIES

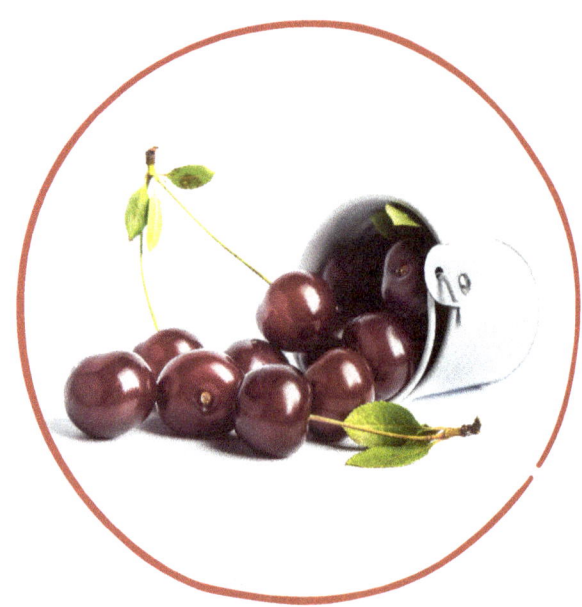

BING [BING]

Bing cherries are named after Ah Bing, the **horticulturist** that developed this popular, sweet, heart-shaped variety. They are extra-large, deep red to black, juicy, **firm**, and very flavorful.

LAMBERT [LAM-BERT]

A purple to red cherry that is firm and sweet. Lambert cherries are smaller in size than Bing cherries. While sweet enough to eat fresh, they are great for baking because they maintain their firm **texture** when cooked.

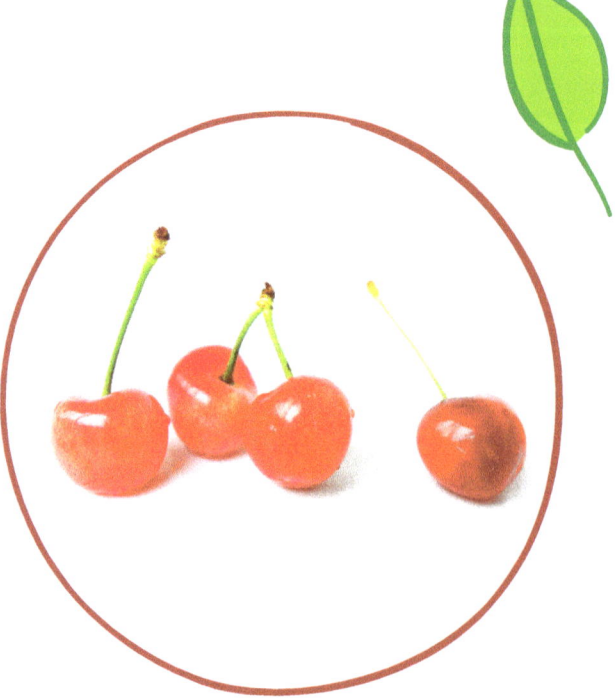

MONTMORENCY [MONT-MUH-REN-SEE]

A bright red cherry that is small and tart. Montmorency cherries are often used for cooking, baking, and juice. They are the most commonly grown type of tart cherry in the United States.

RAINIER [REY-NEER]

Ranier cherries are golden yellow inside and out with a red blush. They have a delicate, sweet **flavor** with a hint of tartness.

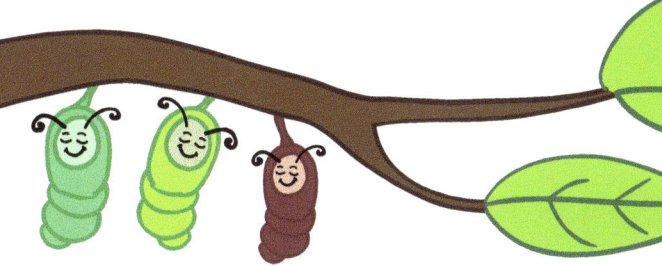

ROYAL ANN | NAPOLEON
[ROI-UHL AN] | [NUH-POH-LEE-UHN]

A light amber to yellow cherry with a red blush. Royal Ann cherries, also known as Napoleon cherries, are firm, juicy and have a sweet flavor. This **variety** is most often dyed and bottled to make maraschino cherries.

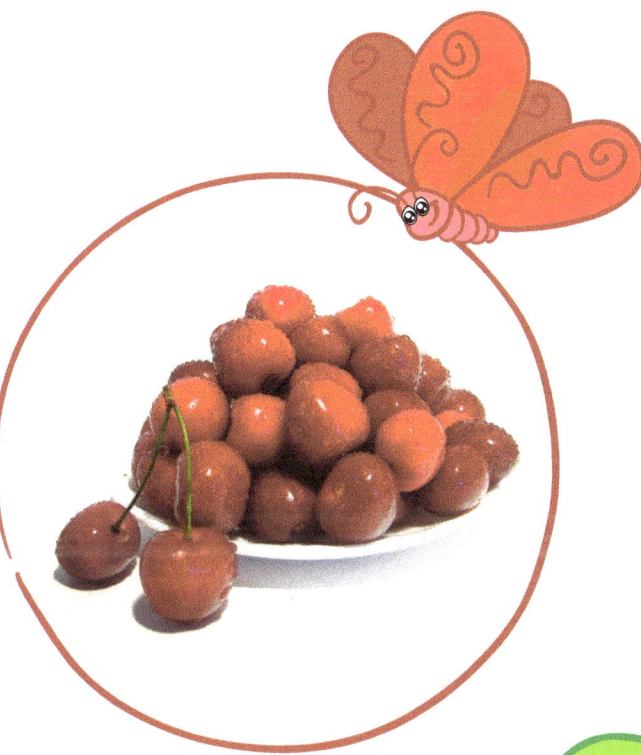

TULARE [TOO-LAIR-EE]

A dark red cherry with a tangy aftertaste. Tulare cherries are tarter, sweet cherries that are slightly less firm than the Bing variety.

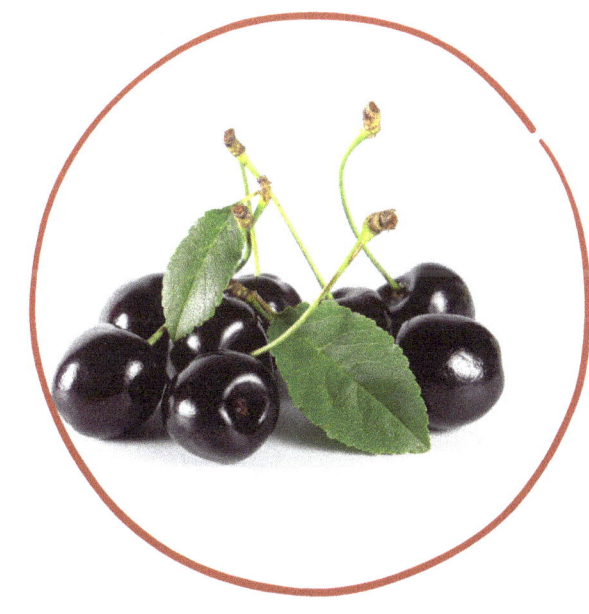

A Book of Fruits

COCONUT

[koh-kuh-nuht]

creamy, dry, meaty, rich, sweet

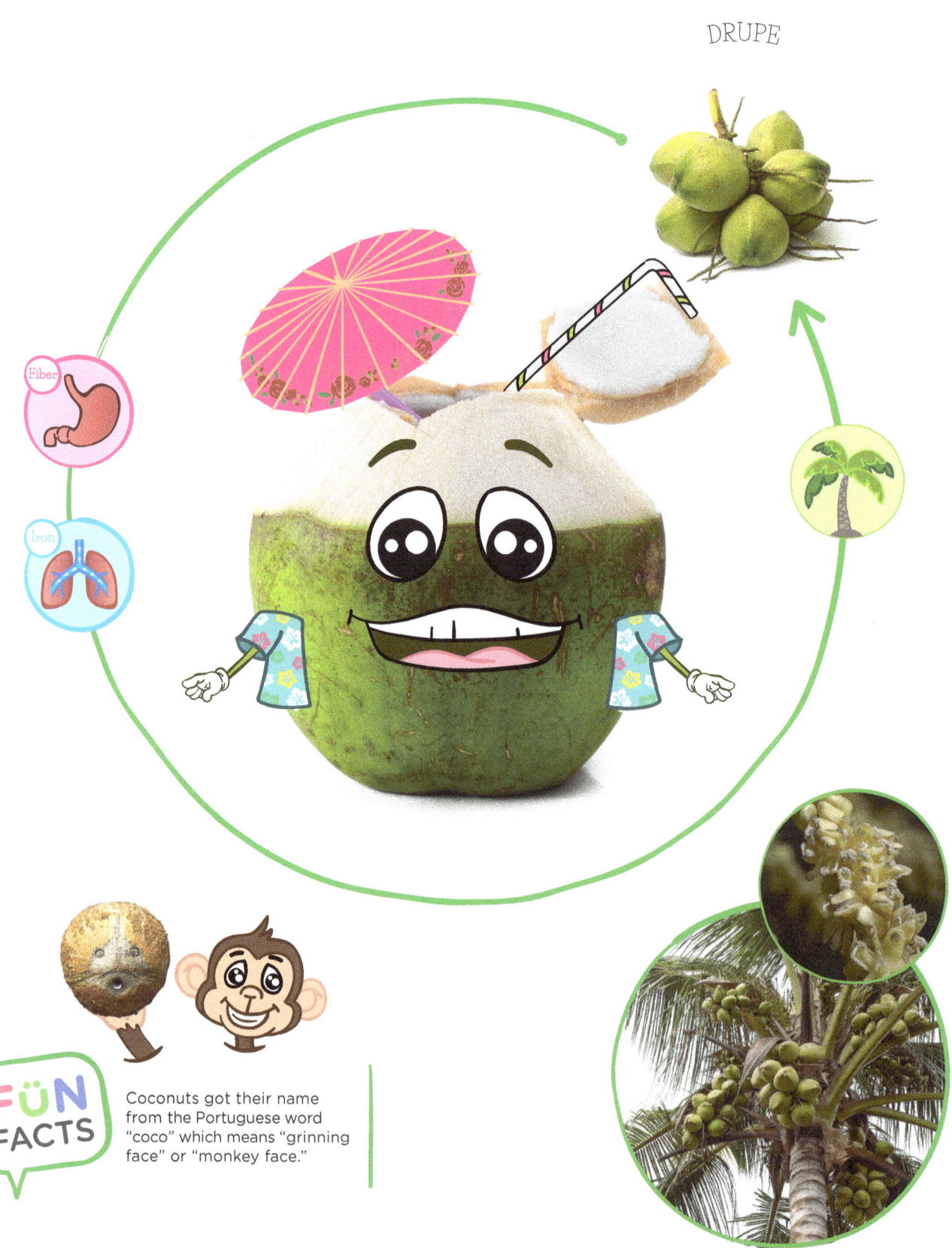

DRUPE

FUN FACTS

Coconuts got their name from the Portuguese word "coco" which means "grinning face" or "monkey face."

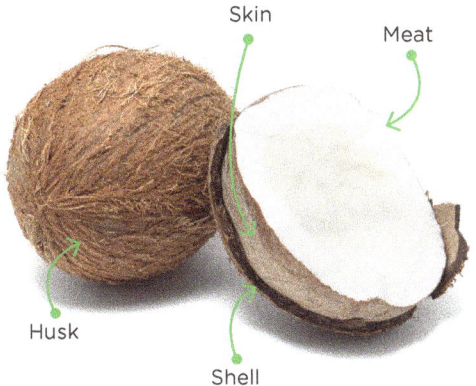

Skin
Meat
Husk
Shell
Eyes

PICK
Pick fruit that feel heavy for their size. Coconuts should be free of cracks and **mold** on the "eyes." Shake coconuts and listen for a splashing sound. Coconuts without coconut water may mean the fruit has spoiled.

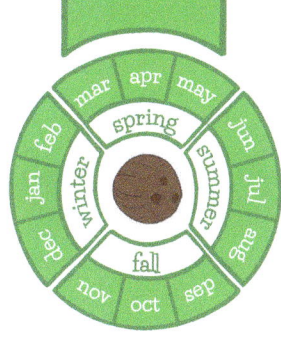

Varieties available year-round; Imported year-round

STORE
Keep whole coconuts at room **temperature** for up to 7 days. Refrigerate whole coconuts for 3-4 weeks or shelled in airtight containers for 4-5 days. Freeze shelled coconuts in airtight containers for up to 6 months. Dried coconuts may be stored in airtight containers for 6-12 months.

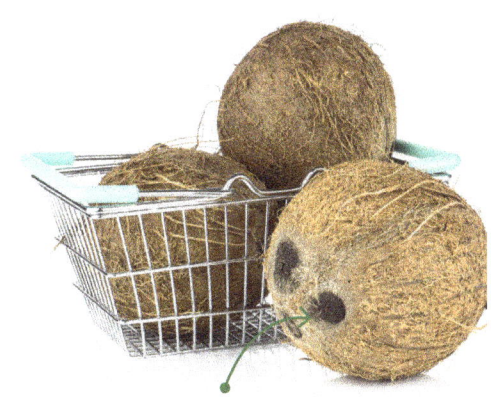

COCONUT TIDBITS

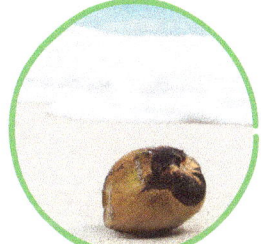

Coconuts are considered a tropical **drift** seed because they float and can survive years at sea. The ocean is a way for coconuts to spread their **seeds** and grow coconut palm trees in new locations.

EAT
You are going to need the help of an adult to cut through this hard shell! Preheat your oven to 350 degrees F. Clean the shell, place the coconut on a hard surface, puncture 2 of the 3 "eyes," and drain the liquid or coconut water into a bowl. Place whole coconut on a foil-lined baking sheet and heat in the oven for 15 minutes to help crack and shrink the meat away from the shell. Then, on a hard surface, split the coconut shell with a hammer where it cracked in the oven or put the coconut in a plastic bag and smash it on concrete. Once split, remove the coconut meat from the shell with a spoon and peel off the brown skin.

Toasted Coconut
Preheat oven to 350 degrees F. Use a potato peeler to cut ribbons of coconut meat and place on a foil-lined baking sheet in the oven for 10-15 minutes. Stir ribbons every five minutes to toast evenly. Coconut should be golden and crisp. Eat as a snack or use as a garnish.

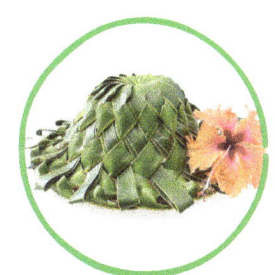

All parts of the coconut plant can be used. The tree trunk can be used as wood, leaves for baskets, and **husks** for ropes.

A Book of Fruits 59

CRANBERRY

[kran-ber-ee]

bitter, chewy, sour, tangy, tart

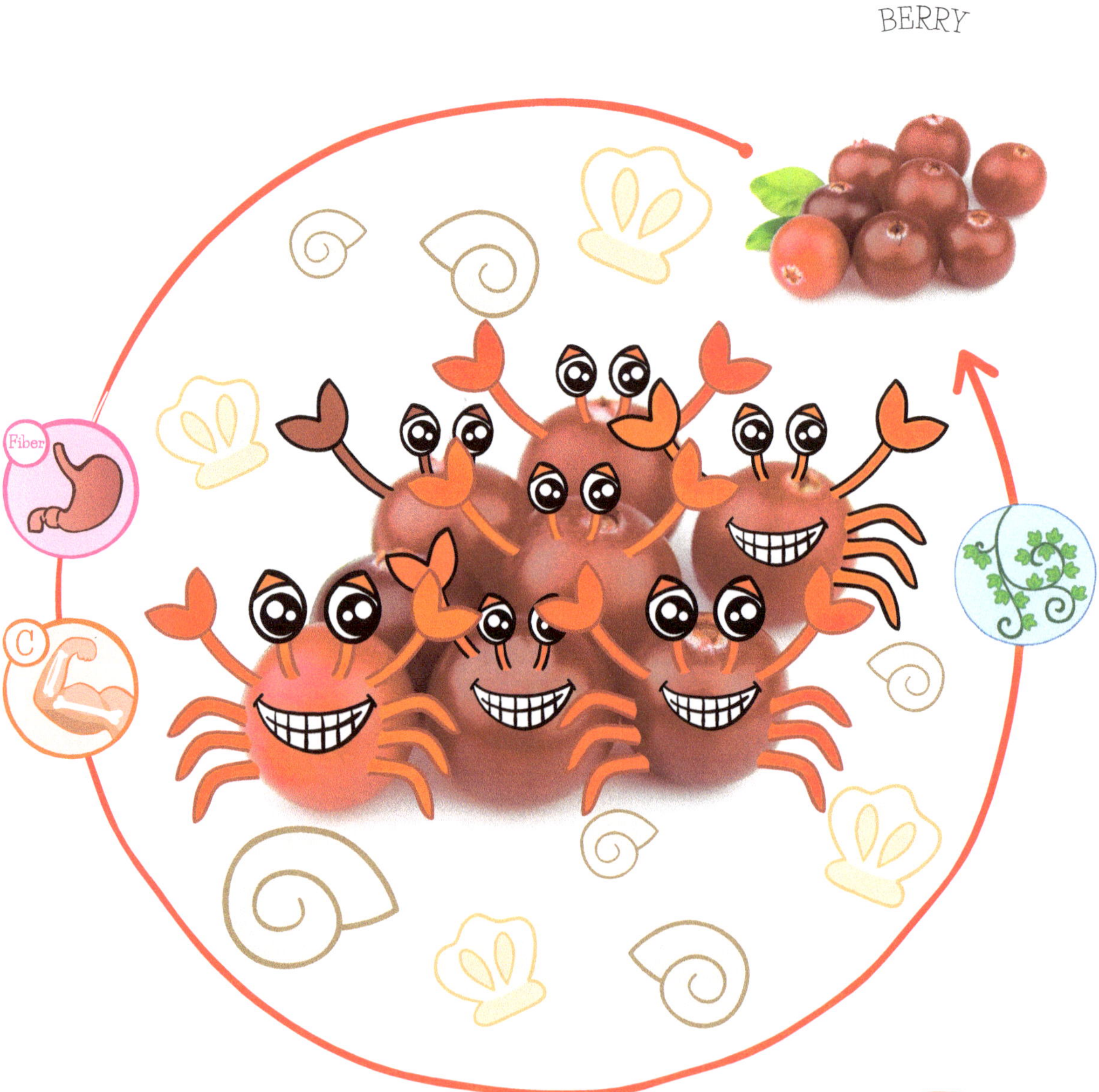

BERRY

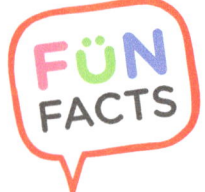

Before **farming technology**, cranberries were rolled down a short flight of stairs for selection. Good cranberries bounce like little rubber balls!

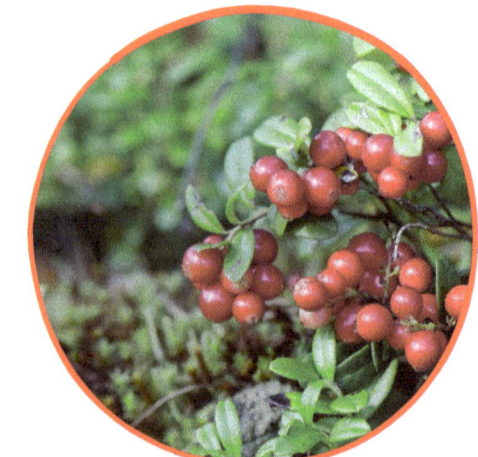

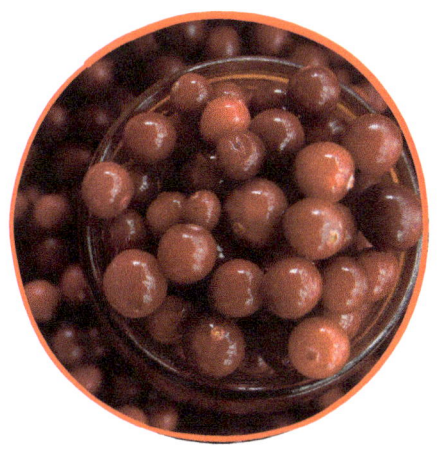

PICK
Pick bright red, **plump**, and **firm** fruit. Avoid cranberries that are soft, crushed, or shriveled.

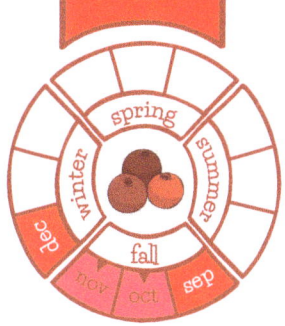

Available September to December

Peak Season
October-November

STORE
Keep cranberries from **spoiling** by storing them in the refrigerator. Refrigerate cranberries in a plastic bag for up to 6 weeks. Refrigerate fresh cranberry sauce in airtight containers for 10-14 days. Freeze cranberries in airtight containers for 10-12 months. Dried cranberries may be stored in airtight containers for 6-12 months.

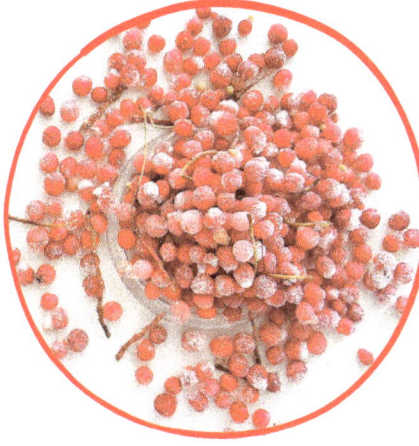

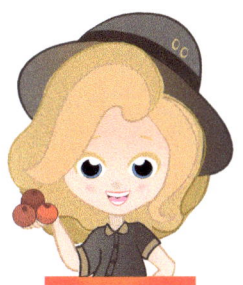

CRANBERRY TIDBITS

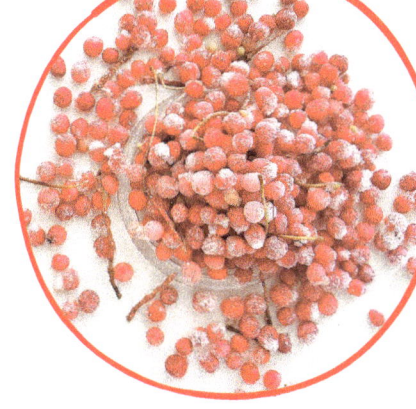

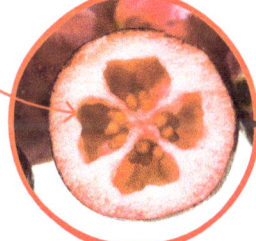

Look at the inside of a cranberry. The four chambers inside the cranberry are filled with air which helps them bounce when **ripe**.

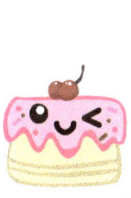

EAT
Clean just before using.

Balsamic Cranberries
Preheat oven to 400 degrees F. Combine 1 cup cranberries, 3 tablespoons maple syrup, 2 tablespoons balsamic vinegar, 1 tablespoon orange juice, 1 tablespoon melted coconut oil, and 1/2 teaspoon orange **zest** in a 8x8 inch, glass baking dish. Cover with foil and roast in the oven for 15-20 minutes or until most of the cranberries have popped. Stir and allow to cool for 5 minutes. Try on sandwiches or as a garnish on top of roasted vegetables such as Brussels sprouts, butternut squash, or sweet potatoes.

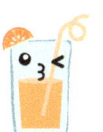

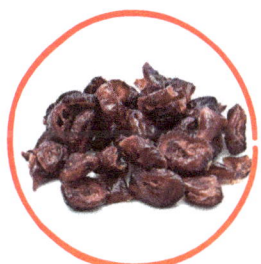

Dried and sweetened cranberries are tasty and can be eaten just like raisins!

CURRANT
CASSIS

[kur-uhnt] | [ka-sees]

aromatic, astringent, pulpy, sweet, tart

BERRY

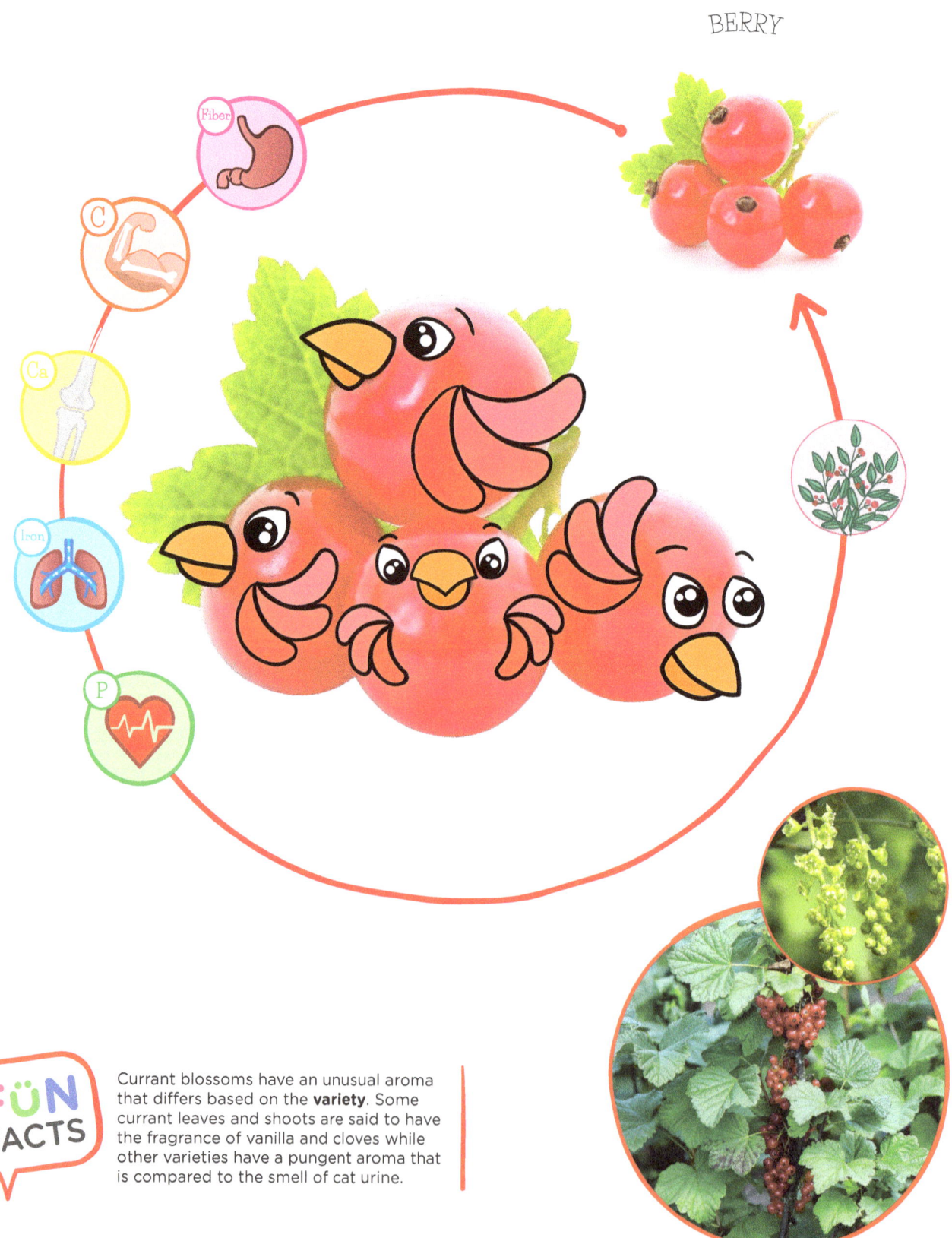

FUN FACTS

Currant blossoms have an unusual aroma that differs based on the **variety**. Some currant leaves and shoots are said to have the fragrance of vanilla and cloves while other varieties have a pungent aroma that is compared to the smell of cat urine.

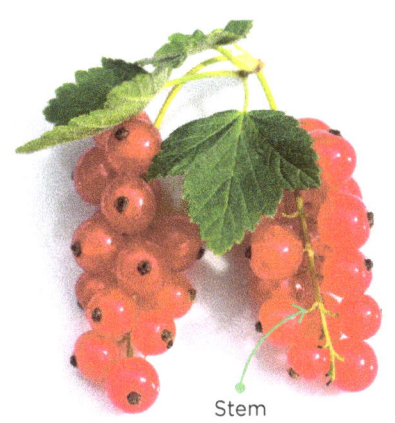
Stem

PICK
Pick deep red or black, glossy, **firm** fruit. Currants should be uniform in size. Check the bottom of the package to make sure there is not any juice or mold and that currants are not crushed.

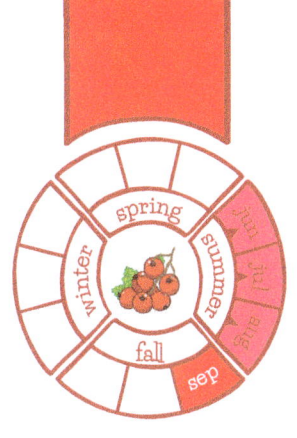

Available June to September

Peak Season
June-August

STORE
Keep currants from **spoiling** by storing them in the refrigerator. Place currants in a shallow container covered with plastic wrap for up to 2 weeks. Freeze currants in airtight containers for 10-12 months. Dried currants may be stored in airtight containers for 6-12 months. Before storing currants, throw away any crushed or **moldy** fruit.

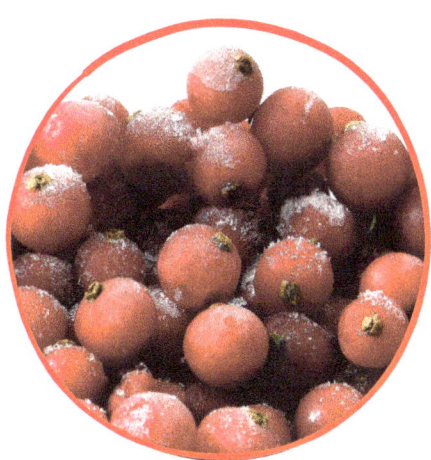

CURRANT TIDBITS

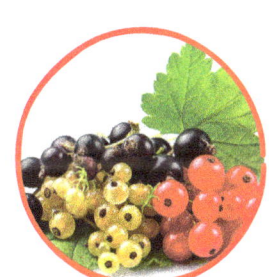

Currants come in three colors: red, white, and black.

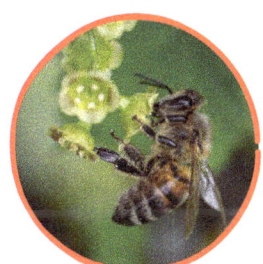

EAT
De-stem and clean just before eating or using.

Black Currant Lemonade
Combine 4 quarts black currants and 1 cup water in a saucepan and simmer for 20 minutes or until fruit is soft. Strain the fruit from the juice and return the juice to the saucepan to make syrup. Stir 1 cup white sugar into the juice and boil until sugar **dissolves**, about 3 minutes. Pour black currant syrup into a glass jar and store in refrigerator for up to 1 month. For lemonade, mix 4 ounces water with 4 ounces black currant syrup, and 1/2 a fresh squeezed lemon.

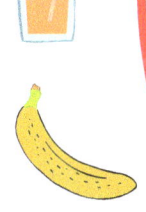

Currant flowers attract honeybees for **pollination** but can **self-pollinate** when insects are not available. This means they can create new **seedlings** without any help.

DATE

[deyt]

caramel-like, chewy, honey-like, sugary, tender

DRUPE

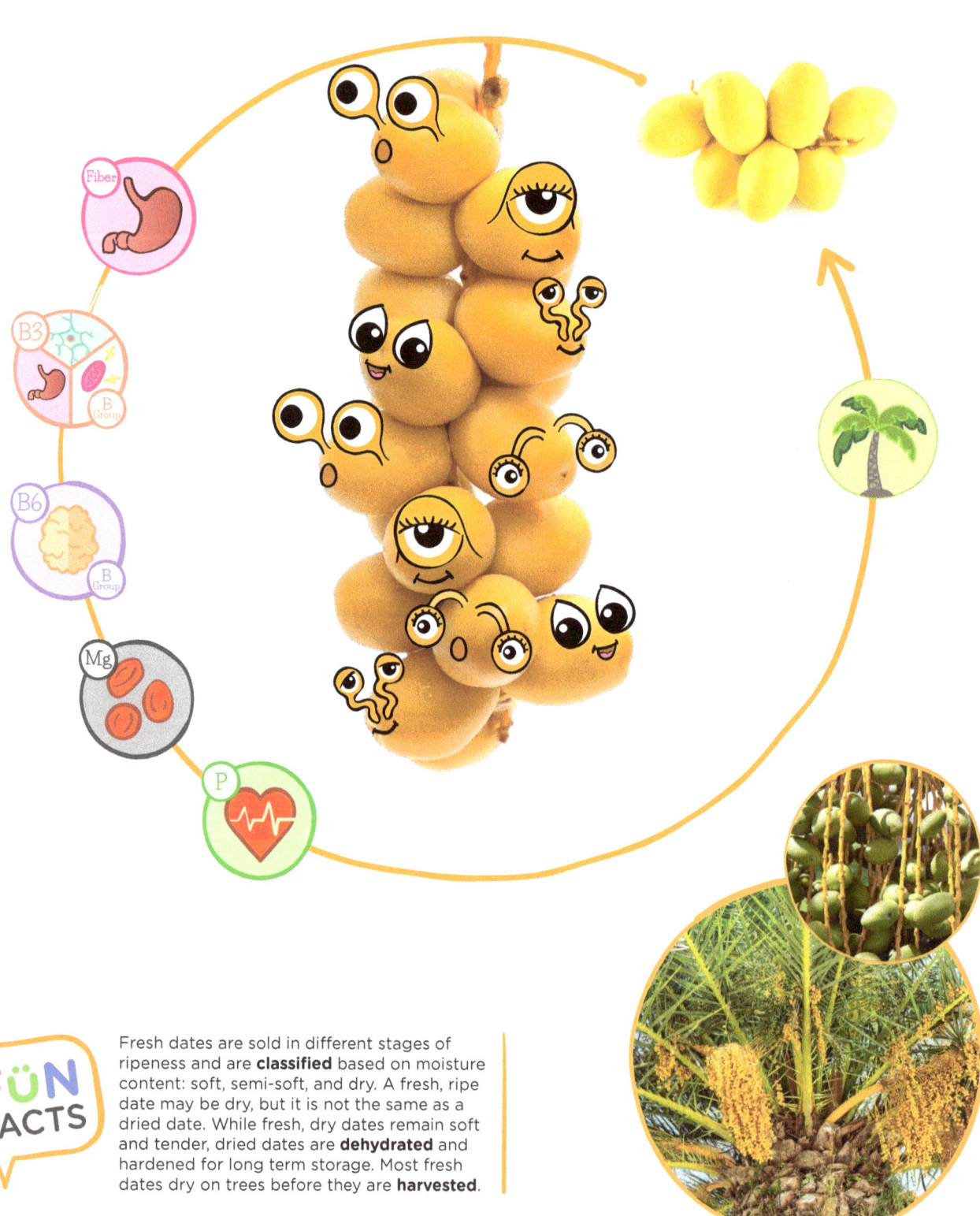

FUN FACTS
Fresh dates are sold in different stages of ripeness and are **classified** based on moisture content: soft, semi-soft, and dry. A fresh, ripe date may be dry, but it is not the same as a dried date. While fresh, dry dates remain soft and tender, dried dates are **dehydrated** and hardened for long term storage. Most fresh dates dry on trees before they are **harvested**.

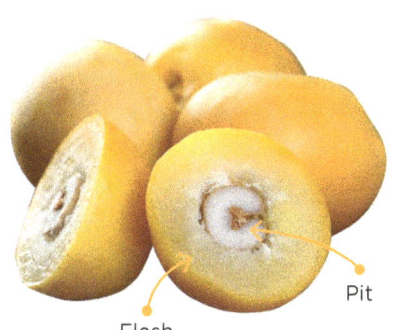

Flesh · Pit

PICK
Pick fresh, underripe, yellow, shiny, **plump** fruit free of cuts and **bruises**. Pick fresh, ripe, brown, shiny, wrinkly fruit that are soft to touch. Fresh dates should be free of hardened spots and sugar crystals on the skin. Dried dates should be free of sticky skin.

Available September to December; Imported year-round

Peak Season
September-November

STORE
Keep **ripe** dates in airtight containers at room **temperature** for up to 1 month and dried dates for up to 2 months. Refrigerate ripe dates in airtight containers for up to 6 months and dried dates for up to 1 year. Freeze dates in airtight containers for 1-2 years. Keep away from foods with strong odors.

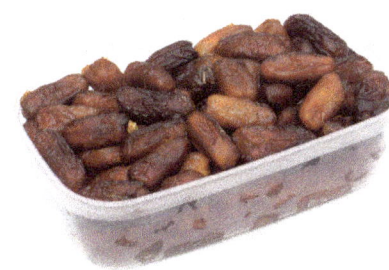

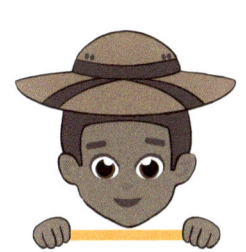

DATES TIDBITS

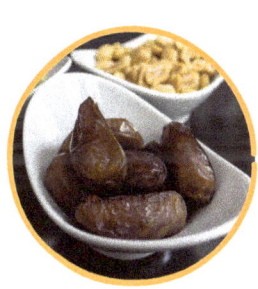

Dates are called the "candy that grows on trees" because they are sweet, chewy, and an easy snack on the go.

EAT
Clean the skin, slice or bite in half, and remove the **pit** from the center. Eat, chop, or slice per recipe.

Date and Pecan Salad with Orange Vinaigrette
Combine 1 cup fresh or dried, pitted, and chopped dates, 1 cup cored and chopped **firm** pear, 1/4 cup dried cherries, and 1/4 cup pecan pieces. To make orange **vinaigrette**, shake together 3 ounces orange juice, 2 tablespoons white balsamic vinegar, 2 tablespoons olive oil, 1 tablespoon Dijon-style mustard, 2 teaspoons honey, and a pinch salt and pepper in a small jar with a lid. Toss fruit and nut mixture with 2 cups of salad greens and orange vinaigrette.

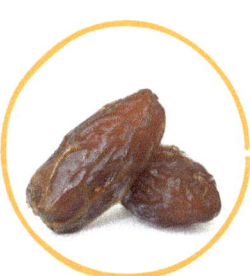

One of the most common varieties of dates is the Medjool date. They are known for their sweet, moist, meaty **texture**.

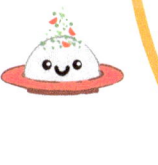

A Book of Fruits

DRAGON FRUIT
PITAHAYA

[drag-uhn froot] | [pit-uh-hahy-uh]

crunchy, juicy, mild, refreshing, tangy

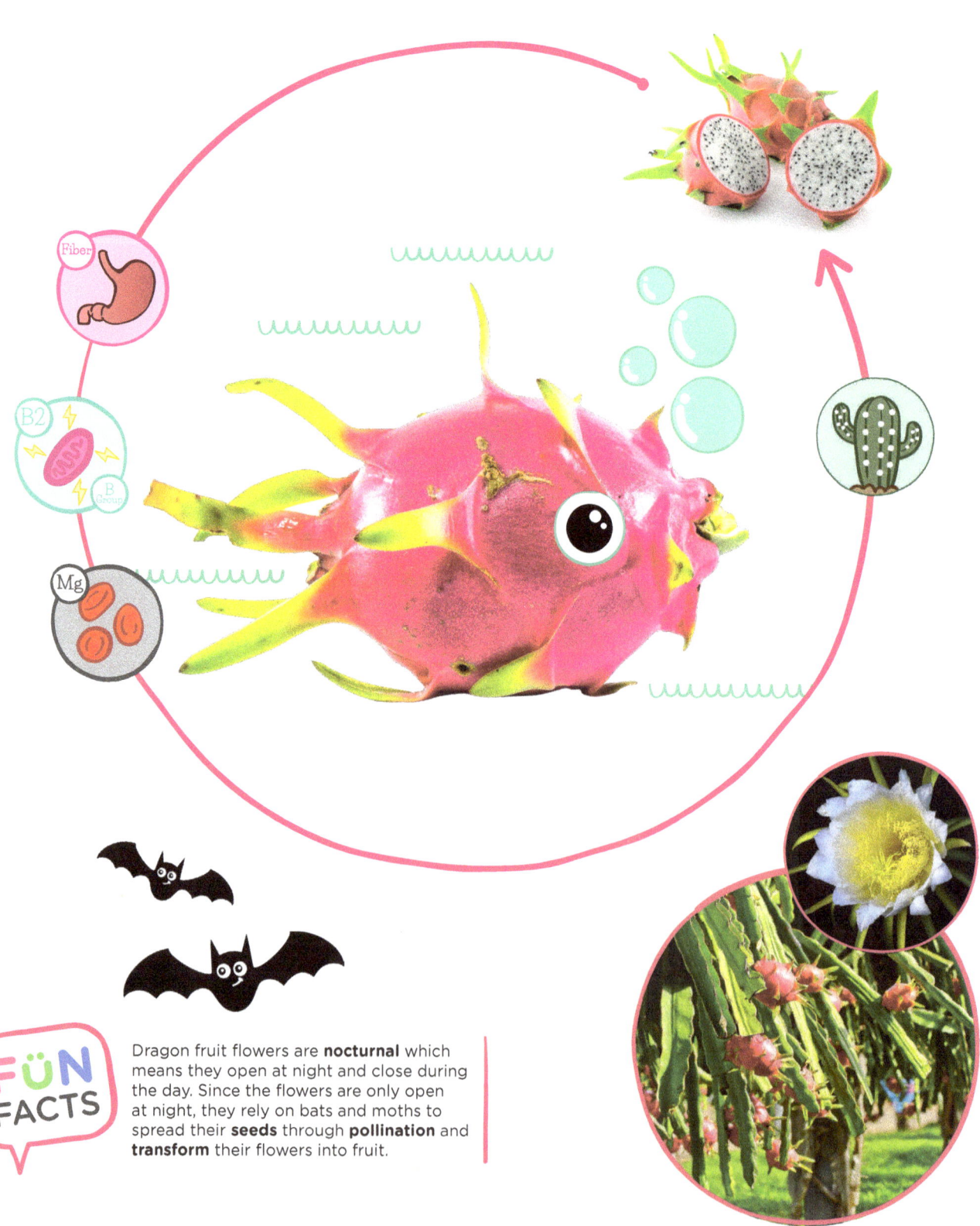

BERRY

FUN FACTS: Dragon fruit flowers are **nocturnal** which means they open at night and close during the day. Since the flowers are only open at night, they rely on bats and moths to spread their **seeds** through **pollination** and **transform** their flowers into fruit.

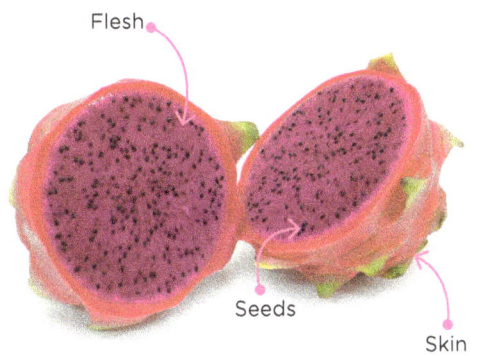

PICK
Pick bright, deep-colored skin that is a fading red to green color on the scaly tips and soft to touch. Dragon fruits should be free of mushy spots.

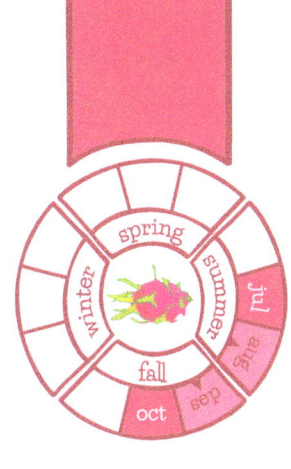

Available July to October; Imported year-round

Peak Season
August-September

STORE
Keep dragon fruits at room **temperature** for up to 3 days. Refrigerate whole dragon fruits in a plastic bag for 5-7 days or sliced in airtight containers for 1-2 days. Freeze dragon fruits in airtight containers for 10-12 months. Keep away from foods with strong odors.

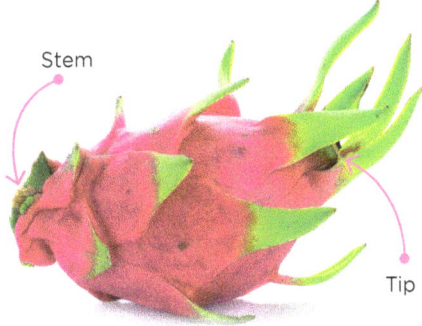

DRAGON FRUIT TIDBITS

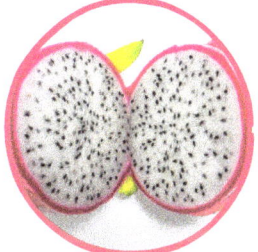

Do you see all the tiny black flecks in the dragon fruit flesh? Those are crunchy seeds that are similar in **texture** to seeds in kiwi.

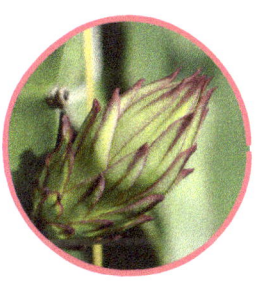

The dragon fruit flower bud is **edible** and can be **prepared** like a vegetable. With a **flavor** similar to asparagus, the flower buds are added to soups, sautéed, or eaten battered and fried.

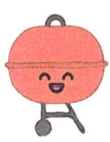
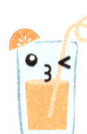

EAT
Clean the skin, slice in half stem to tip or around the center of the fruit, spoon out the **flesh**.

Dragon Fruit Star-Shaped Garnish
Slice the fruit in half around the center of the fruit and spoon out the flesh. Slice fruit into 1 inch slices. You should be able slice 4 to 6 slices from one dragon fruit. Then press a star-shaped cookie cutter **firmly** into the fruit flesh, pop out the dragon fruit, and use it to top fruit salads, fruit kabobs, or add a stick to the bottom and freeze into star popsicles.

A Book of Fruits 67

DURIAN

[door-eeuhn]

aromatic, custard-like, rich, succulent, sweet

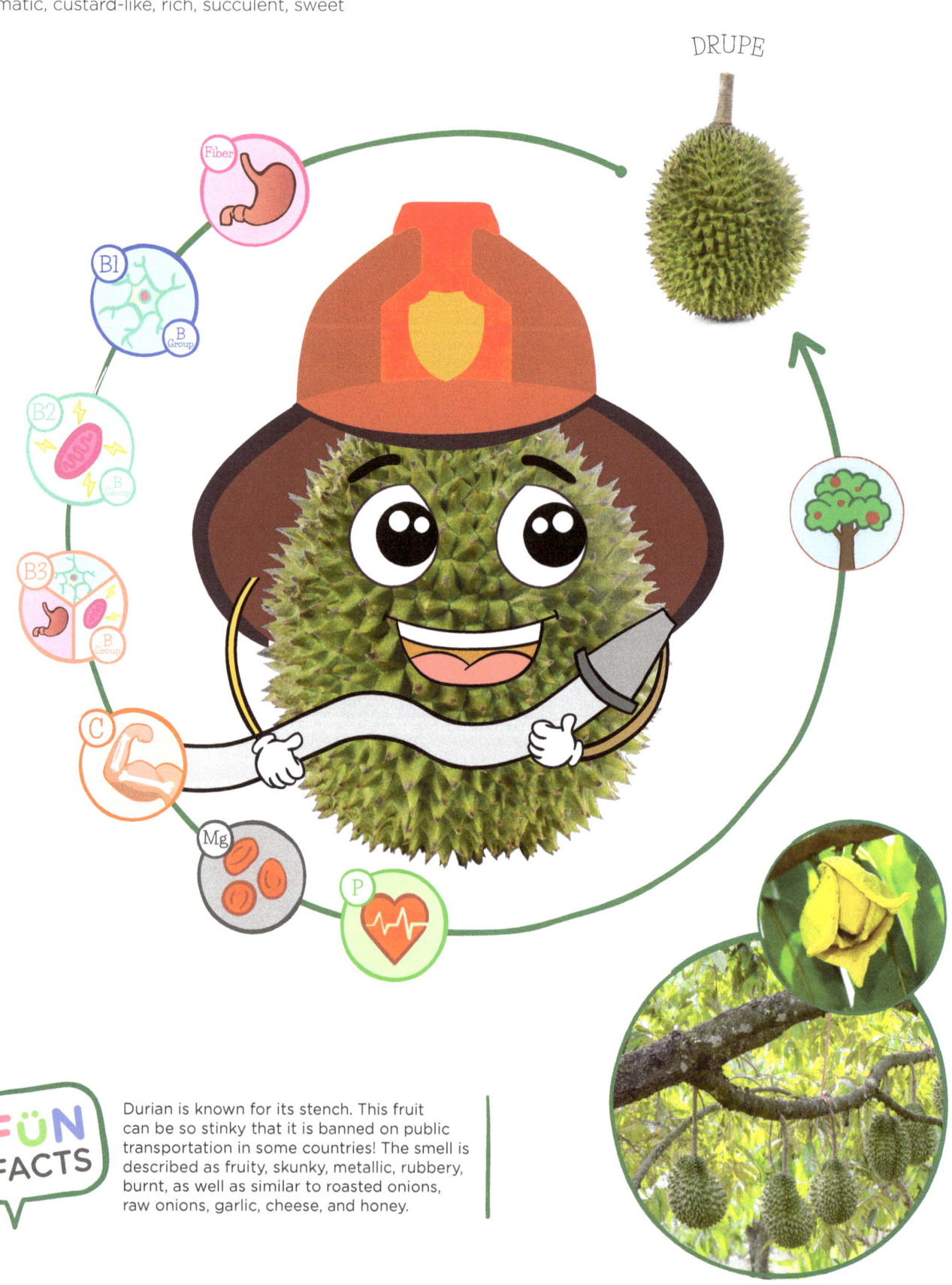

DRUPE

FUN FACTS: Durian is known for its stench. This fruit can be so stinky that it is banned on public transportation in some countries! The smell is described as fruity, skunky, metallic, rubbery, burnt, as well as similar to roasted onions, raw onions, garlic, cheese, and honey.

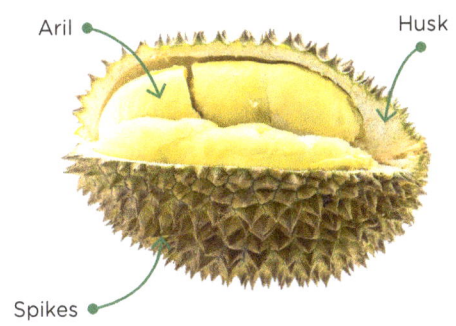

PICK
Pick dark green **husks** covered with sharp spikes and large solid stems. Durians should feel light for their size with a strong aroma. Avoid durian that smell sour.

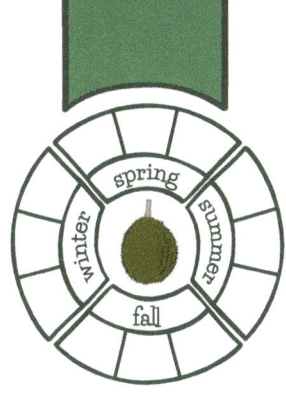

Available imported March to August

STORE
Keep whole durians at room **temperature** for up to 3 days. Refrigerate whole durians away from other food or in a plastic bag for up to 14 days and deseeded **flesh** in airtight containers for up to 7 days. Freeze whole durians or the flesh in airtight containers for 1-2 years.

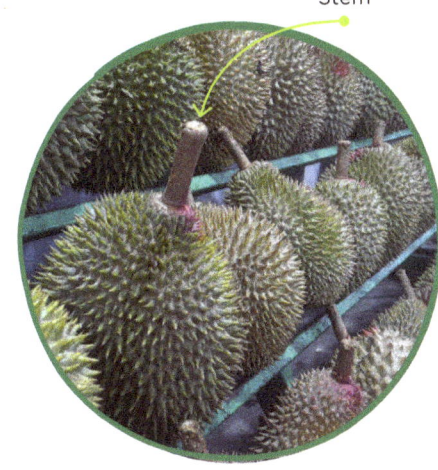

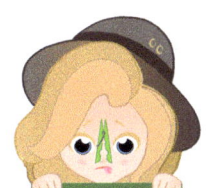

DURIAN TIDBITS

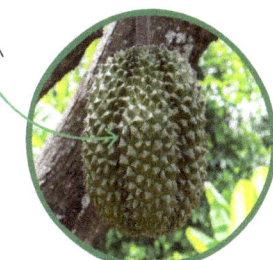

Durian fruit is technically not a **drupe** but a fleshy aril from an **indehiscent capsule**, meaning the fruit does not split open when they are **ripe**. When durians are fully ripe, they fall from trees to the ground.

EAT
You are going to need the help of an adult to cut through this spikey husk. You may want to use a towel to protect your hands from the spikes! Clean the husk, slice off the stem, and place the stem end down on the cutting board. Look for the natural seams or lines on the fruit and use a knife to slice from the tip all the way around, scoring the skin. Use your hands to pull apart the husk at the seams and pull out the cream-colored **arils**. Slice open the arils and throw away the large black **seeds**.

Fresh Durian
Refrigerate freshly opened durian **flesh** in an airtight container for 2 hours, then sample fruit fresh. You can also try blending 4 ounces durian flesh, 2 cups Greek yogurt, and 1/2 cup sugar and refrigerating overnight.

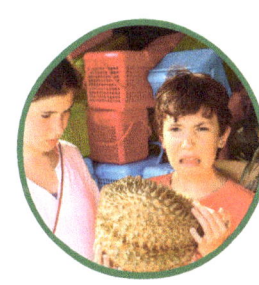
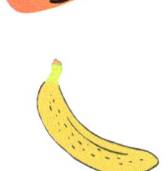

Researchers believe that the strong scent of the durian developed over time to attract animals to eat the fruit and spread its seeds.

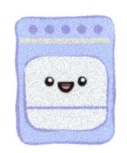

A Book of Fruits 69

ELDERBERRY

[el-der-ber-ee]

astringent, bitter, bright, fruity, sweet-tart

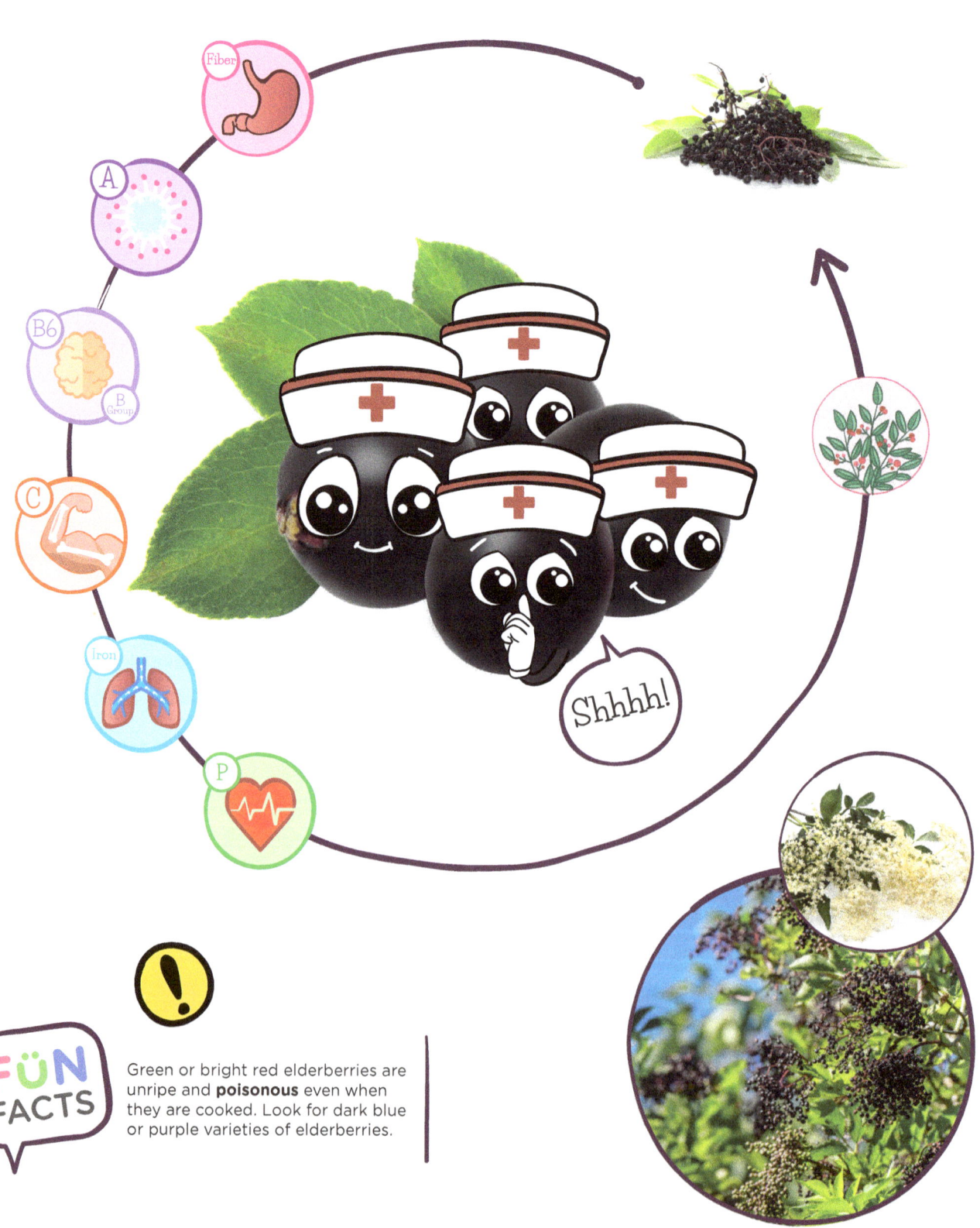

BERRY

Shhhh!

FUN FACTS: Green or bright red elderberries are unripe and **poisonous** even when they are cooked. Look for dark blue or purple varieties of elderberries.

70 | Where Do Bananas Come From?

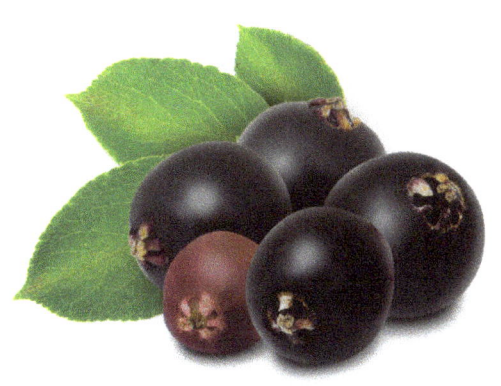

PICK
Pick dark purple to black fruit that are soft to touch. Check the bottom of the package to make sure there is not any juice or mold and that elderberries are not crushed.

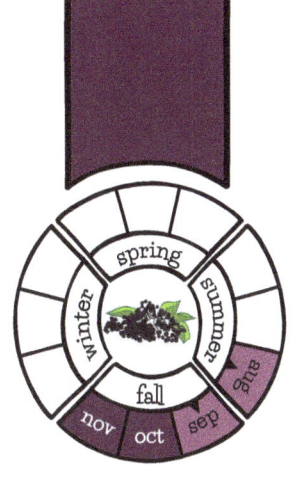

Available August to November

Peak Season
August-September

STORE
Keep elderberries from **spoiling** by storing them in the refrigerator. Refrigerate elderberries in a shallow container covered with plastic wrap for up to 3 days. Freeze elderberries in airtight containers for 10-12 months. Dried elderberries may be stored in airtight containers for 6-12 months. Before storing elderberries, throw away any crushed or **moldy** fruit.

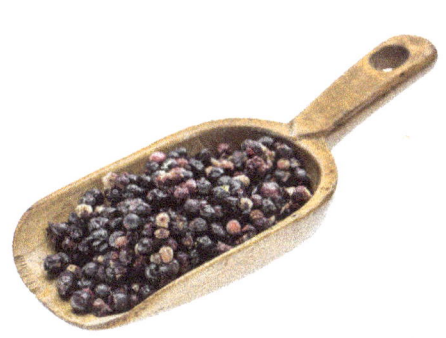

ELDERBERRY TIDBITS

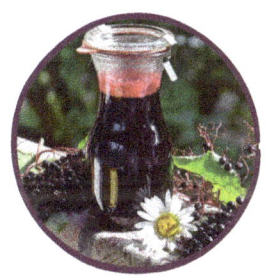

Elderberry syrup has long been used as a natural way to boost immunity and as a remedy for colds and the flu.

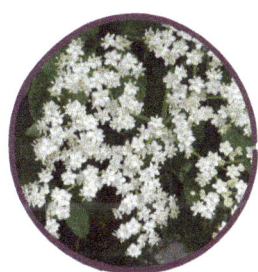

Elderberry flowers attract flies for **pollination** but can **self-pollinate** when insects are not available. This means they can create new **seedlings** without any help.

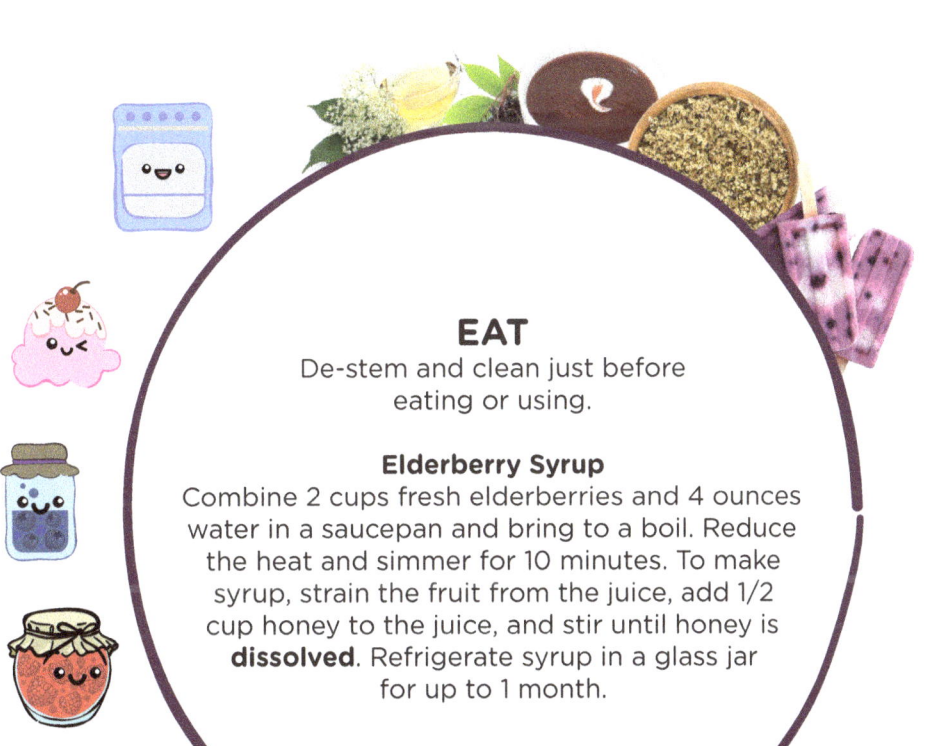

EAT
De-stem and clean just before eating or using.

Elderberry Syrup
Combine 2 cups fresh elderberries and 4 ounces water in a saucepan and bring to a boil. Reduce the heat and simmer for 10 minutes. To make syrup, strain the fruit from the juice, add 1/2 cup honey to the juice, and stir until honey is **dissolved**. Refrigerate syrup in a glass jar for up to 1 month.

A Book of Fruits

FIG

[fig]

chewy, grainy, honey-like, nutty, sweet

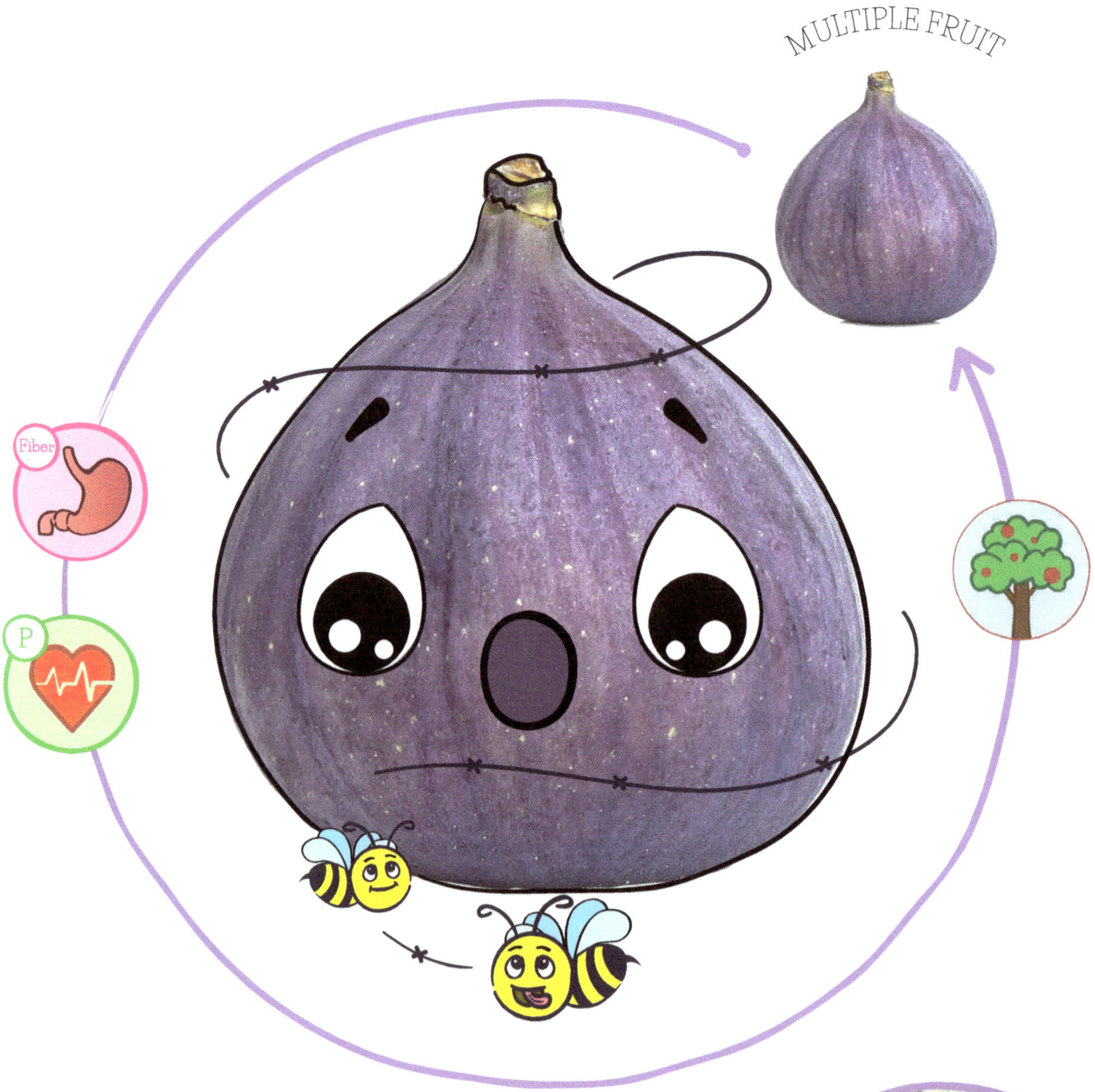

MULTIPLE FRUIT

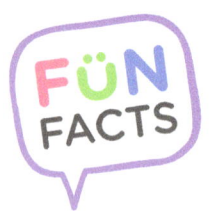

Figs are considered the sweetest fruit. They have a natural sugar content of 55%! Have you ever tried a fig for dessert?

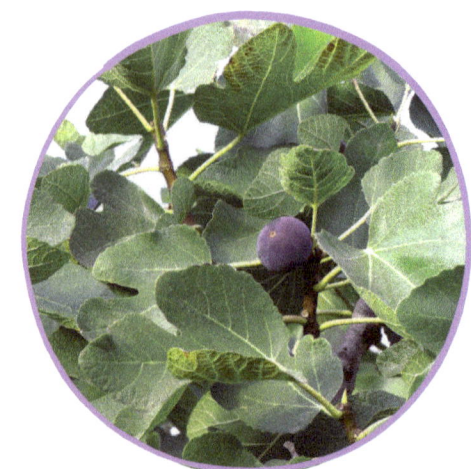

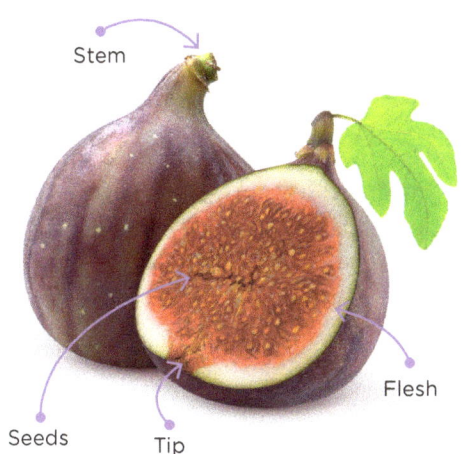
Stem · Flesh · Seeds · Tip

PICK
Pick greenish-yellow to purple fruit with smooth, dry skin that is soft to touch. Figs should be free of mushy spots.

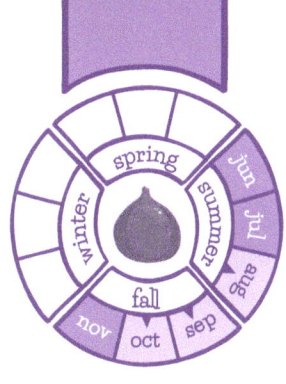

Available June to November

Peak Season
August-October

STORE
Refrigerate figs in a plastic bag for up to 2 days. Freeze figs in airtight containers for 10-12 months. Dried figs may be stored in airtight containers for 6-12 months.

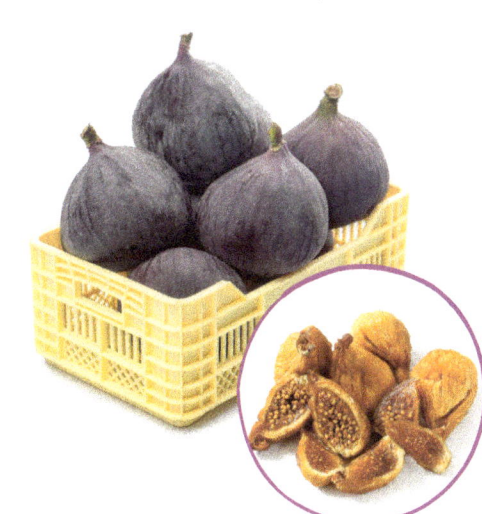

FIG TIDBITS

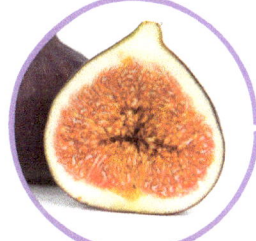

Figs are inverted flowers. This means that fig trees do not flower like apples and bananas. Instead, their flowers **bloom** inside the pear-shaped pod which turns into the fruit we eat.

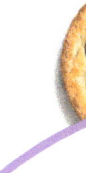
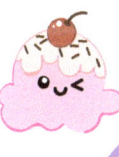

EAT
Clean the skin and slice or twist off the stem. Eat, chop, or slice per recipe.

Sautéed Figs
Slice 6 figs in half from stem to tip. Melt 1 tablespoon butter and 1 tablespoon honey in a small frying pan on medium heat and place figs cut-side down. Spoon butter and honey over the top of the figs and cook until figs start to brown, about 5 minutes. Serve over vanilla yogurt or ice cream.

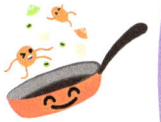
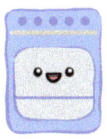

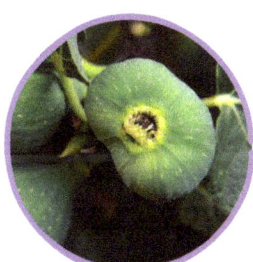

Figs are pollinated by a special type of wasp which enters the fig through a tiny passage in the bottom of the fruit.

A Book of Fruits

GOJI BERRY
WOLFBERRIES

[go-gee ber-ee] | [woolf ber-ee]

chewy, sour, sweet, tangy, tart

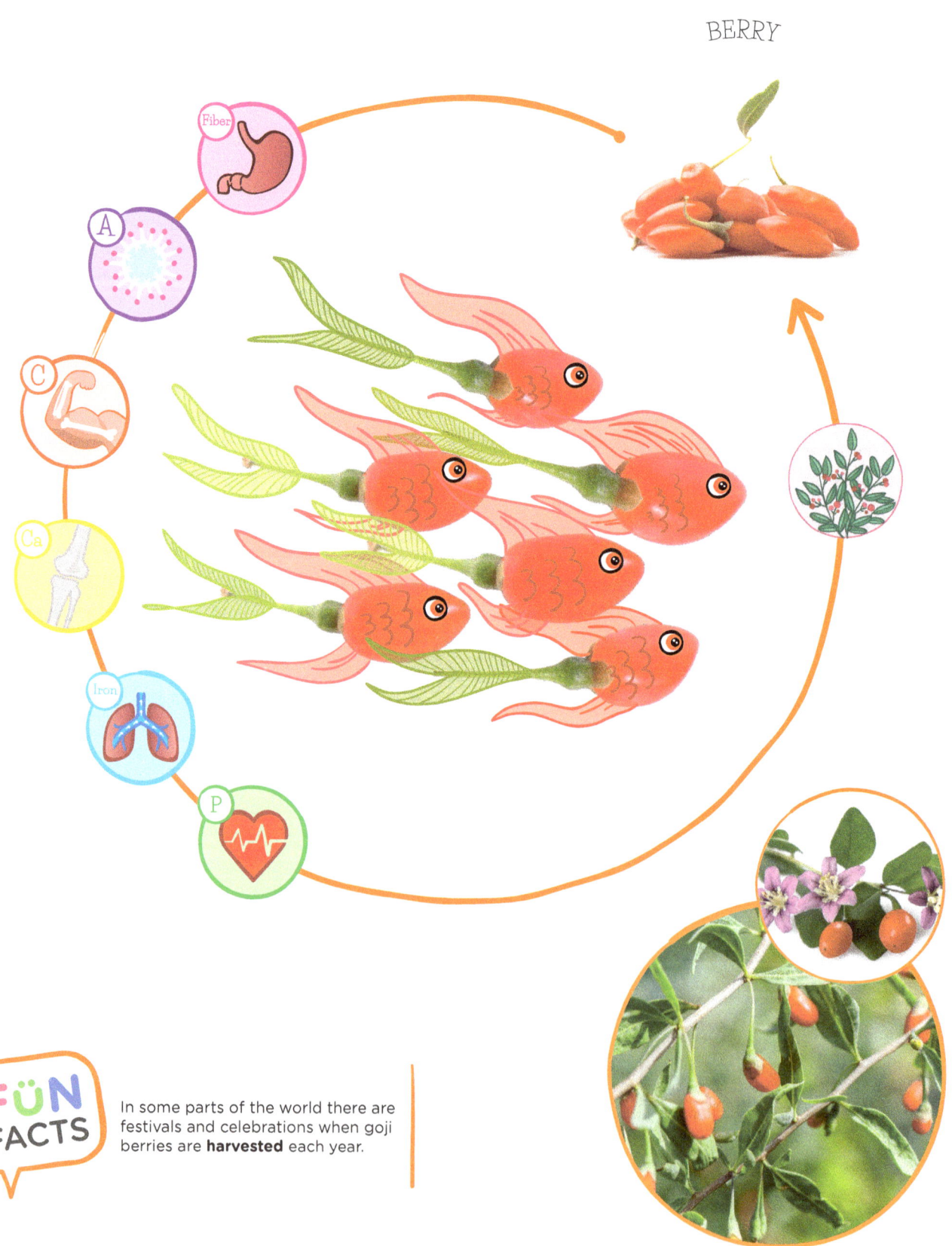

BERRY

FUN FACTS: In some parts of the world there are festivals and celebrations when goji berries are **harvested** each year.

74 | Where Do Bananas Come From?

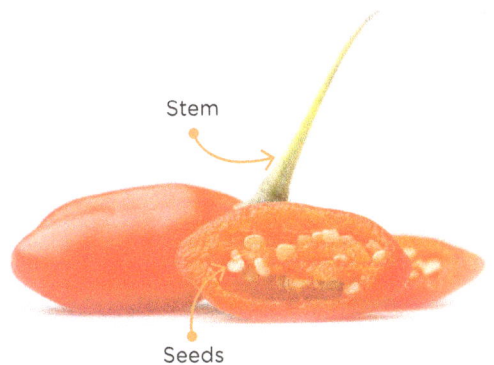
Stem
Seeds

PICK
Goji berries are typically sold dried outside of the countries where they grow because they **spoil** very quickly. Fruit should be dark red with wrinkled skin that is similar to raisins.

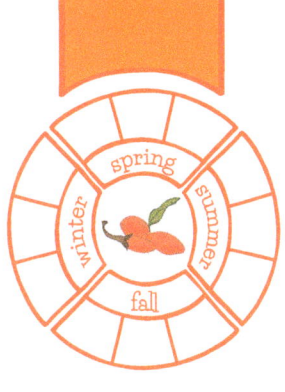

Available imported year-round

STORE
Store per packaging.

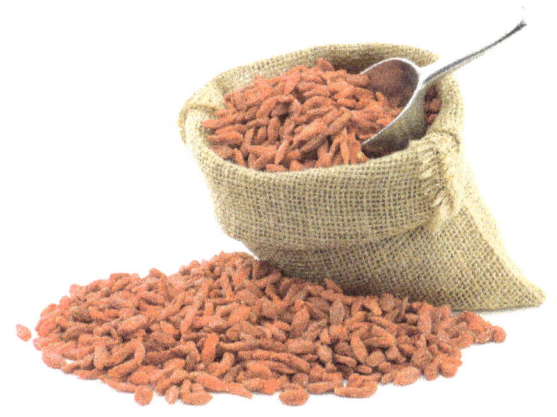

EAT
Goji berries are typically sold dried or as a powder.

Dried Goji Berries
Take goji berries for a snack on the go, add to cereal, top yogurt, or bake into muffins the same way you would use raisins.

GOJI BERRY TIDBITS

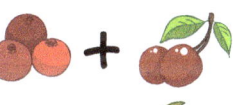

The **flavor** of goji berries is often compared to a cross between a cranberry and a cherry.

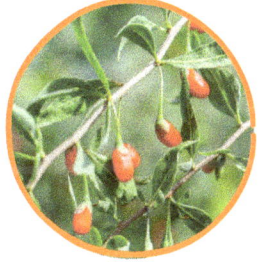

The shoots and leaves of goji berries have a slightly bitter, spinach-like taste and can be cooked and eaten like a leaf vegetable.

A Book of Fruits 75

GRAPE

[greyp]

chewy, juicy, refreshing, sweet, sweet-tart

BERRY

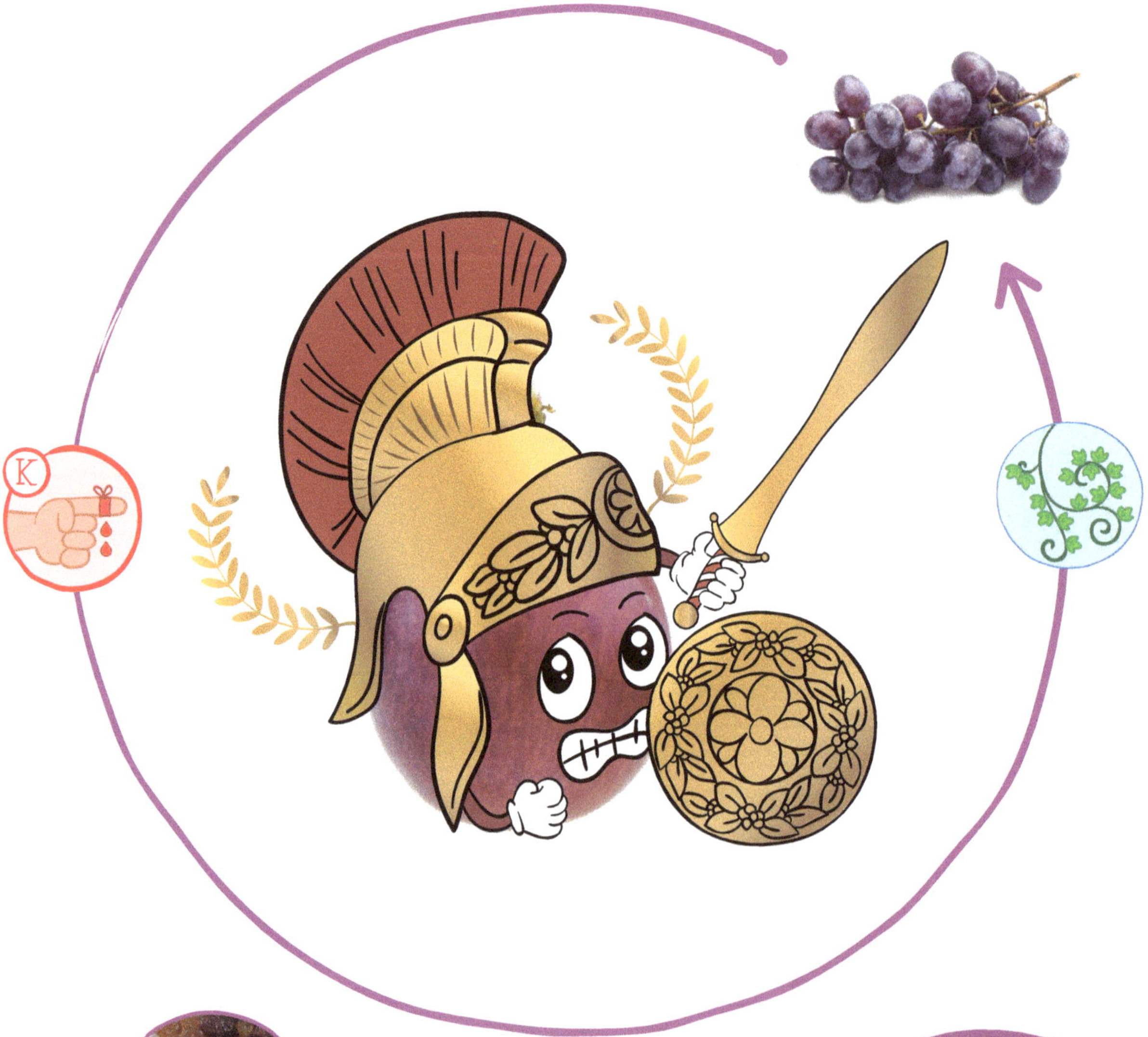

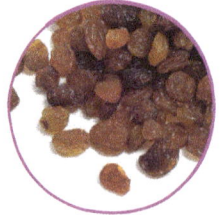

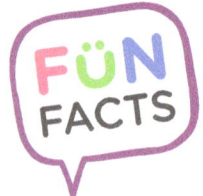

FUN FACTS: Dried grapes are called raisins. In ancient Rome, raisins were highly valued and used as a form of **currency**.

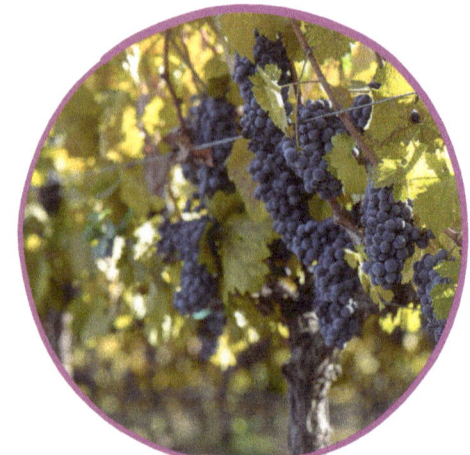

Where Do Bananas Come From?

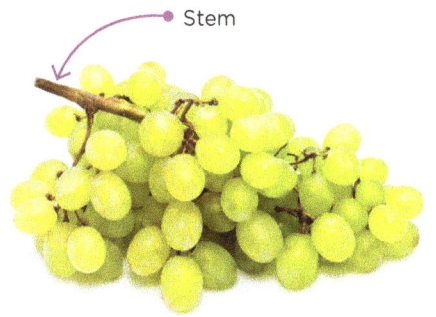
Stem

PICK
Pick deep-colored, **plump**, **firm** fruit with fresh green stems attached. Grape varieties should be free of soft spots and mold. Colors differ depending on **variety**.

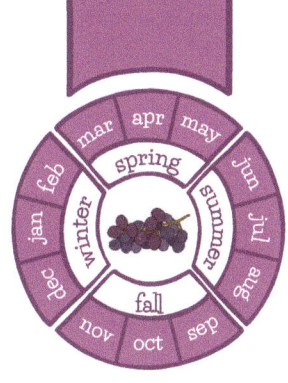

Varieties available year-round;
Imported year-round

Peak Season
Varies based on variety

STORE
Grapes kept at room **temperature** should be eaten the same day. Refrigerate grapes in their **perforated** plastic bag or place loosely in a shallow container covered with plastic wrap for up to 14 days. Freeze grapes in airtight containers for 10-12 months. Dried grapes, or raisins, may be stored in airtight containers for 6-12 months. Before storing grapes, throw away any crushed or **moldy** fruit. Keep away from foods with strong odors.

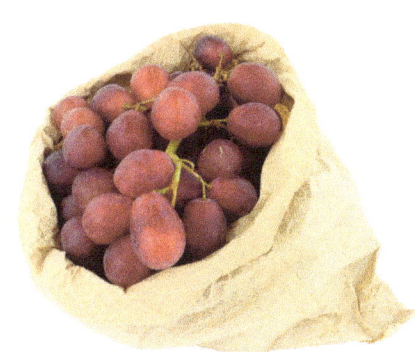

GRAPE TIDBITS

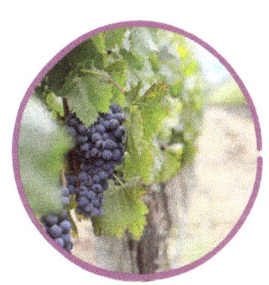

Viticulture, a branch of **horticulture**, is the art and science of growing and **harvesting** grapes. Viti comes from the Latin word for vine and grapes grow on vines.

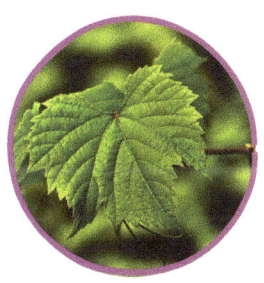

Young, tender grape leaves are **edible** and can be stuffed with a variety of savory fillings including rice, meat, and cheese.

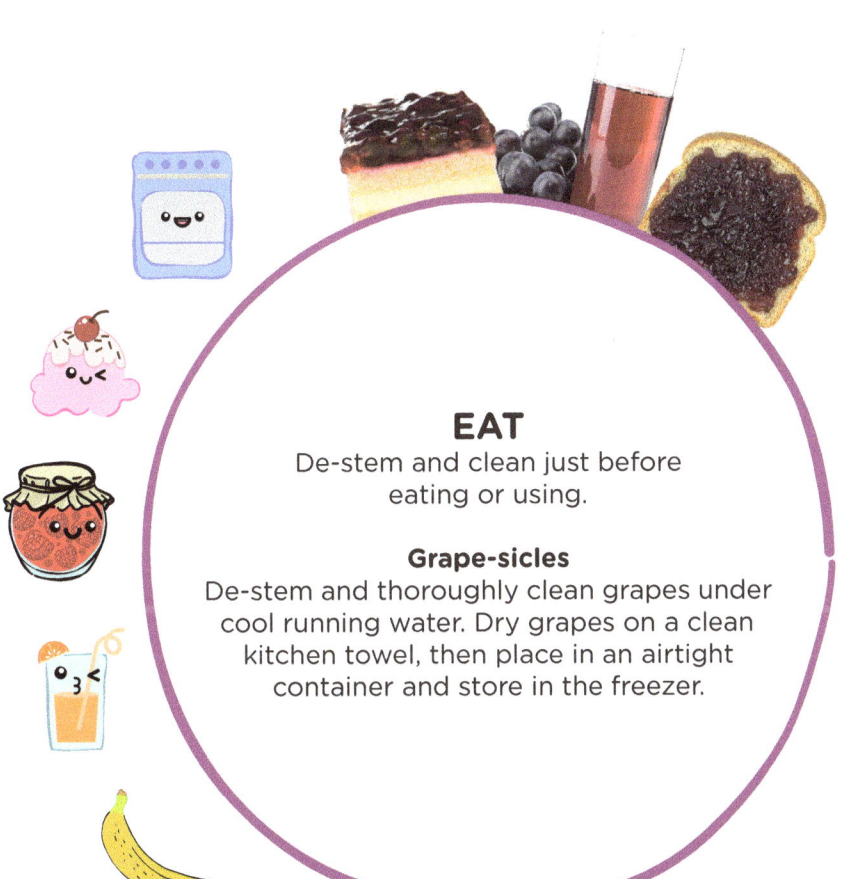

EAT
De-stem and clean just before eating or using.

Grape-sicles
De-stem and thoroughly clean grapes under cool running water. Dry grapes on a clean kitchen towel, then place in an airtight container and store in the freezer.

A Book of Fruits

GRAPE VARIETIES

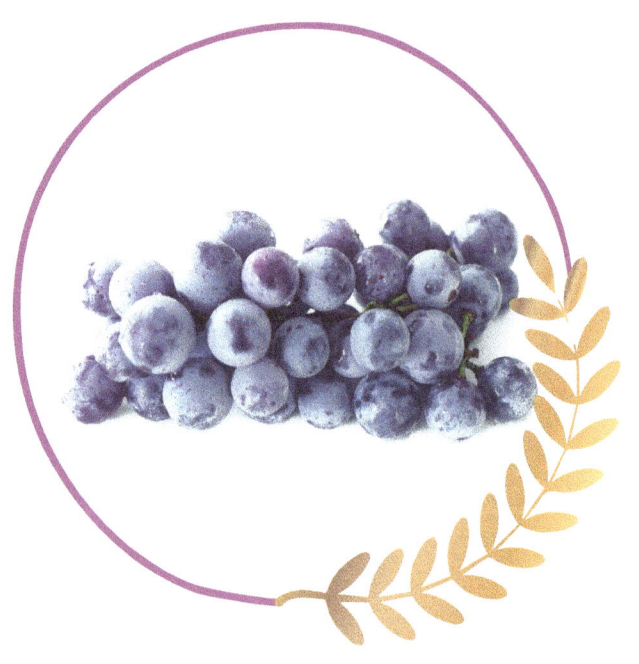

CONCORD [KON-KAWRD]

A dark blue-black or purple grape that is round, medium to large in size, and seeded. Concord grapes are fragrant, have tough skin, and sweet-tart juicy **flesh**. They are eaten fresh, made into jelly, and pressed for juice.

COTTON CANDY [KOT-N KAN-DEE]

A light green grape that is **plump**, juicy, and seedless. Cotton Candy grapes taste exactly like cotton candy and are perfect fresh or frozen.

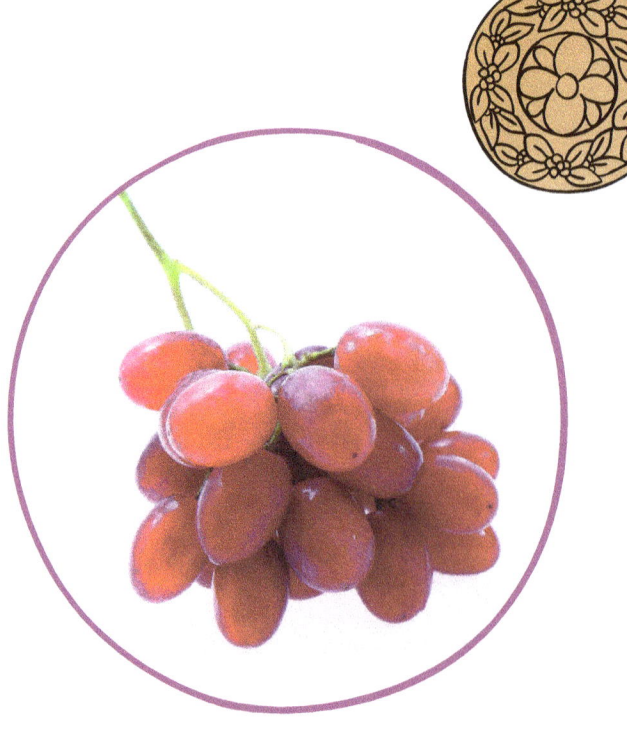

FLAME TOKAY | RED FLAME
[FLEYM TOK-AY] | [RED FLEYM]

A bright red, beautiful, long grape. Flame Tokay grapes may be seeded or seedless. They are **firm**, juicy, and very sweet with a strong grape **flavor**. Try them fresh or dried into extra-large raisins.

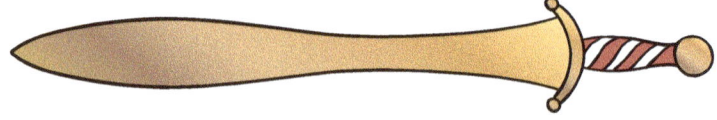

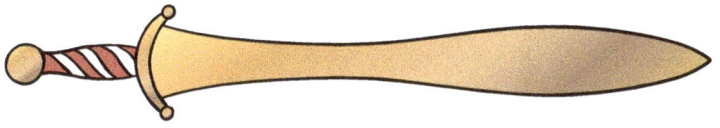

MONUKKA | BLACK MONUKKA
[MON-U-KA H] | [BLAK MON-U-KA H]

A purple to black grape that is crisp with a rich, robust grape flavor. Monukka grapes are twice as large as Thompson Seedless grapes. They are seedless and grown for drying into raisins.

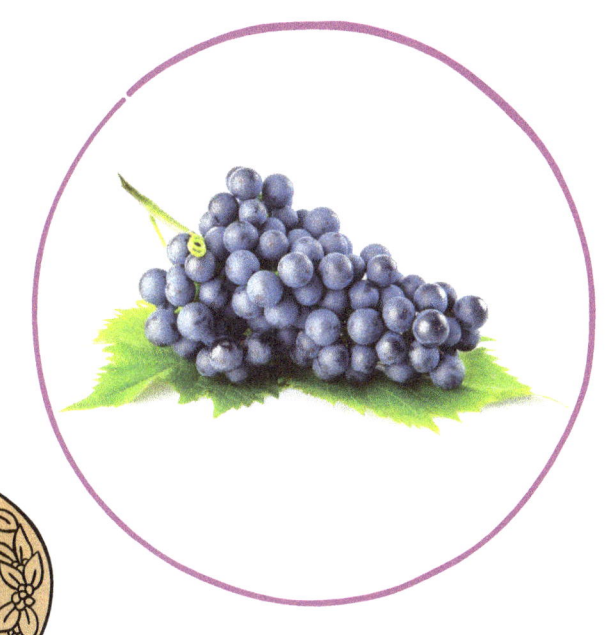

MUSCAT [MUHS-KAT]

A green-yellow or a deep purple grape with a distinct musky, fruity flavor. Muscat grapes are a large, round, seeded **variety**. They are eaten fresh or dried and can be used to make juice.

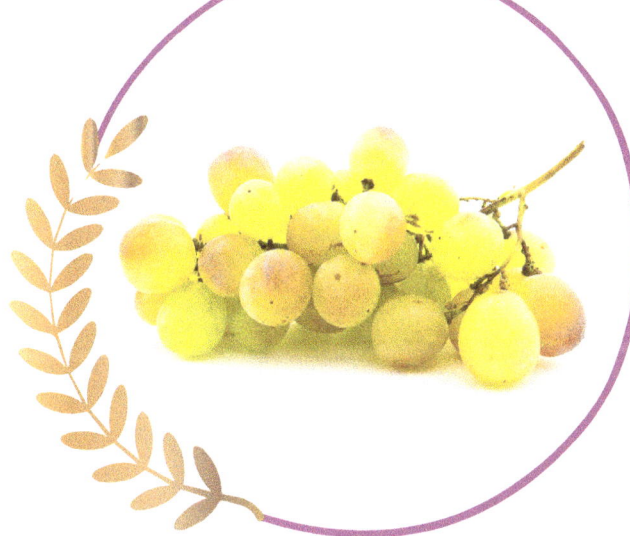

THOMPSON | SULTANA
[TOMP-SUHN] | [SUHL-TAN -UH]

A light green grape that is medium in size, with an oval shape, and seedless. Thompson grapes are the most common variety of grape. They are firm yet tender with juicy sweet flesh and slightly tart skin. When dried they are called golden raisins.

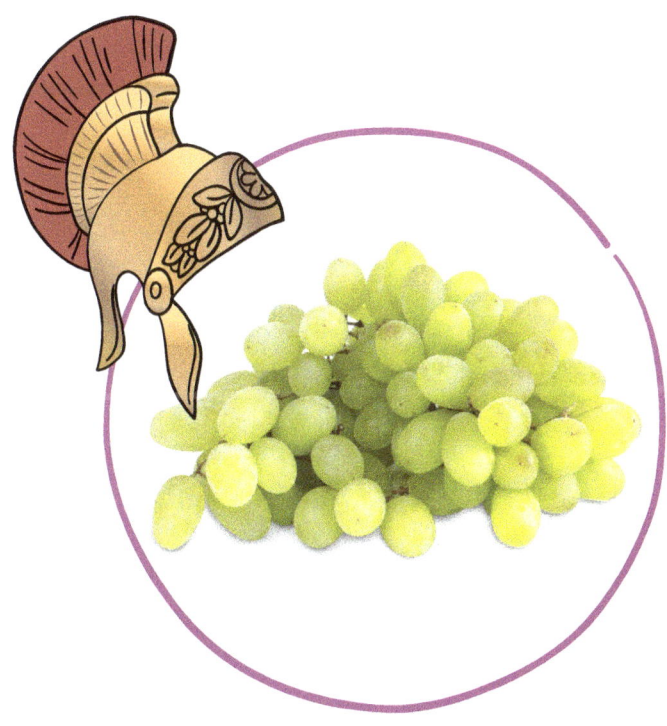

A Book of Fruits 79

GUAVA

[gwah-vuh]

exotic, fragrant, gritty, musky, sweet

BERRY

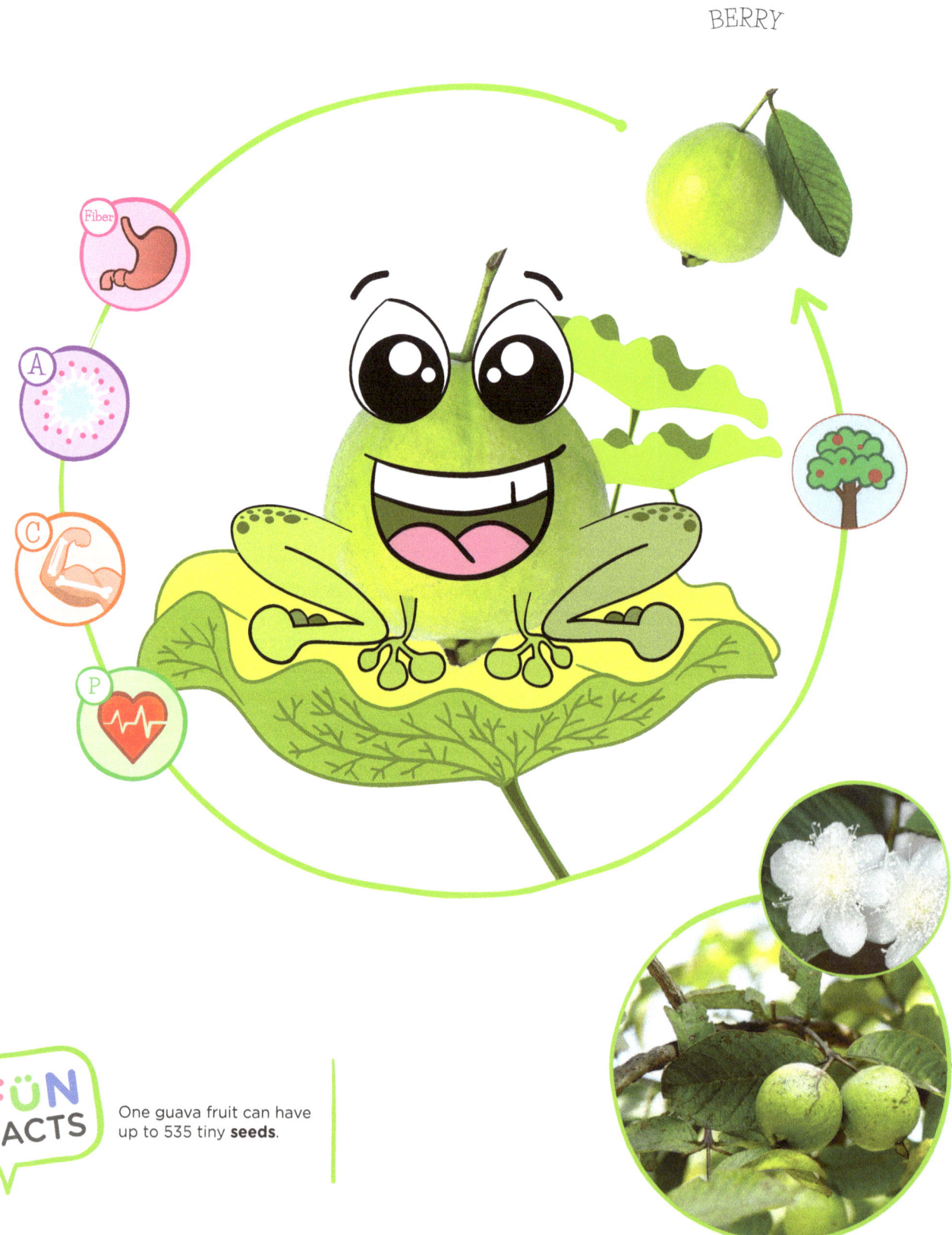

FUN FACTS One guava fruit can have up to 535 tiny **seeds**.

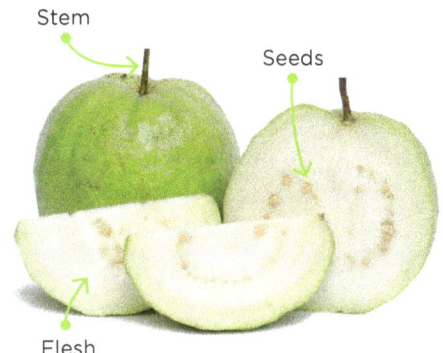

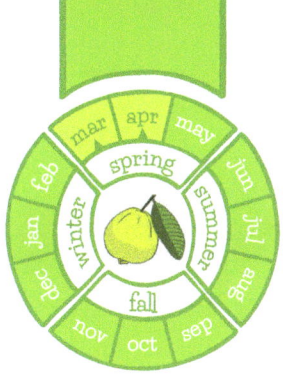

PICK
Pick yellow, maroon, or green fruit that are soft to touch with a floral aroma. Guavas should be free of **bruises** and mushy spots.

Varieties available year-round;
Imported year-round

Peak Season
March-April

STORE
Keep guavas at room **temperature** for up to 5 days or until **ripe**. Refrigerate whole guavas in a plastic bag for 3-4 days or cut up in airtight containers for 3-4 days. Freeze guavas in airtight containers for 10-12 months. Dried guavas may be stored in airtight containers for 6-12 months.

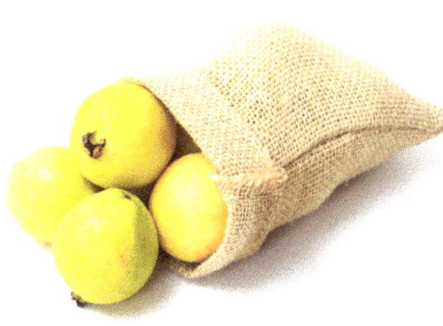

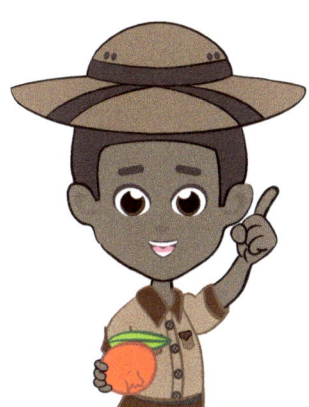

GUAVA TIDBITS

In Hawaii, the strawberry guava is considered an **invasive species** because it grows and spreads quickly damaging the native forest.

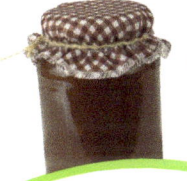

EAT
Clean the skin and eat, chop, or slice per recipe.

Guava Jam
Combine 1 ½ pounds chopped guava and 2 cups water in a saucepan and boil until fruit is soft and mushy, about 15 minutes. Mash the fruit with a potato masher then strain the seeds from the pulp and juice. To make jam, return the pulp and juice to the saucepan, stir in 1 cup sugar and 2 tablespoons lemon juice, and bring to a boil. Reduce heat and simmer for 10 minutes stirring every few minutes until jam **thickens**. Check that the temperature of the jam reaches 220 degrees F to ensure it gels properly. Cool for 10 minutes and pour into a glass jar. Refrigerate jam in a glass jar for up to 1 month.

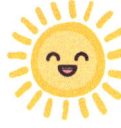
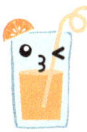

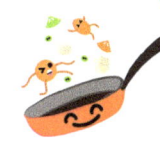

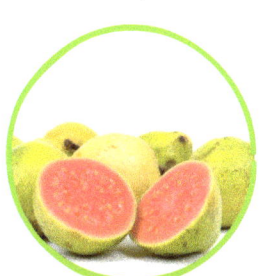

There are over 100 different varieties of guavas with varying sizes, colors, **textures**, and **flavors**.

A Book of Fruits

JACKFRUIT

[jak-froot]

candy-like, mild, pulpy, starchy, tangy

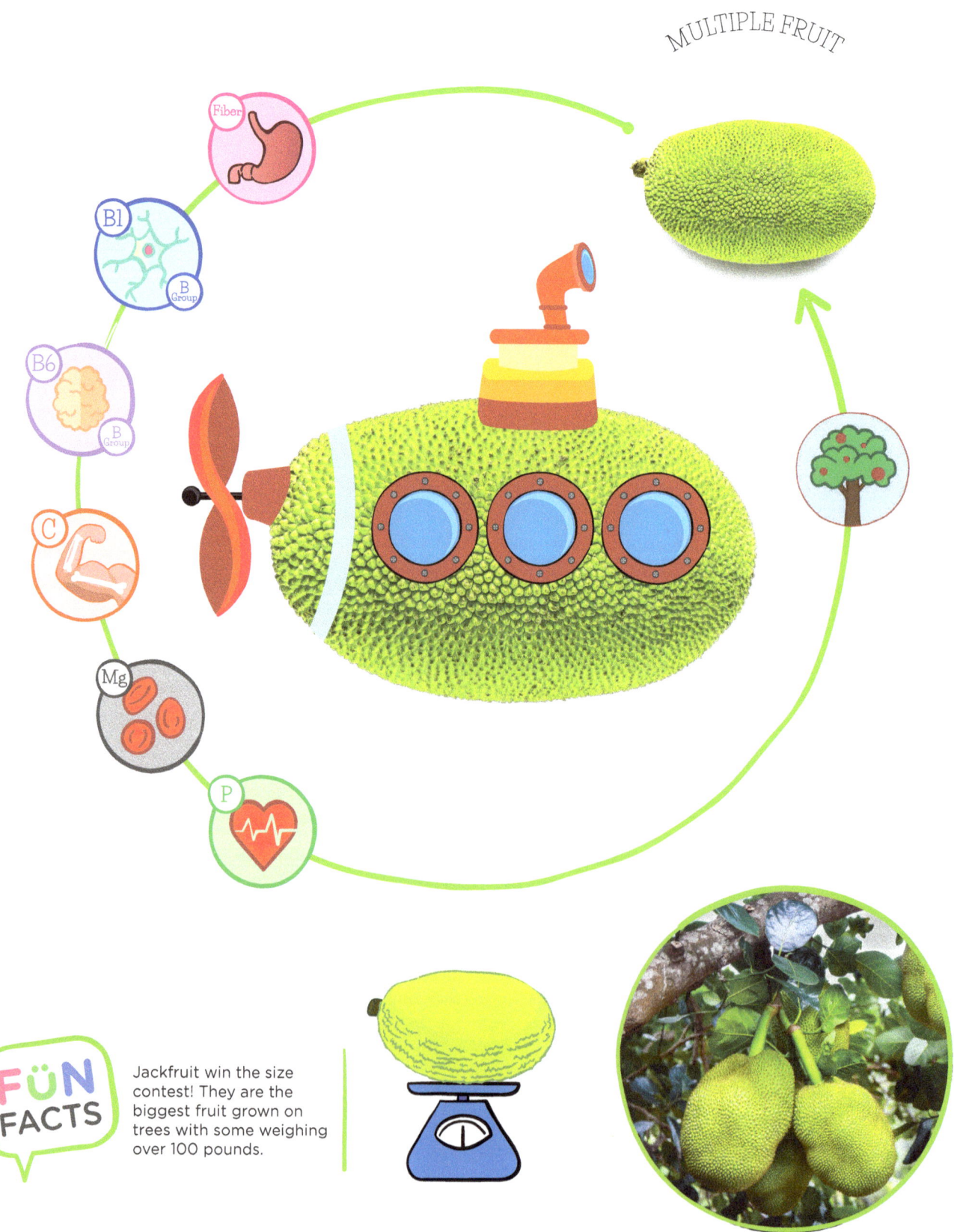

MULTIPLE FRUIT

FUN FACTS Jackfruit win the size contest! They are the biggest fruit grown on trees with some weighing over 100 pounds.

82 | Where Do Bananas Come From?

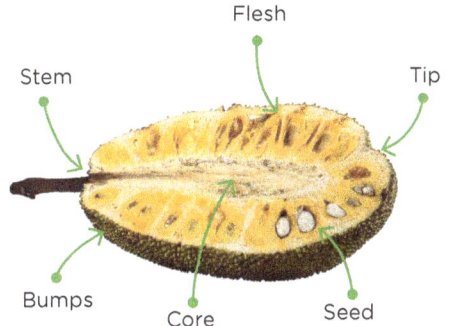

PICK
Pick fruit that are turning from green to yellow with bumps that are soft to touch. Jackfruits should have a sweet aroma and be free of **bruises** and mushy spots.

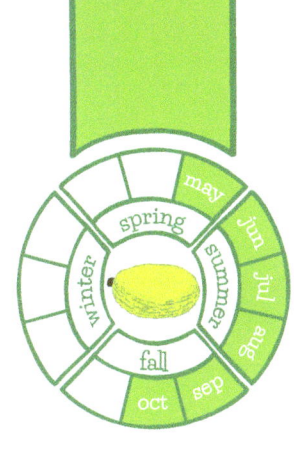

Available May to November; Imported year-round

STORE
Keep jackfruits at room **temperature** for up to 10 days. Refrigerate whole jackfruits for 1 week or cut up in airtight containers for 3-4 days. Freeze jackfruit **arils** in airtight containers for 10-12 months.

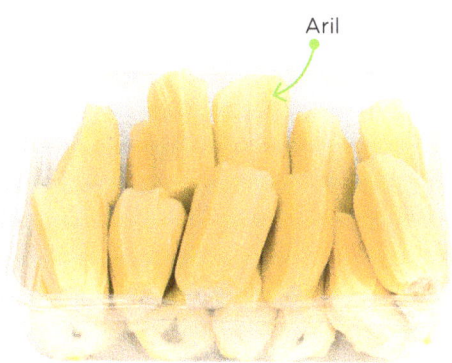

JACKFRUIT TIDBITS

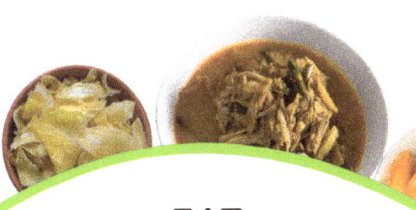

EAT
You are going to need the help of an adult to cut through this bumpy skin. Clean the skin, coat a sharp knife with oil, and slice the fruit in half from stem to tip. Next, slice the fruit from stem to tip into quarters. Slice out the **thick** inner core on the quarters and pull out the **fleshy** cream-colored arils. Pull apart the arils and remove the **seed**. Eat, chop, or slice per recipe.

BBQ Jackfruit
Heat 4 tablespoons olive oil in a skillet over medium heat and sauté 1/2 cup chopped yellow onion and 4 minced cloves garlic until **translucent**, about 3 minutes. Add 3 pounds jackfruit to the skillet and cook for 10 minutes or until lightly browned. Turn down heat to medium-low, add 2 cups barbeque sauce, 1 cup water, 1/2 teaspoon chili powder, and cook for 2 hours or until the jackfruit is tender and easily shreds with a fork.

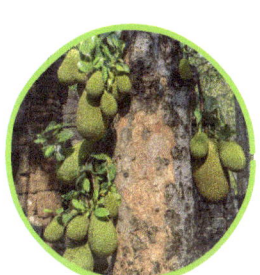

Jackfruit is a **cauliflory** plant. This means that the pods grow from the trunk of the tree rather than on the overhanging branches. The location of the pods close to the ground allows animals that cannot climb or fly to pollinate and disperse seeds.

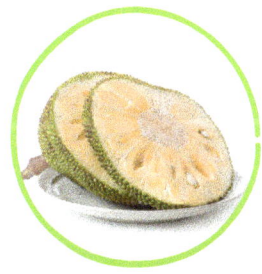

This fruit is served **ripe** as a sweet fruit or unripe as a vegetable or meat substitute.

A Book of Fruits

KIWI
CHINESE GOOSEBERRY

[kee-wee] | [chahy-neez goos-ber-ee]

fuzzy, gritty, juicy, sweet, tart

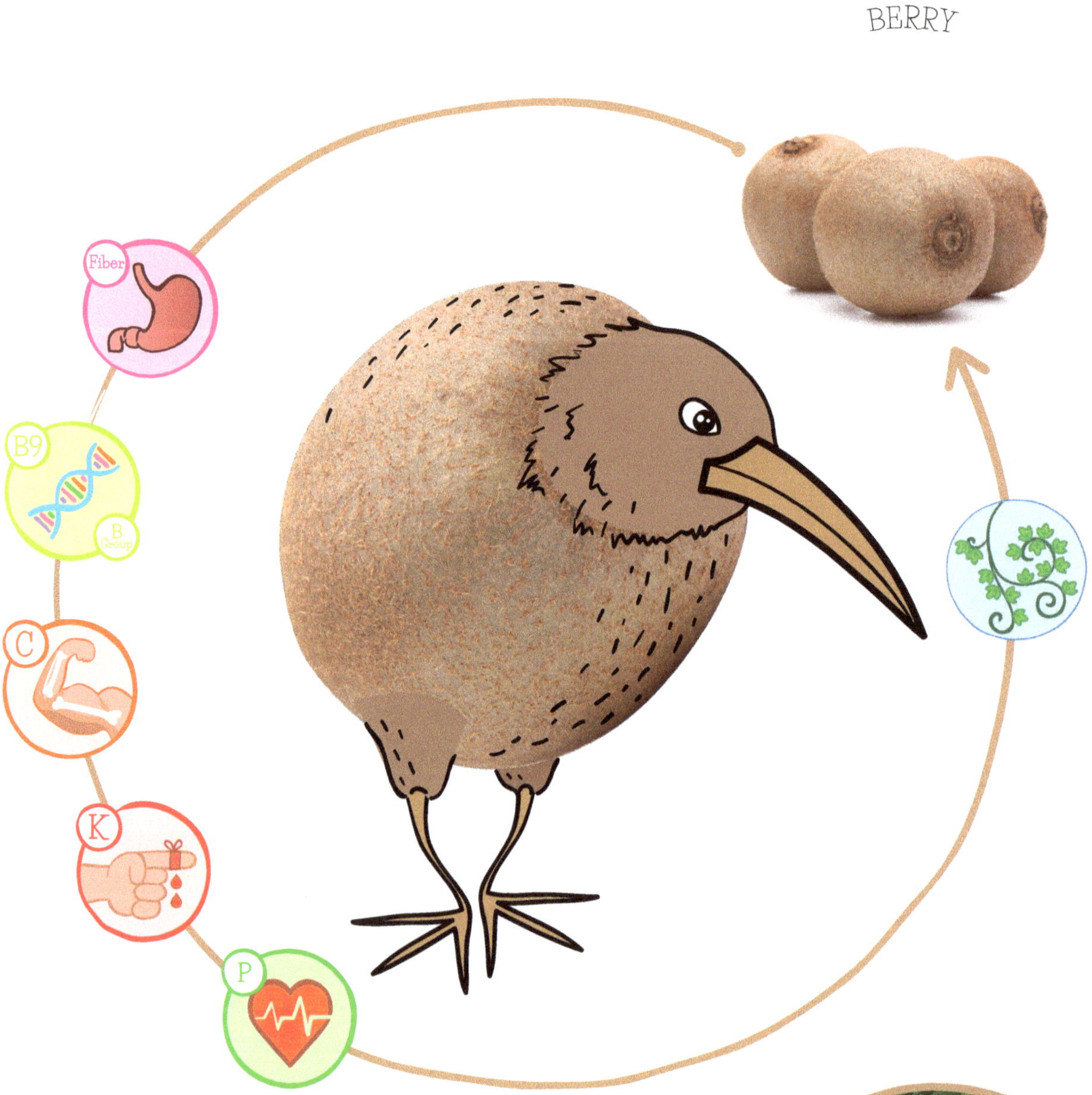

BERRY

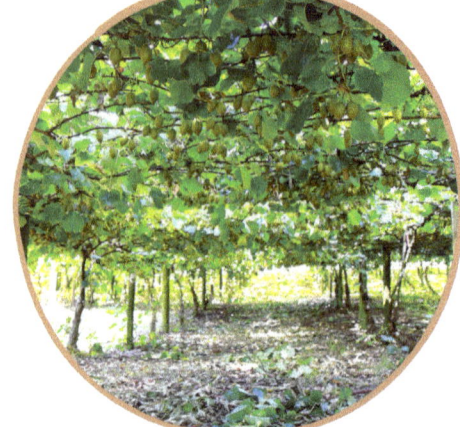

FUN FACTS: Kiwi fruit was originally called a gooseberry. It was renamed to "kiwi" because the **berry** is **imported** from New Zealand and resembles their fuzzy, brown national bird, the kiwi!

84 | Where Do Bananas Come From?

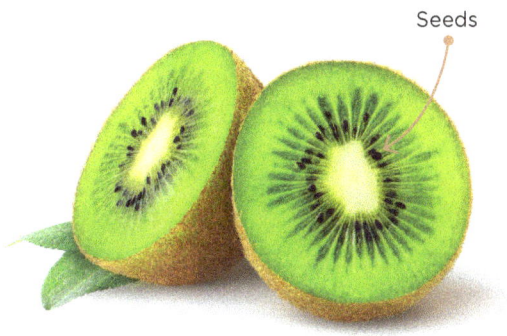
Seeds

PICK
Pick brown, fuzzy fruit that are soft to touch. Kiwis should be free of wrinkles and mushy spots.

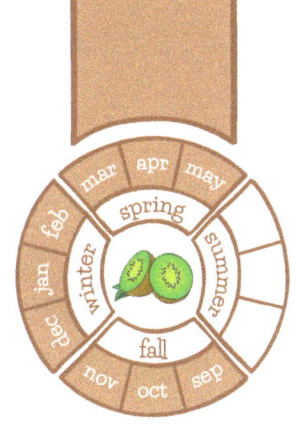

Available September to May; Imported year-round

STORE
Keep kiwis at room **temperature** for up to 5 days or until **ripe**. Refrigerate whole kiwis in a plastic bag for 3-6 weeks or sliced in airtight containers for 3-4 days. Freeze kiwis in airtight containers for 6-12 months. Dried kiwis may be stored in airtight containers for 6-12 months.

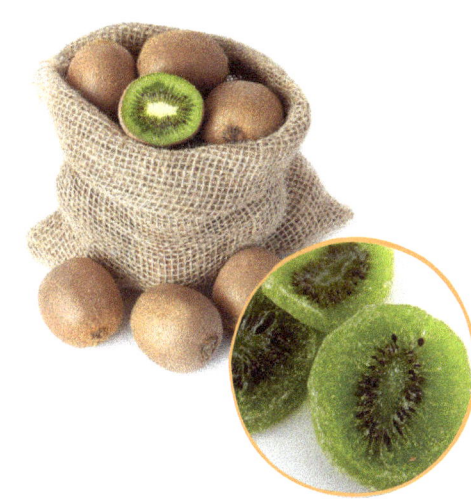

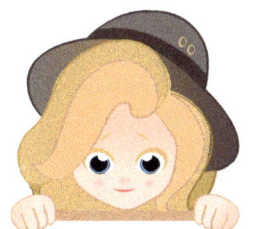

KIWI TIDBITS

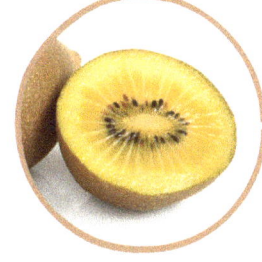

Kiwi flesh ranges from bright green to bright yellow. Which kinds have you tried? Is one more sweet and one more sour?

EAT
Clean the skin, peel, and eat, chop, or slice per recipe.

Fresh Fruit Kabob
Clean and prep fresh fruit such as kiwi, melon, berries, mango, and pineapple and place on a skewer. You can even use cookie cutters to cut out fun shapes! Serve plain or with a yogurt dipping sauce.

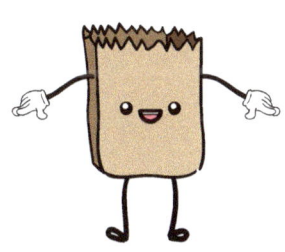

Place unripe kiwi in a paper bag to ripen more quickly.

A Book of Fruits 85

KUMQUAT

[kuhm-kwot]

aromatic, bitter, sweet, tangy, tart

HESPERIDIUM

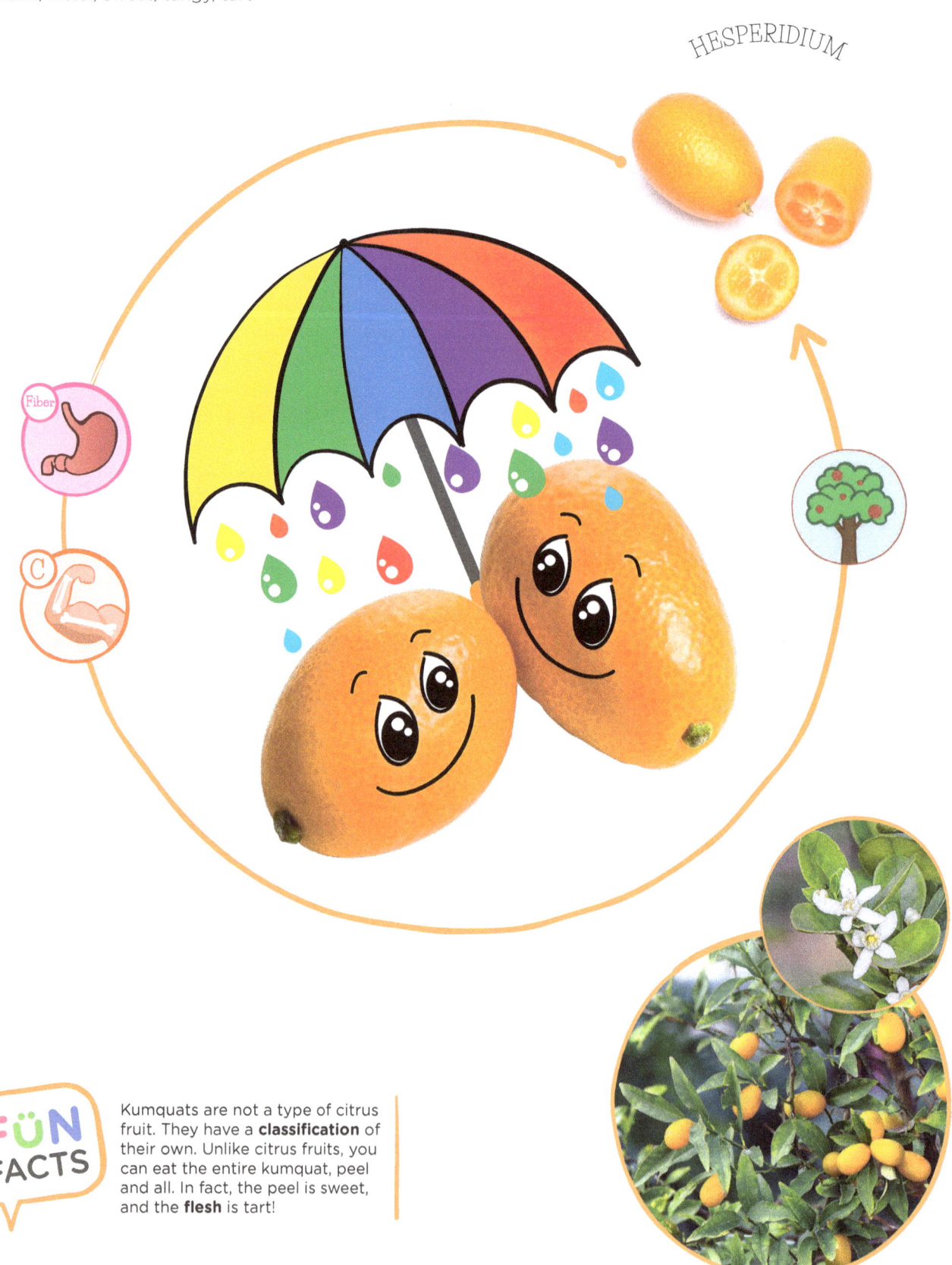

FUN FACTS

Kumquats are not a type of citrus fruit. They have a **classification** of their own. Unlike citrus fruits, you can eat the entire kumquat, peel and all. In fact, the peel is sweet, and the **flesh** is tart!

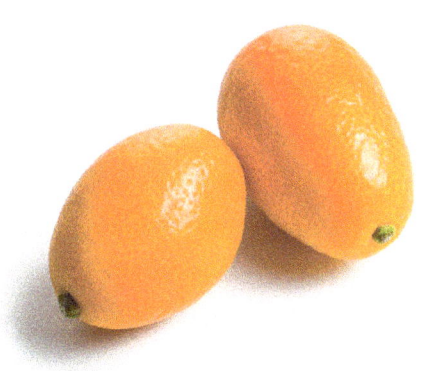

PICK
Pick golden orange, **plump**, **firm**, smooth fruit. Kumquats should be free of soft spots.

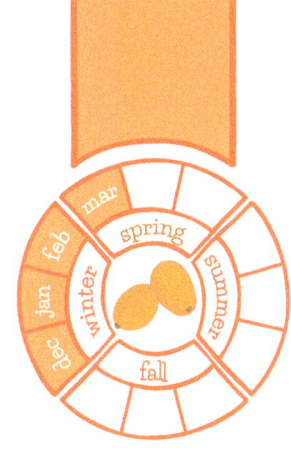

Available December to March; Imported year-round

STORE
Keep kumquats at room **temperature** for up to 5 days. Refrigerate kumquats in a plastic bag for 2-3 weeks. Freeze kumquats in airtight containers for 10-12 months.

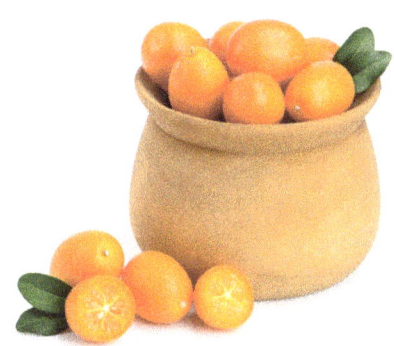

KUMQUAT TIDBITS

The two most common varieties of kumquats are meiwa and nagami. Meiwa are more rounded in shape and have a sweeter **flavor** than the oval-shaped nagami.

***

Kumquats are about the size of your thumb.

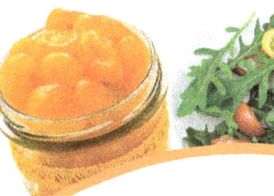

EAT
Clean the skin, squeeze the kumquat in-between your fingers to release the juice and eat, chop, or slice per recipe.

Kumquat Marmalade
Slice kumquats into slivers until you have 1 cup chopped fruit and juice, discard **seeds**. Add fruit and juice, 1 cup water, 1/2 cup sugar, and the juice and **zest** of one small lemon to a saucepan. Allow the mixture to sit at room temperature for 2-3 hours or in the refrigerator overnight to soften. Heat saucepan with fruit mixture to a boil, then simmer for 10 minutes stirring occasionally. Reduce heat to medium-low and continue cooking for 30-40 minutes, stirring occasionally, until the mixture is **thickened**. Check that the temperature of the marmalade reaches 220 degrees F to ensure it gels properly. Cool for 10 minutes and pour into a glass jar. Refrigerate marmalade for up to 1 month.

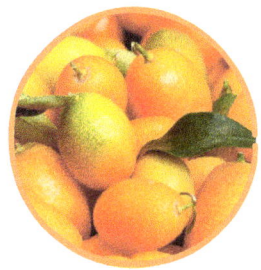

Kumquats are native to China. The English name for the fruit is translated from a word in Cantonese which means golden tangerine.

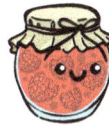
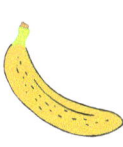
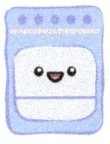
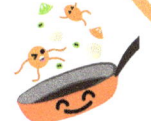

A Book of Fruits 87

LEMON

[lem-uhn]

acidic, fresh, juicy, sour, zippy

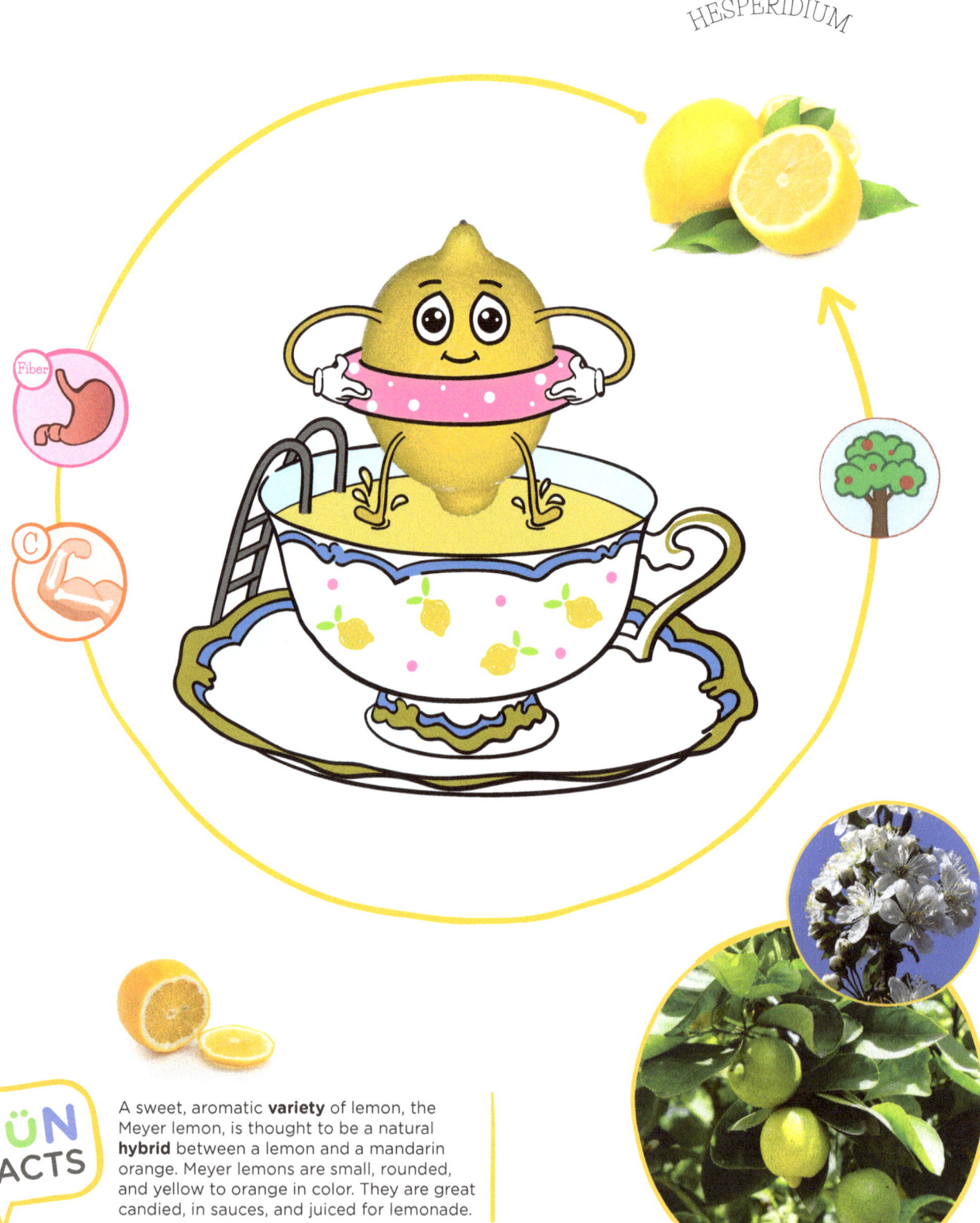

HESPERIDIUM

Fun Facts: A sweet, aromatic **variety** of lemon, the Meyer lemon, is thought to be a natural **hybrid** between a lemon and a mandarin orange. Meyer lemons are small, rounded, and yellow to orange in color. They are great candied, in sauces, and juiced for lemonade.

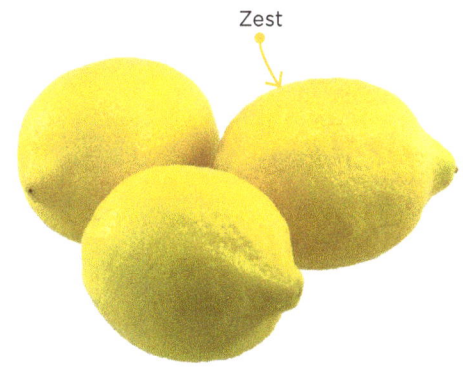
Zest

PICK
Pick golden yellow, **firm**, smooth fruit that feel heavy for their size. Lemons should be free of dark or soft spots.

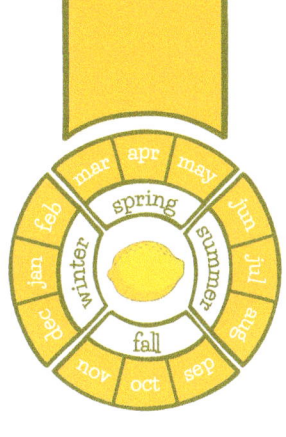

Varieties available year-round;
Imported year-round

STORE
Keep lemons at room **temperature** for up to 7 days. Refrigerate whole lemons in a plastic bag for 3-4 weeks or sliced in airtight containers for 3-4 days. Freeze lemons in airtight containers for 3-4 months.

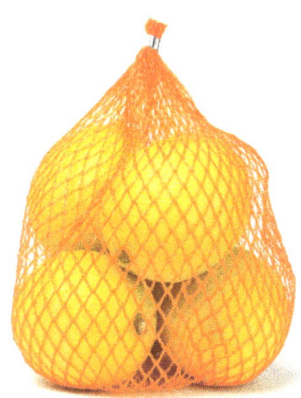

LEMON TIDBITS

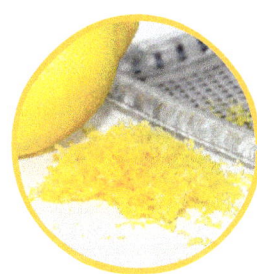

The entire lemon can be used in many ways from baking to cooking and even cleaning! The skin can be zested and used as a garnish and the juice can be used to tenderize meat, add **flavor** to vegetables, and enhance baked goods. You can even use lemon juice to remove **stains** from clothes.

EAT
Clean the skin and roll the fruit on a flat surface under the palm of your hand to release the juices. Slice, juice, or **zest** per recipe.

Lemon Cake
Preheat oven to 350 degrees F and line a 1 pound bread loaf tin with parchment paper. **Cream** together 1 cup softened unsalted butter and 1 cup sugar until they are light and fluffy. Add 4 eggs, mixing in one at a time. Sift in 1 3/4 cup self-rising flour, zest of one lemon, and mix until well combined. Spoon mixture into bread loaf tin and bake in oven for 45-50 minutes until a toothpick comes out clean. Mix together 3/4 cup powdered sugar and the juice of 1 1/2 lemons to make a glaze. Once cooled, remove cake from tin, place on a plate, and use a fork to prick holes in the cake top. **Drizzle** glaze over the top.

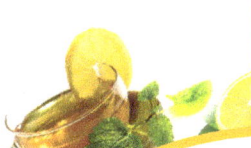

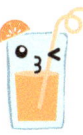
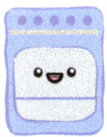
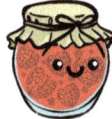

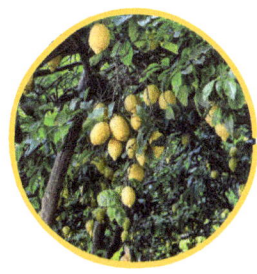

A single lemon tree can produce up to 3,000 lemons per year.

A Book of Fruits 89

LIME

[lahym]

acidic, floral, piney, refreshing, tangy

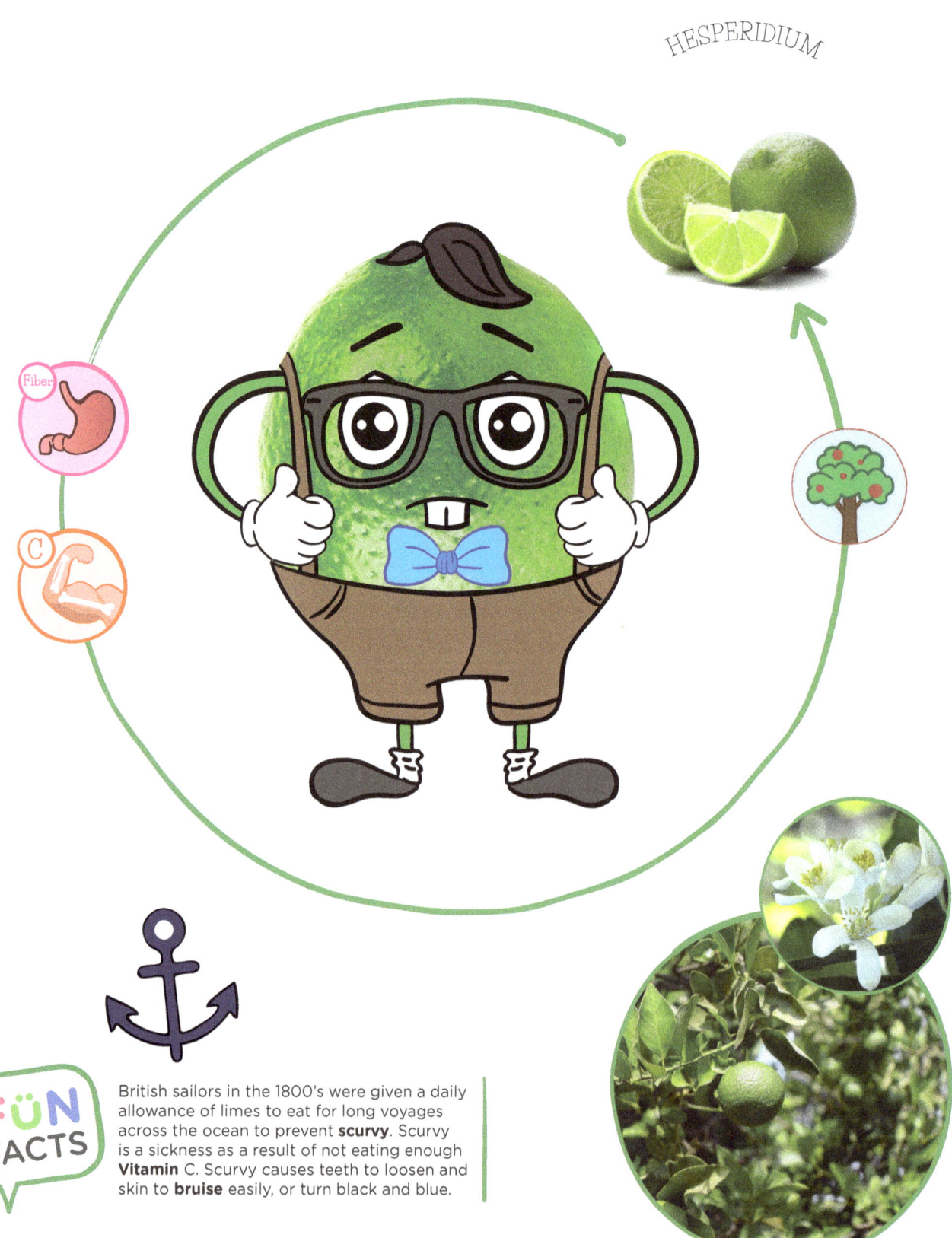

HESPERIDIUM

FUN FACTS: British sailors in the 1800's were given a daily allowance of limes to eat for long voyages across the ocean to prevent **scurvy**. Scurvy is a sickness as a result of not eating enough **Vitamin** C. Scurvy causes teeth to loosen and skin to **bruise** easily, or turn black and blue.

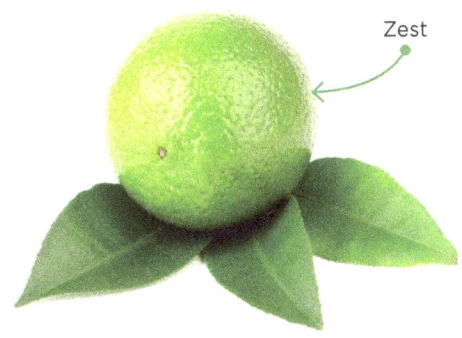
Zest

PICK
Pick bright green, **firm**, smooth fruit that feel heavy for their size. Limes should be free of yellowing or soft spots.

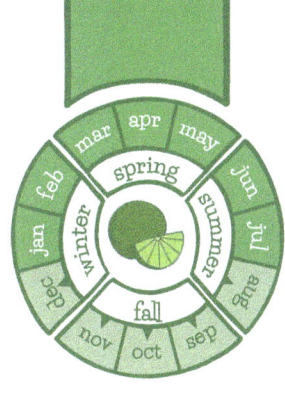

Varieties available year-round; Imported year-round

Peak Season
August-December

STORE
Keep limes at room **temperature** for up to 7 days. Refrigerate whole limes in a plastic bag for 3-4 weeks or sliced in airtight containers for 3-4 days. Freeze limes in airtight containers for 3-4 months.

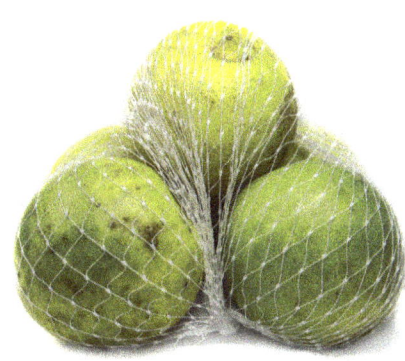

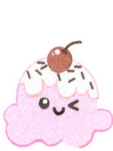

LIME TIDBITS

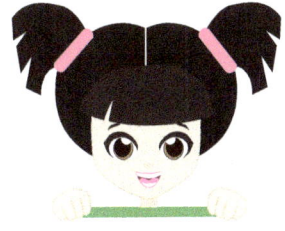

EAT
Clean the skin and roll the fruit on a flat surface under the palm of your hand to release the juices. Slice, juice, or **zest** per recipe.

One-Pot Lime Chicken Soup
Chop and sauté 4 green onions and a deseeded poblano pepper over medium heat in a large pot with olive oil for 5 minutes. Add 2 large chopped tomatoes and sauté another 5 minutes. Pour sautéed veggies into a bowl and set aside. Chop and sauté 5 chicken breasts, 1 large red onion, and 5 cloves garlic in the same pot with olive oil for 5 minutes. Add 9 cups chicken broth, 2 teaspoons dried oregano, 1 teaspoon pepper, 1/2 teaspoon dried thyme, and bring to a boil. Reduce heat to medium-low and simmer until chicken breast is cooked throughout, about 15 minutes. Add in sautéed veggies, juice of 5 limes, and simmer another 10 minutes. Top with cilantro, avocado, and plain Greek yogurt.

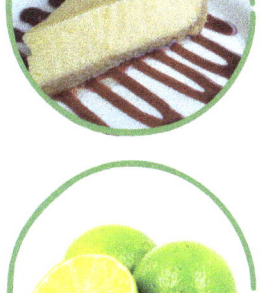

Have you ever heard of a key lime pie? The name comes from a small, seeded, aromatic **variety** of lime called key lime. Key lime is smaller in size than the common lime and has tart and floral juice.

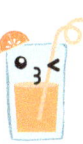

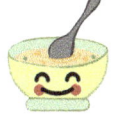

LOQUAT
JAPANESE PLUM

[loh-kwot] | [jap-uh-neez pluhm]

floral, succulent, sweet, sweet-tart, tangy

POME

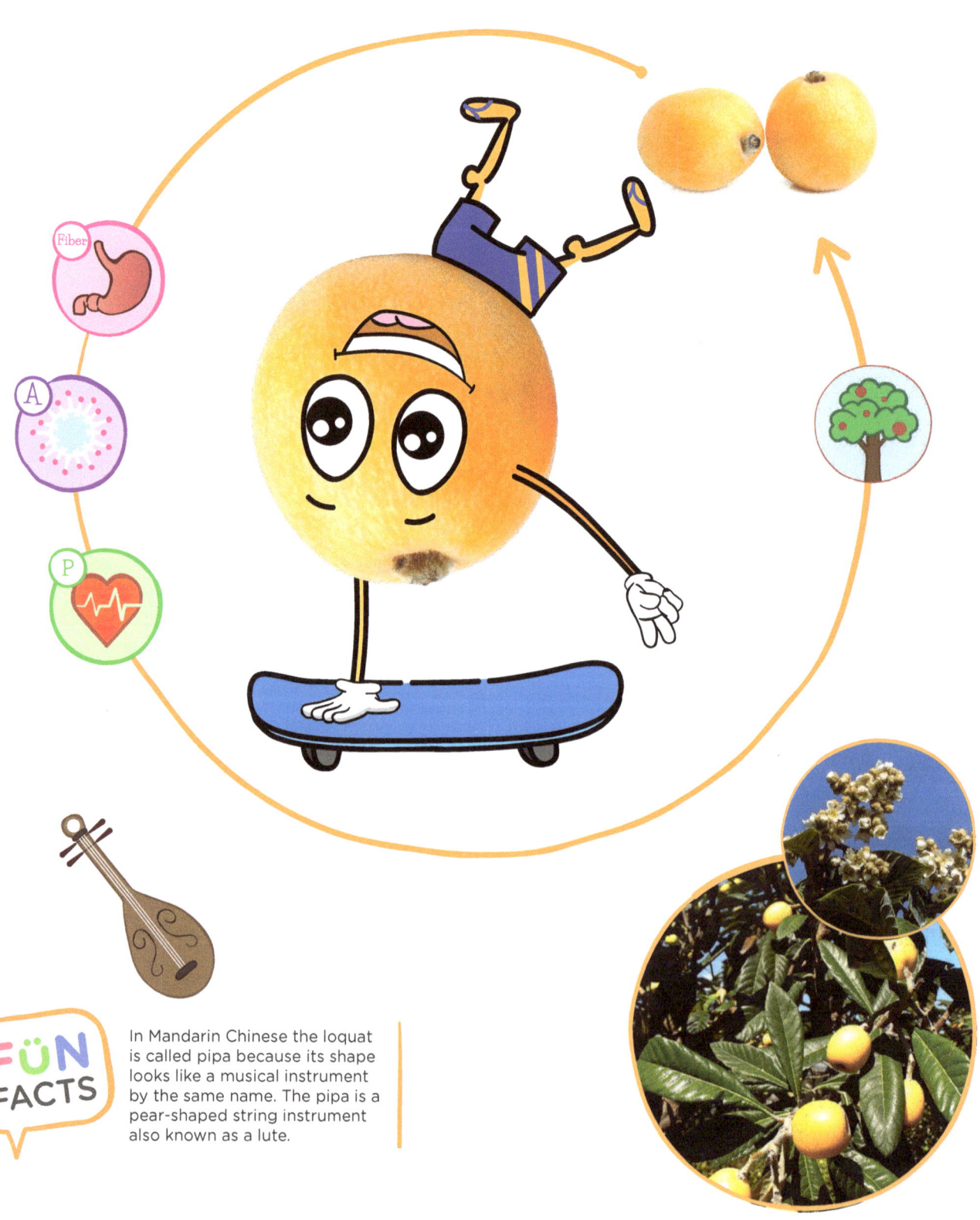

FUN FACTS: In Mandarin Chinese the loquat is called pipa because its shape looks like a musical instrument by the same name. The pipa is a pear-shaped string instrument also known as a lute.

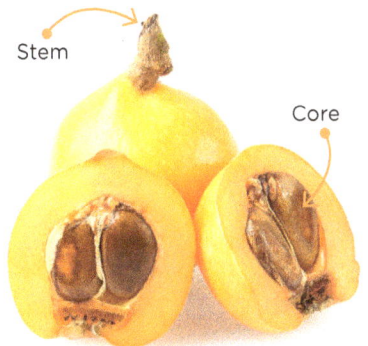
Stem
Core

PICK
Pick yellow or orange to golden **firm**, smooth fruit that have a sweet aroma. Some fruit may have brown, freckled surfaces. Loquats should be free of **bruises** and soft spots.

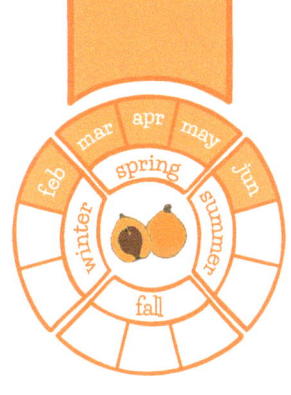

Available February to June; Imported January to May

STORE
Keep loquats at room **temperature** for up to 3 days. Refrigerate whole loquats in a plastic bag for 1-2 weeks or sliced in airtight containers for 3-4 days. Freeze loquats in airtight containers for 10-12 months.

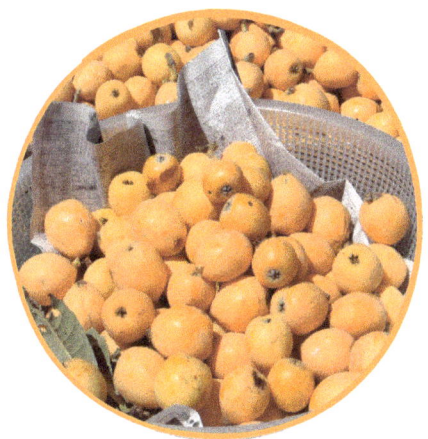

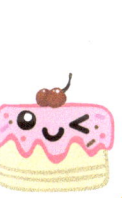
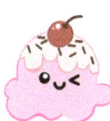
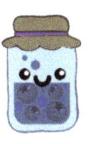
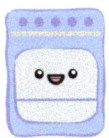

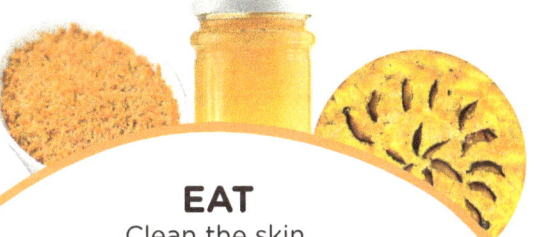

EAT
Clean the skin, remove the core, and chop or slice per recipe.

Loquat Crumble
Preheat oven to 375 degrees F. Place 13 x 9-inch baking dish with 1/2 cup of butter in oven while its preheating. Slice 4 cups of loquats and mix with 3/4 cup brown sugar, 1 tablespoon lemon juice, 2 teaspoons cornstarch, 1 teaspoon vanilla extract, then pour mixture on top of the melted butter in the baking dish, and place back in the oven for 5 minutes. Meanwhile, combine and mix 1 cup flour, 1 cup white sugar, 1 tablespoon baking powder, a pinch of salt. Then add 1 cup milk and mix until dry ingredients are just moistened. Pour batter over the fruit, but do not mix. Bake for 40-45 minutes until golden brown.

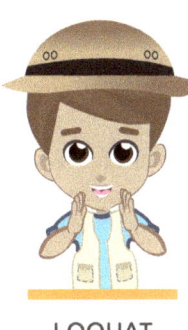

LOQUAT TIDBITS

The **flavor** of a loquat is often compared to a plum, cherry, or grape. The **texture** of the flesh is similar to an apricot while the skin is similar to a peach.

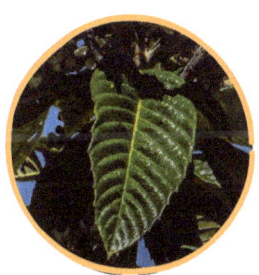

Dried loquat leaves are used to make **herbal** tea that tastes mild, earthy, and sweet.

A Book of Fruits 93

LYCHEE

[ly-chee]

aromatic, crisp, floral, juicy, sweet

DRUPE

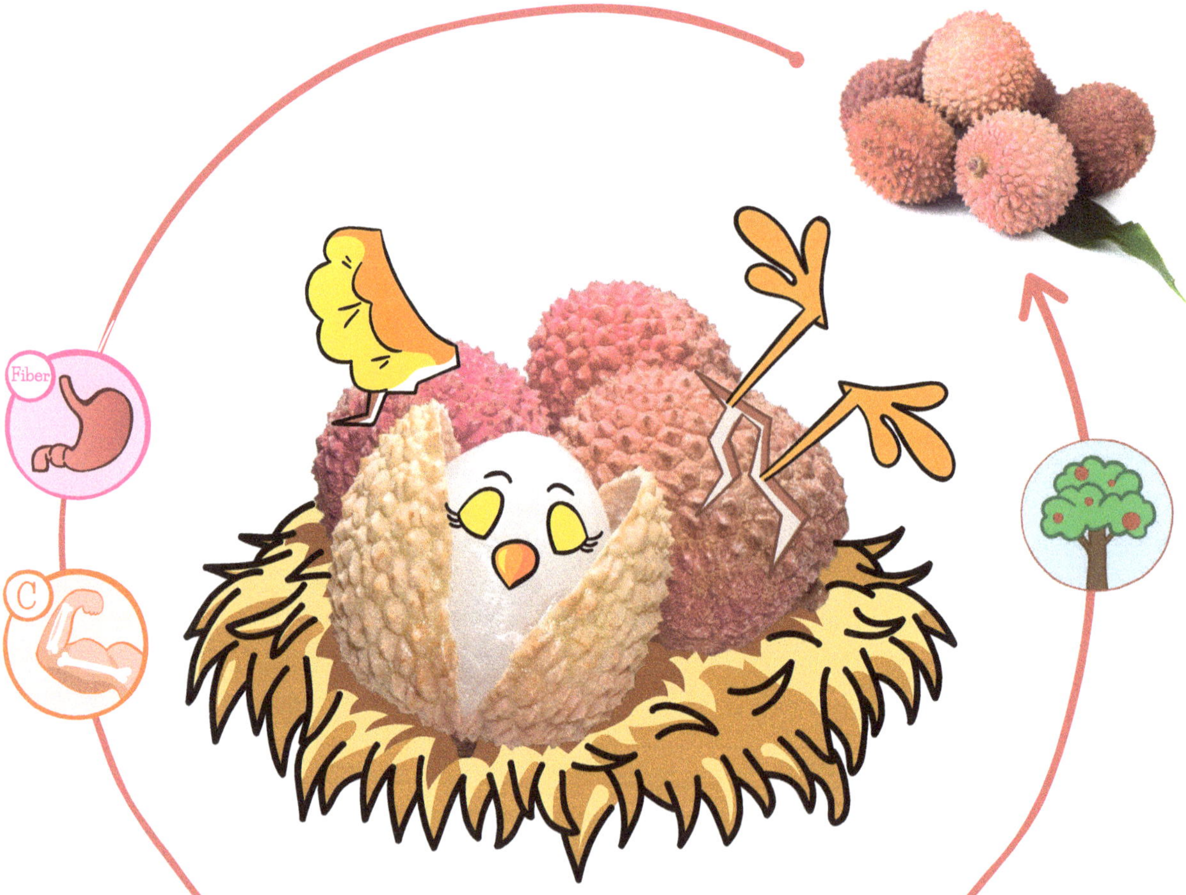

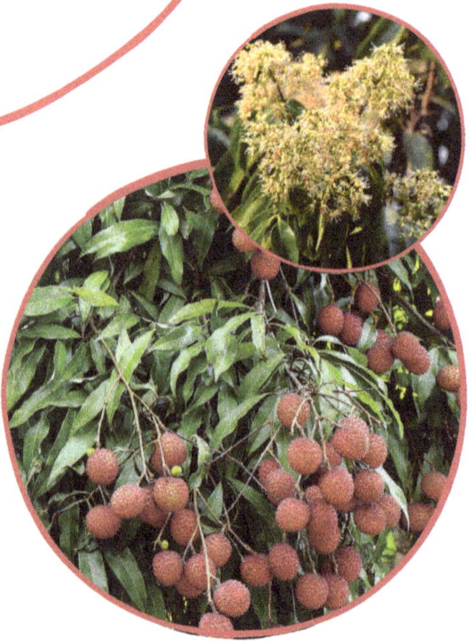

FUN FACTS: The sweet flesh of the lychee fruit is **translucent**. This means that light can pass through the fruit but you cannot see what is on the other side.

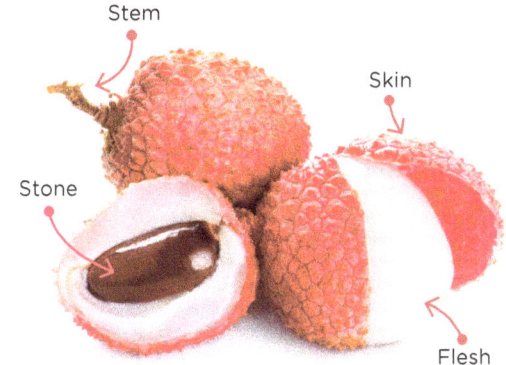

Stem
Skin
Stone
Flesh

PICK
Pick pink, **plump**, semi-**firm**, fruit with tight leathery skin and a sweet, flowery aroma. Lychees should be free of leaking cracks and mold. Avoid lychees with a sour aroma.

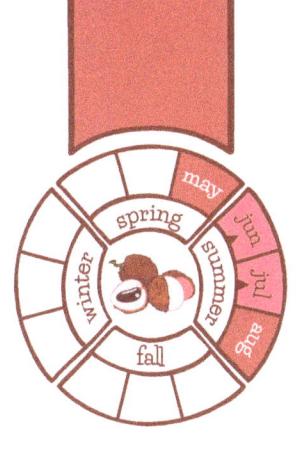

Available May to August; Imported May to July

Peak Season
June-July

STORE
Keep lychees from **spoiling** by storing them in the refrigerator. Refrigerate lychees in a plastic bag for up to 7 days. Freeze lychees in airtight containers for 10-12 months. Dried lychees may be stored in airtight containers for 6-12 months.

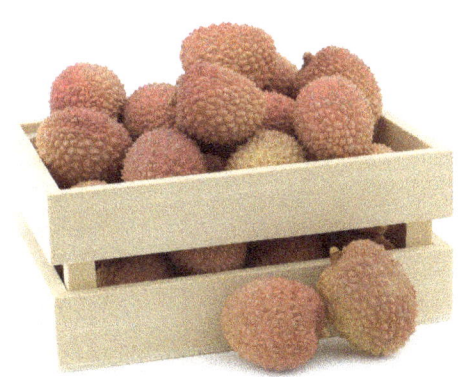

LYCHEE TIDBITS

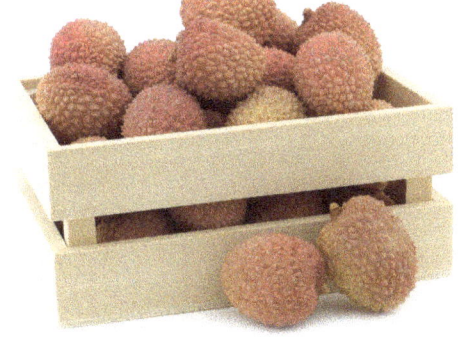

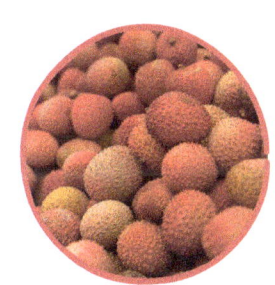

While fruit production can vary, some exceptional trees have produced more than 1,500 pounds of lychee fruit per year which would equal over 20,000 fruit from one tree!

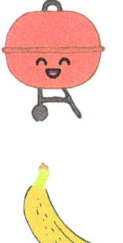

EAT
Clean the skin, pinch the leathery skin at one end, and squeeze the white **fleshy** part out. Slice or bite in half to remove the **stone** from the center. Eat, chop, or slice per recipe.

Tropical Fruit Salad
Mix 4 ounces coconut milk, 1/2 a juiced lime, and 1 tablespoon sugar in a bowl. Add chopped fruit from 10 lychee, 1 mango, 1 papaya, 3 kiwi, and 1/2 pineapple then toss in coconut milk. Garnish with finely sliced mint leaves.

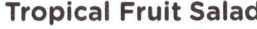

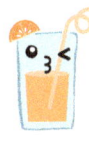

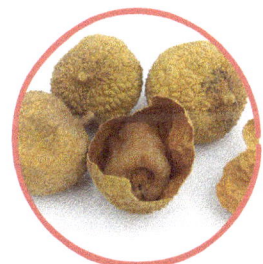

Dried lychees can be eaten like raisins or used in tea as a sweetener in place of sugar.

MAMONCILLO
SPANISH LIME

[mah-muhn-see-oh] | [span-ish lahym]

acidic, gelatinous, juicy, sweet, tangy

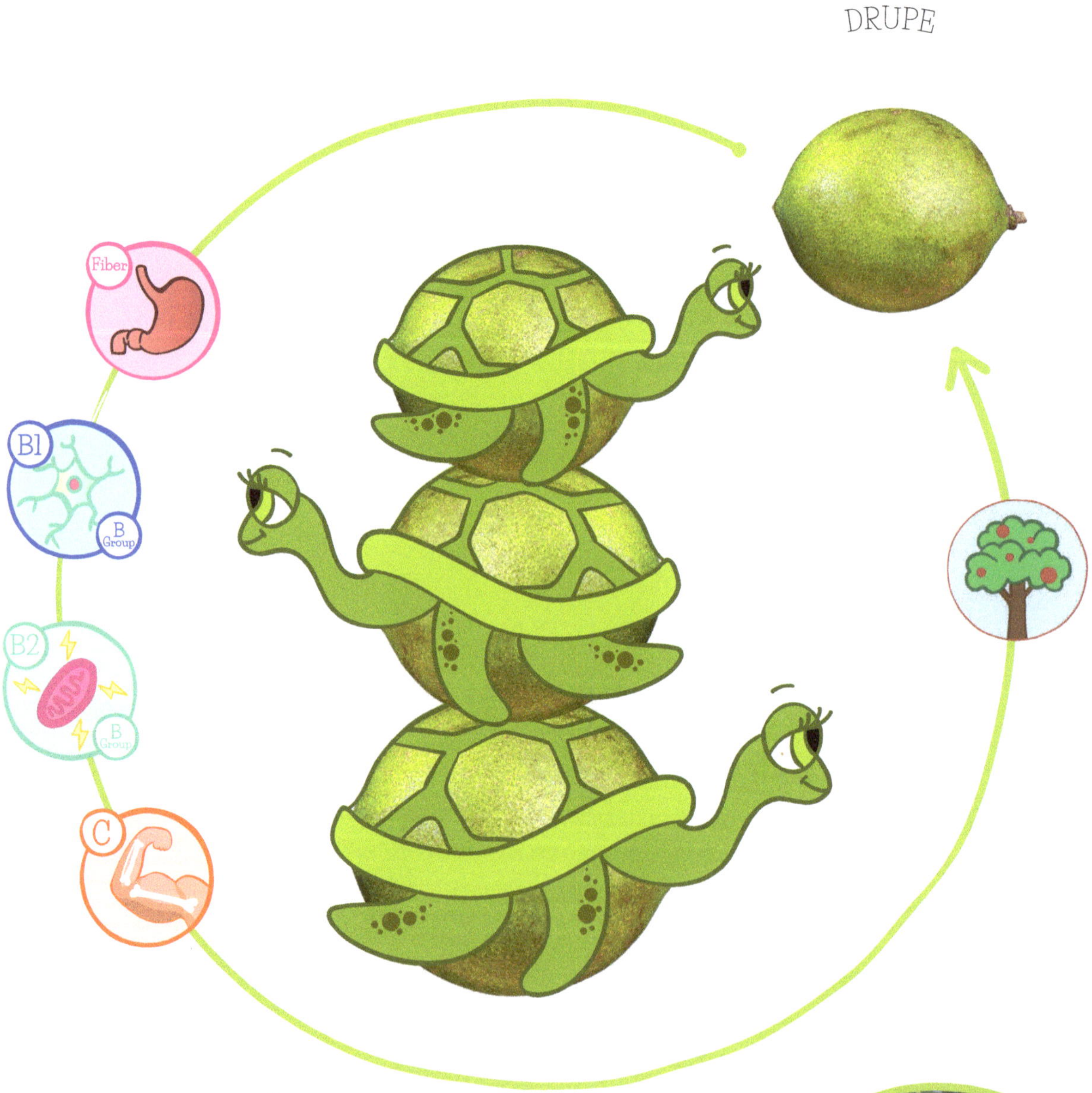

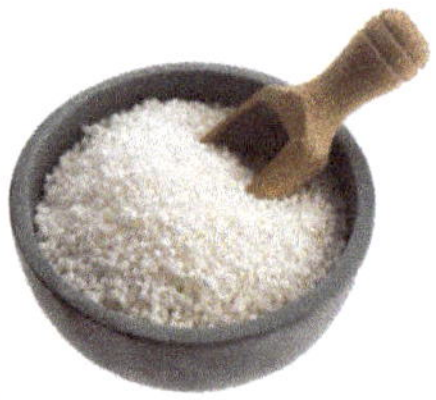

DRUPE

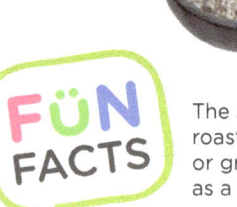

FUN FACTS — The seeds of mamoncillo can be roasted and eaten like chestnuts or ground into a flour and used as a substitute for cassava flour.

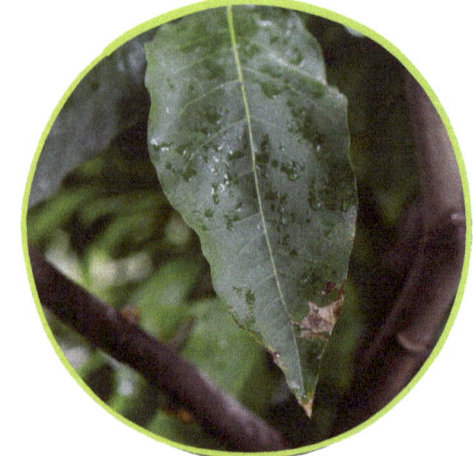

96 | Where Do Bananas Come From?

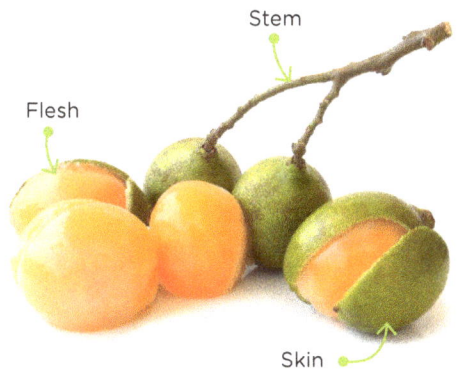

Stem · Flesh · Skin

PICK
Pick green, **plump**, semi-**firm**, fruit with tight leathery skin. Mamoncillos do not change color, their **ripeness** is determined by fruit size and **flavor**.

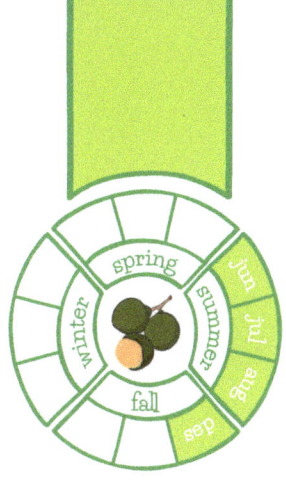

Available June to September; Imported June to August

STORE
Keep mamoncillos at room **temperature** for up to 3 days. Refrigerate whole mamoncillos in a plastic bag for 5-7 days or cut up in airtight containers for 3-4 days.

MAMONCILLO TIDBITS

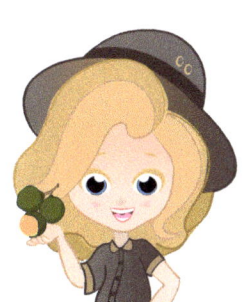

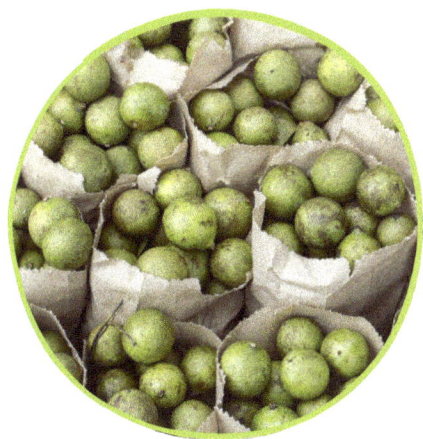

EAT
Clean the skin, puncture the peel, and remove the skin. Slice to remove the **stone** from the center. Eat, chop, or slice per recipe.

Fresh Mamoncillo
Peel the skin, pop the whole fruit into your mouth, and suck the juicy pulp from the **seed**.

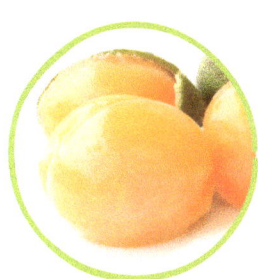

With its green leathery skin, mamoncillo looks like a small lime from the outside. Mamoncillo have salmon to yellow, **translucent** flesh and look like a lychee or rambutan on the inside.

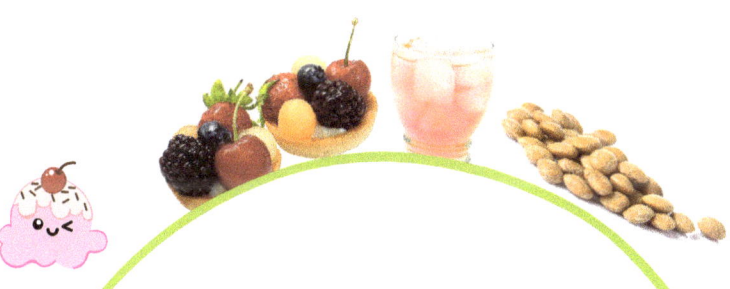

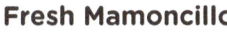
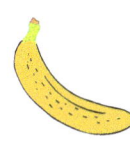
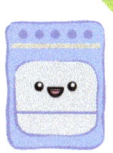

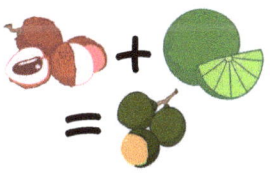

The flavor of mamoncillo is often compared to a cross between a lime and a lychee.

A Book of Fruits

MANGO

[mang-goh]

creamy, fibrous, fragrant, rich, succulent

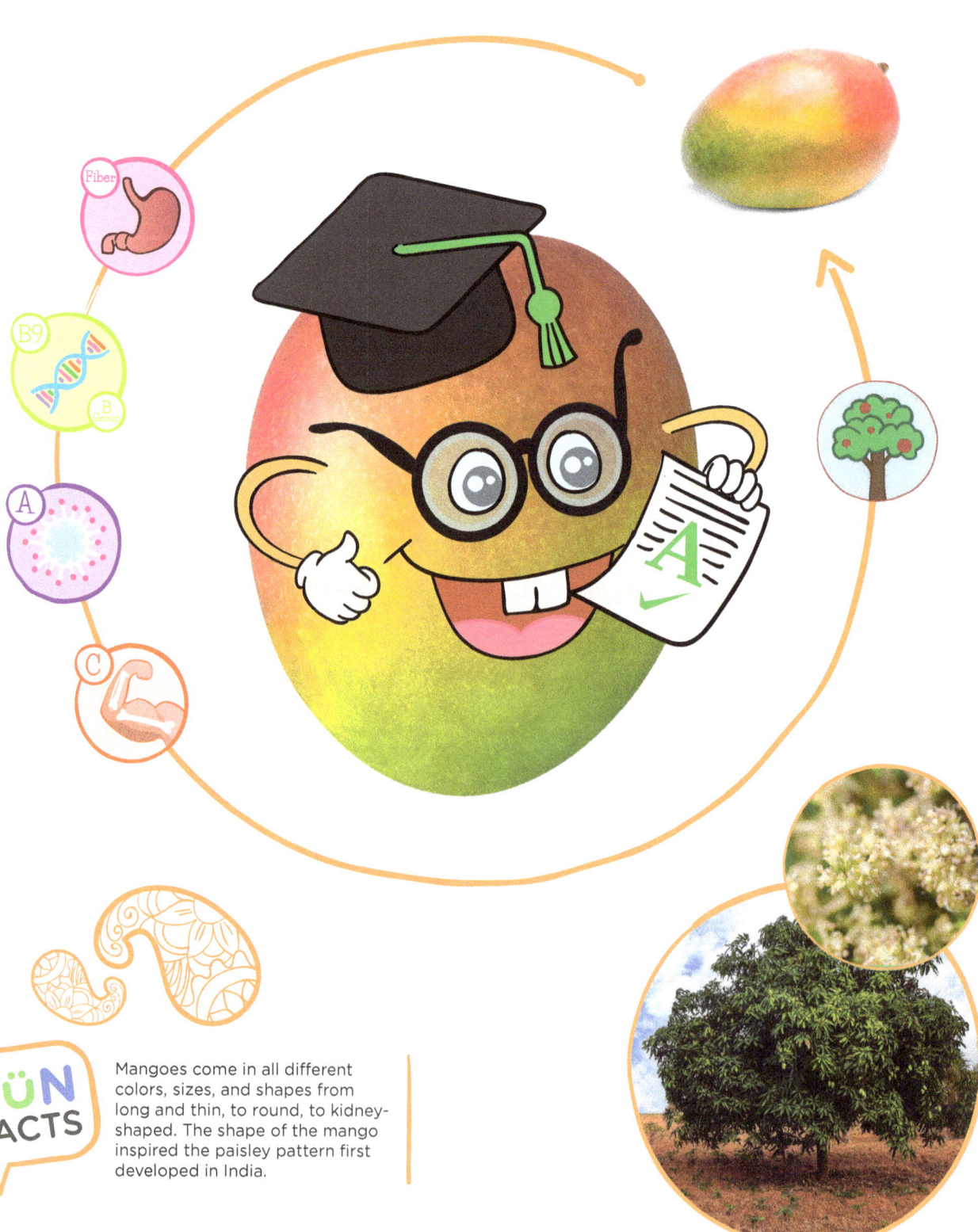

DRUPE

FUN FACTS: Mangoes come in all different colors, sizes, and shapes from long and thin, to round, to kidney-shaped. The shape of the mango inspired the paisley pattern first developed in India.

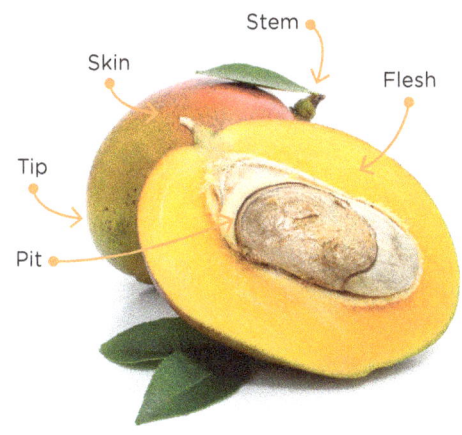

Stem, Skin, Flesh, Tip, Pit

PICK
Pick fruit that are soft to touch, feel heavy for their size, and have a sweet aroma. Mango varieties should be free of dark, mushy spots, and sticky sap on the skin. Colors, shapes, and sizes differ depending on **variety**.

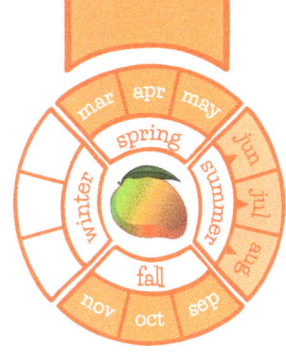

Available March to November; Imported year-round

Peak Season
June-August

STORE
Keep mangoes at room **temperature** for up to 5 days or until **ripe**. Refrigerate whole mangoes in a plastic bag for 5-7 days or cut up in airtight containers for 3-4 days. Freeze mangoes in airtight containers for 10-12 months. Dried mangoes may be stored in airtight containers for 6-12 months.

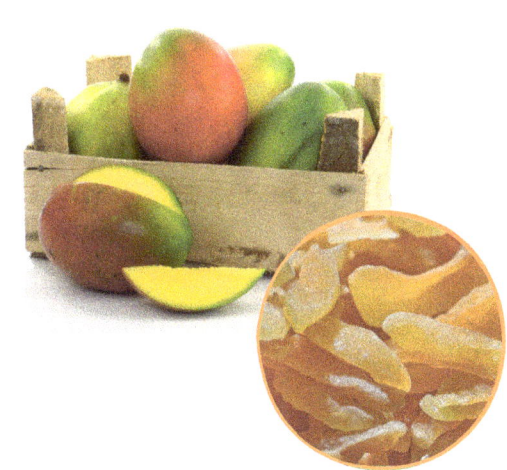

MANGO TIDBITS

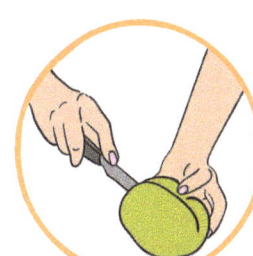
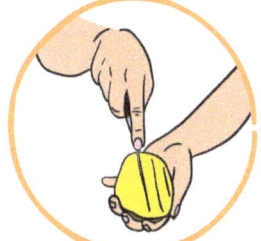
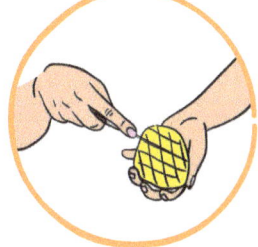

EAT
Ask an adult for help with slicing mangoes. Clean the skin and place mango on its side on a cutting board with the stem side up. Slice stem to tip 1/4 inch away from the center at the widest section of the fruit to remove the **pit**. Repeat on the other side. Next, cut vertical and horizontal lines in the **flesh** in a grid-like pattern being careful not to cut through the skin. Then flip the skins inside out. Eat the cubes off the skin or slice off the cubes.

Mango Salsa
In a bowl, combine 2 large, diced mangoes, 1 small deseeded and minced jalapeno, 1/2 cup chopped of the following: red pepper, cucumber, and red onion, 1/4 cup chopped cilantro leaves, 1 large juiced lime, and 1/2 teaspoon salt.

A Book of Fruits 99

MANGO VARIETIES

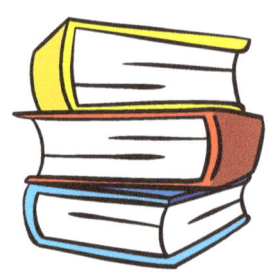

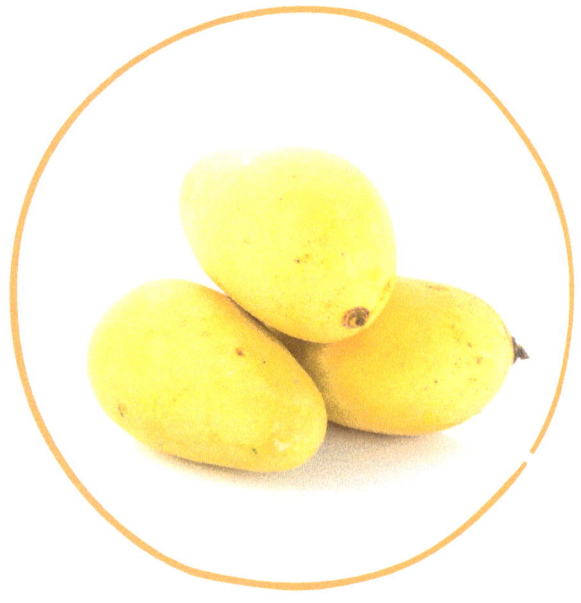

ATAULFO | HONEY
[AT-ALL-FO] | [HUHN-EE]

A bright yellow, small, oval-shaped mango that is sweet and creamy with **firm flesh**. Ataulfo, or honey mangoes, have a high flesh to **pit** ratio. A high flesh to pit ratio means there is more fruit than pit. They are great fresh, grilled, or roasted. This **variety** is also called Champagne mango.

EGG OF THE SUN | IRWIN
[EG OF THE SUHN] | [UR-WIN]

An aromatic, juicy, sweet-tart, ruby red mango with very little fiber that is said to melt in your mouth. The "Egg of the Sun" mango is grown in Japan. It is the same common variety grown in Florida known as an Irwin mango. However, due to the unique growing and **harvesting** conditions, Egg of the Sun mangoes have sold for more than $3,500 for two fruits.

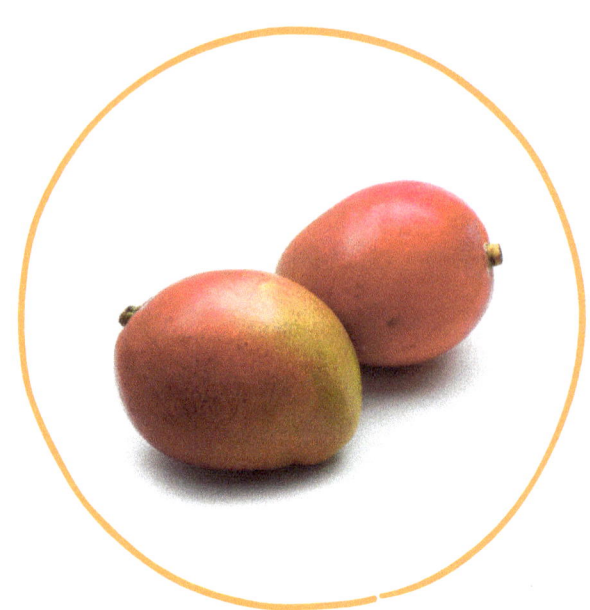

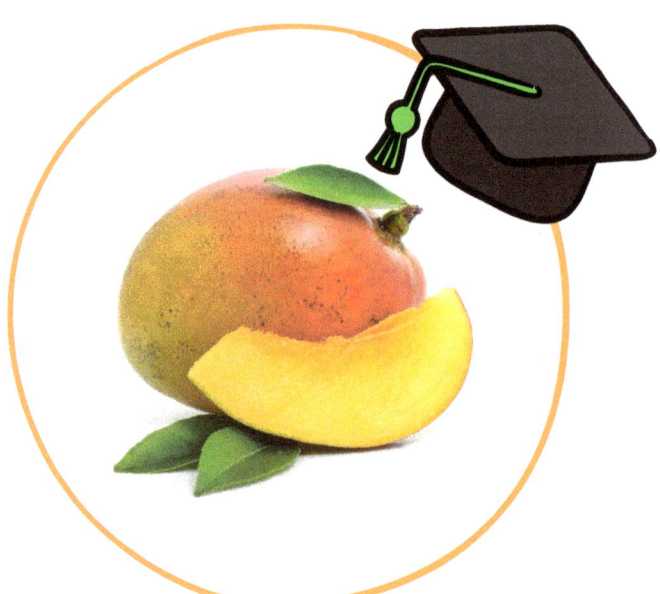

HADEN [HEYD-N]

A bright red, green, and yellow mango that has **firm** flesh with fine fibers and a floral aroma. Haden mangoes are medium to large in size, oval to round in shape, and have a rich, sweet **flavor**. This variety started the large-scale mango industry in Florida in 1910.

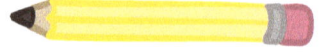

KEITT [KEET]

A medium to dark green mango with a pink blush and an oval shape. Keitt mangoes remain green even when **ripe**. This juicy variety is not fibrous and can be eaten fresh when ripe or enjoyed pickled underripe.

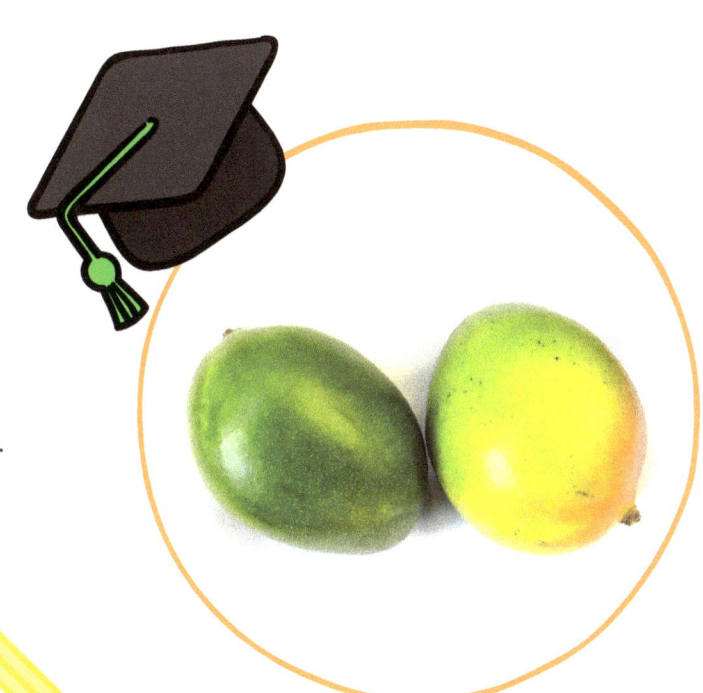

KENT [KENT]

A dark green with a red blush mango with an oval shape. Kent mangoes are juicy, tender, and not very fibrous. This variety is best juiced or dried.

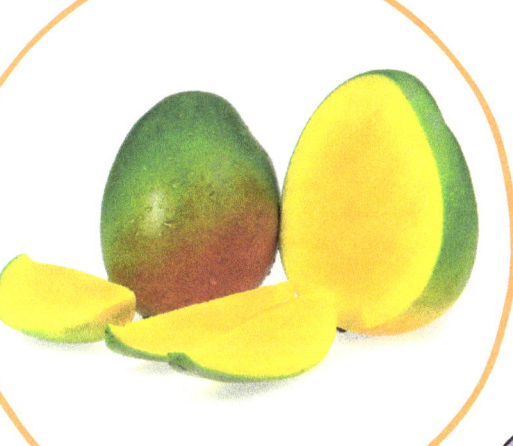

TOMMY ATKINS [TOM-EE AT-KINZ]

A mango with a dark red blush and green to yellow accents. Tommy Atkins mangoes are medium to large in size, have an oval shape, and a mild, sweet flavor. This fibrous variety is the most readily available mango in the United States and is perfect for recipes that require slow cooking such as braises, curries, and stews.

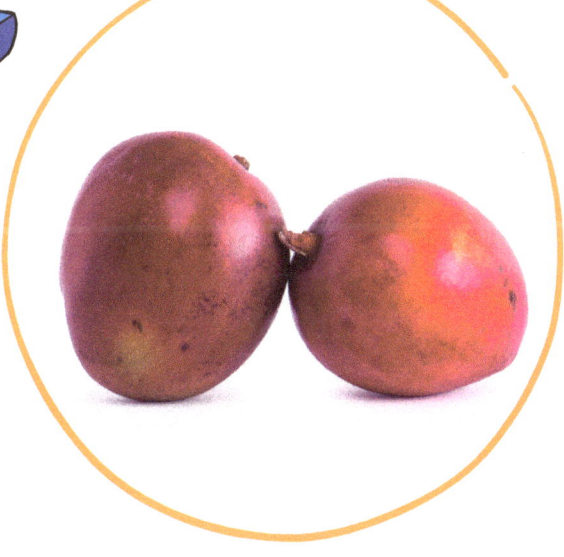

A Book of Fruits

MANGOSTEEN

[mang-guh-steen]

floral, juicy, milky, sweet, tangy

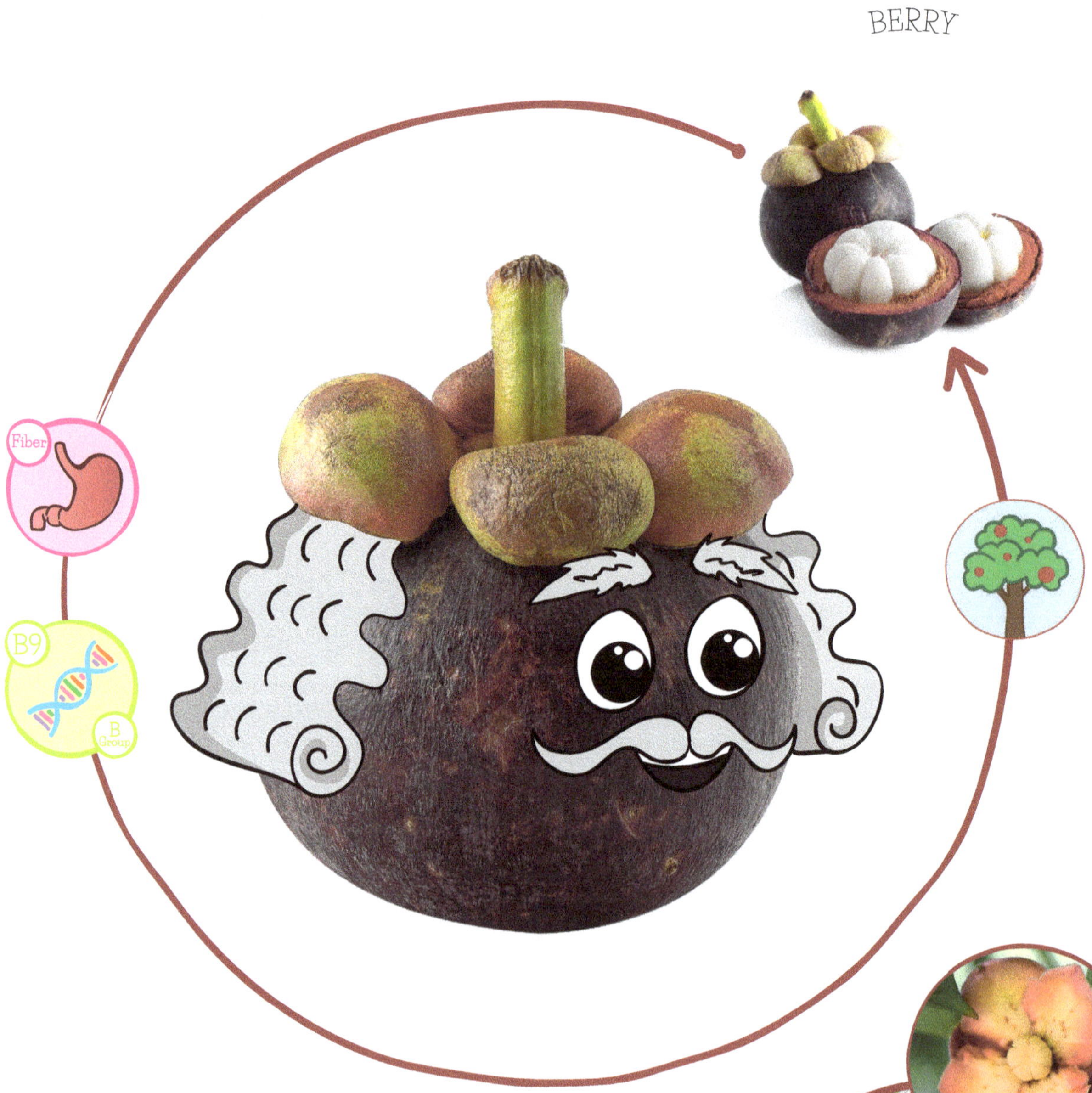

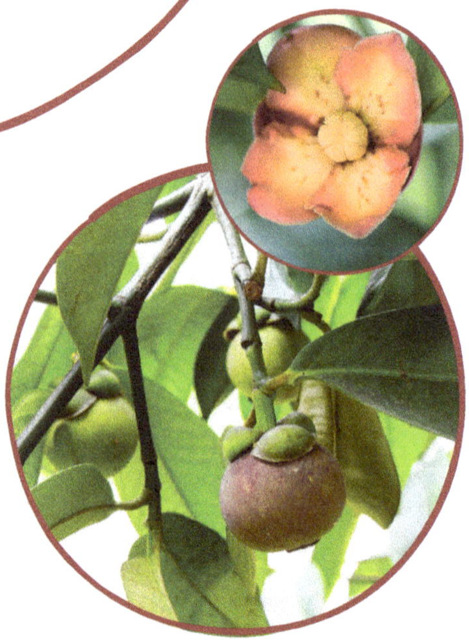

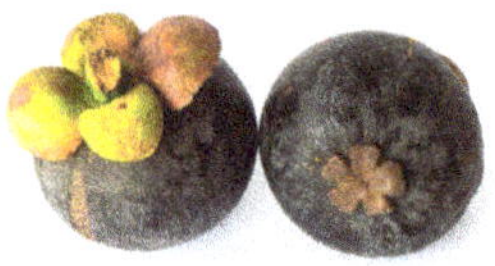

BERRY

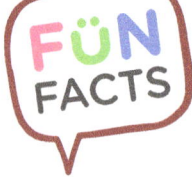

FUN FACTS: Turn a mangosteen upside-down and count the number of petals on the bottom. Each petal tells you how many segments or pieces of fruit you will find inside! Most small segments will not have **seeds** so the more petals the better!

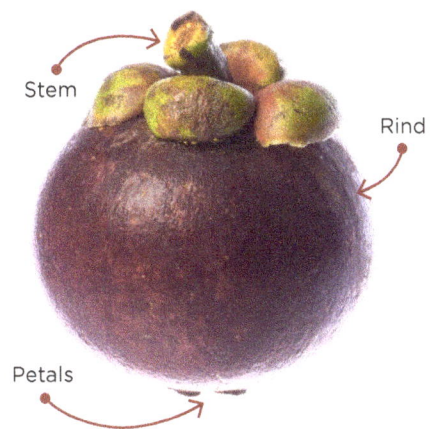

PICK
Pick red-purple, **firm** but not hard, fruit that feel heavy for their size and have fresh green stems that are still attached. Mangosteens should be free of dry or dark spots on their skin.

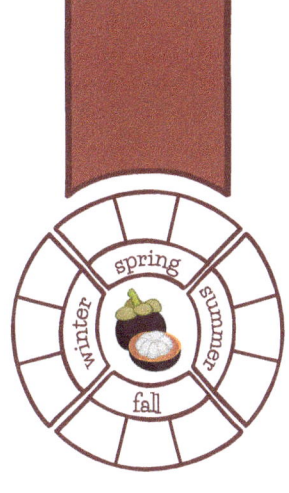

Available imported June to December

STORE
Keep mangosteens at room **temperature** for up to 3 days. Refrigerate whole mangosteens for 5-7 days or the flesh in airtight containers for 3-4 days. Freeze mangosteens in airtight containers for 10-12 months.

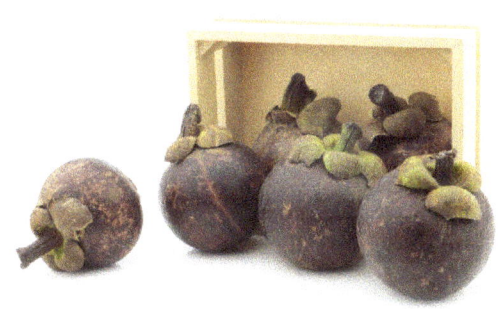

EAT
Clean the skin and use a knife to **score** the skin around the center of the fruit, being careful not to slice the **flesh**. Pull the stem and blossom end apart to reveal the fleshy fruit. Or, break off the stem with your fingers, press the top of the fruit where the stem was with your thumb, then squeeze and pull the two sides of the mangosteen apart, similar to opening a snack bag. Remove the segments with your hands and slice or bite in half, to remove the seed from the center. Eat, chop, or slice per recipe.

Fresh Mangosteen
Peel the skin and taste a fruit segment. Be careful, some segments may have seeds.

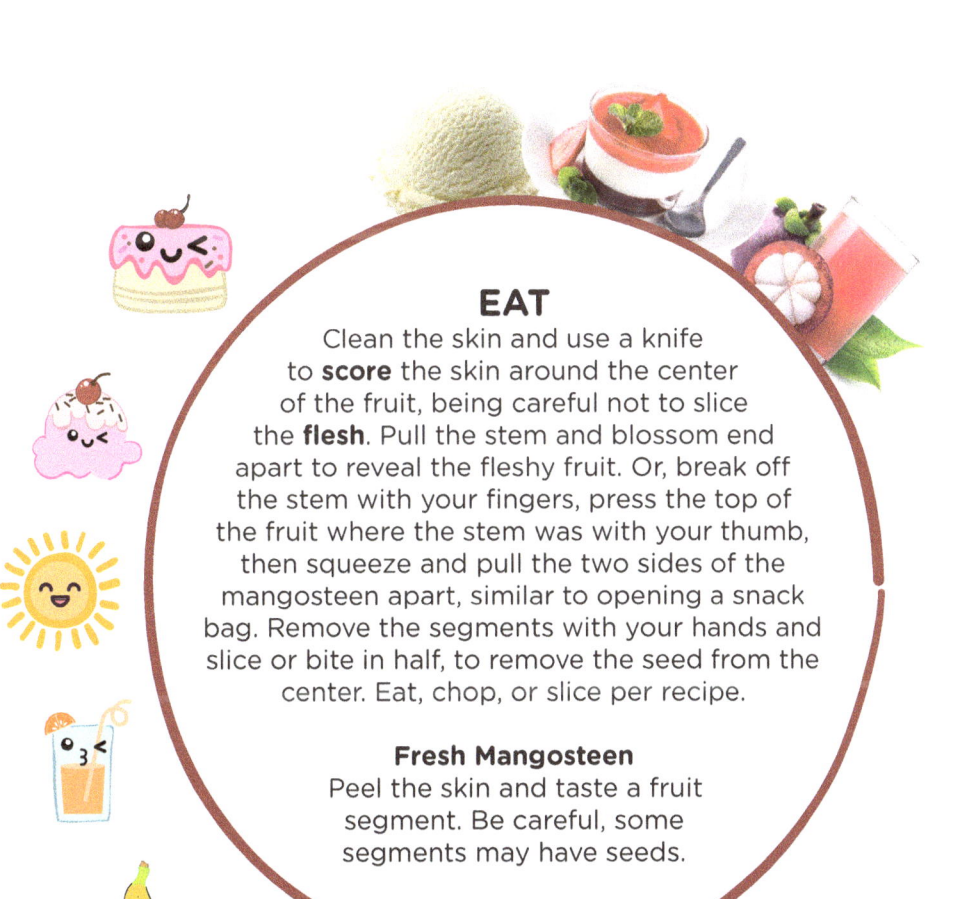

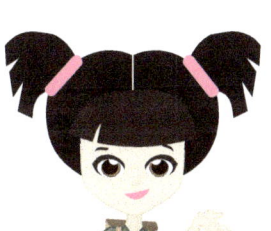

MANGOSTEEN TIDBITS

Mangosteen trees may take 10-15 years to produce fruit.

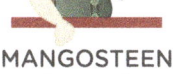

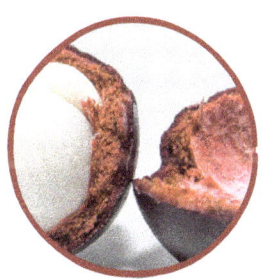

The purple **rind** of the mangosteen can **stain** hands and clothes. In fact, the rind is used to tan or color leather in China.

A Book of Fruits 103

MELON

[mel-uhn]

aromatic, juicy, refreshing, sweet, tender

PEPO

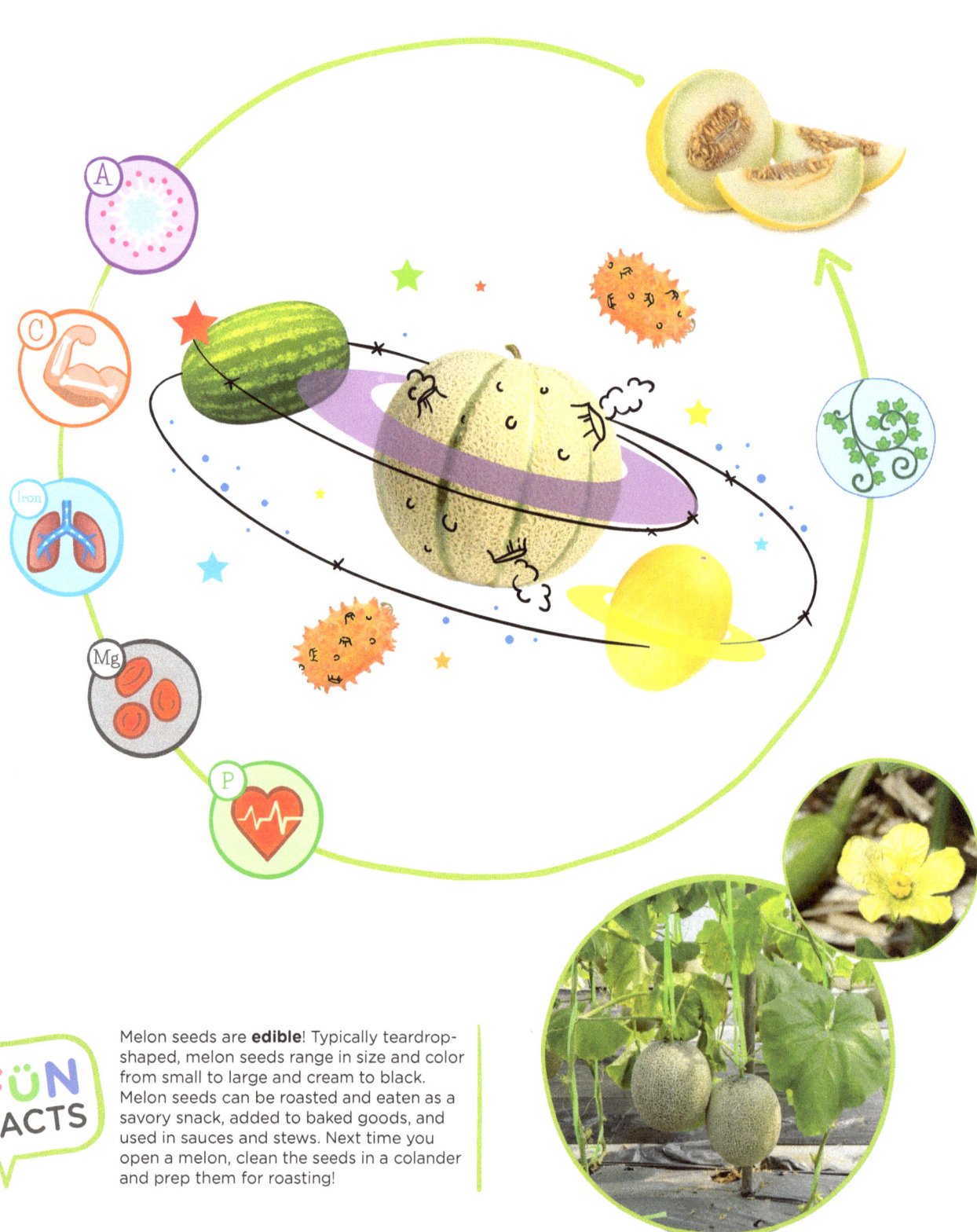

FUN FACTS

Melon seeds are **edible**! Typically teardrop-shaped, melon seeds range in size and color from small to large and cream to black. Melon seeds can be roasted and eaten as a savory snack, added to baked goods, and used in sauces and stews. Next time you open a melon, clean the seeds in a colander and prep them for roasting!

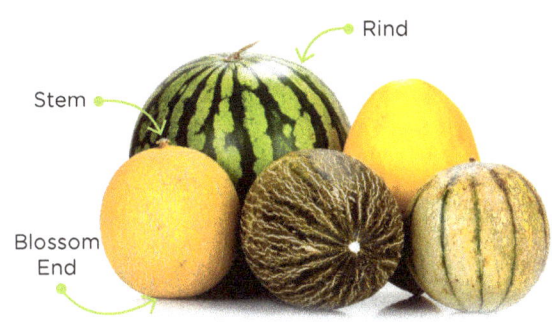

PICK
Pick **symmetrical** fruit with soft blossom ends, feel heavy for their size, and have a sweet aroma. Melon varieties should be free of **bruises**, cuts, and mushy spots. Colors, shapes, sizes, and **textures** differ depending on **variety**.

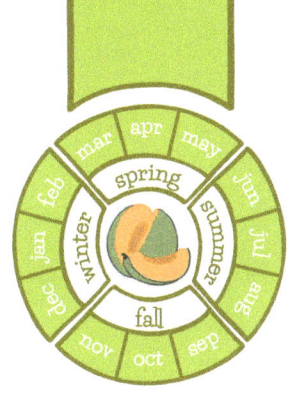

Varieties available year-round;
Imported year-round

Peak Season
Varies based on variety

STORE
In general, keep melons at room **temperature** from 2-10 days. This includes kiwano and Piel de Sapo. Other varieties of melon can be kept at room temperature as follows: cantaloupe 1-2 days; honeydew 2-4 days; and watermelon 7-10 days. Refrigerate most whole melons for 3-14 days. Refrigerate cantaloupe for 3-5 days, bitter melon 4-5 days, honeydew for 5-7 days, and watermelon for 7-14 days or all melons can be cut up in airtight containers for 3-5 days. Freeze melons in airtight containers for 10-12 months.

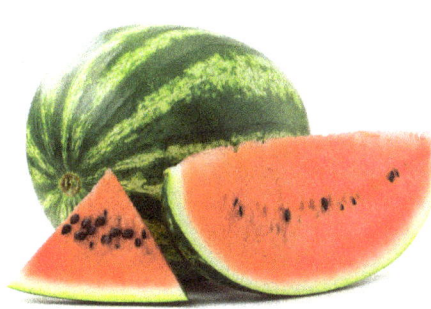

MELON TIDBITS

Melon seeds are located in the middle of the fruit. Can you name a food eaten as a vegetable that has seeds in the center? I'll give you a hint: We carve a variety of this veggie during Halloween. Answer: Pumpkin, a type of squash!

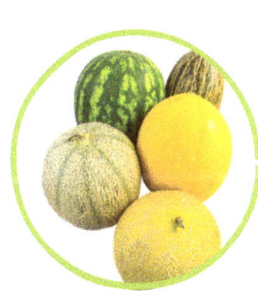

There are numerous varieties of melons that differ in color, shape, size, texture, and sweetness of the fruit.

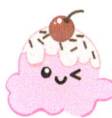

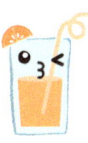
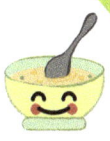

EAT
For most melons, clean the skin, slice in half lengthwise stem to blossom end, and scoop out the **seeds** in center. Then slice each half into small wedges. Next, make slices in the **flesh** of each wedge of fruit. Then take your knife parallel and close to the **rind** and slice off the fleshy pieces.

Roasted Cantaloupe Seeds
Clean the seeds in a strainer to remove the pulp. Place seeds on a clean kitchen towel and allow them to dry overnight. Preheat oven to 320 degrees F. Toss the seeds with 1 1/2 teaspoons olive oil and seasoned salt then spread on a parchment paper-lined baking sheet. Place the seeds in the oven for about 20 minutes or until they turn golden. Eat as a snack or use as savory a garnish.

MELON VARIETIES

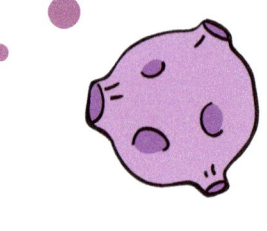

BITTER MELON
[BIT-ER MEL-UHN]

A melon with rough, green, and warty skin. Bitter melon is similar in shape to a cucumber and has off-white, **translucent**, crisp, and bitter seeded **flesh**. Bitter melon is often eaten as a vegetable in stir-fry and curry. It is considered the most bitter of all fruits and it is eaten green when the fruit is unripe. Bitter melon becomes more bitter as the skin turns orange. This melon does not need to be peeled.

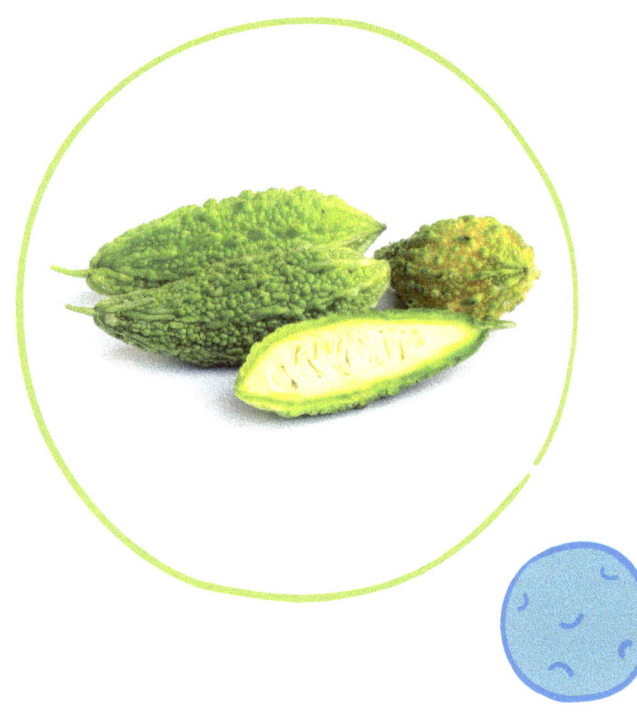

CANTALOUPE | MUSKMELON
[CAN-TA -LOUP] | [MUHSK-MEL-UHN]

A round melon with a green **rind** covered in a rough cream netting. Cantaloupe melon has dense, orange to coral, aromatic flesh that is juicy, tender, and musky.

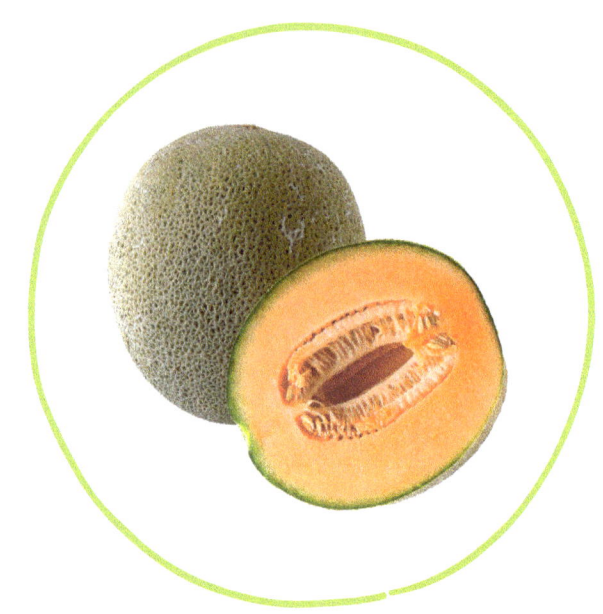

HONEYDEW [HUHN-EE-DOO]

A melon with a whiteish-yellow smooth rind that is oval in shape. Honeydew melon has crisp, pale green, fragrant flesh that is succulent, sweet, and refreshing. Other varieties of honeydew may have golden skin or orange flesh.

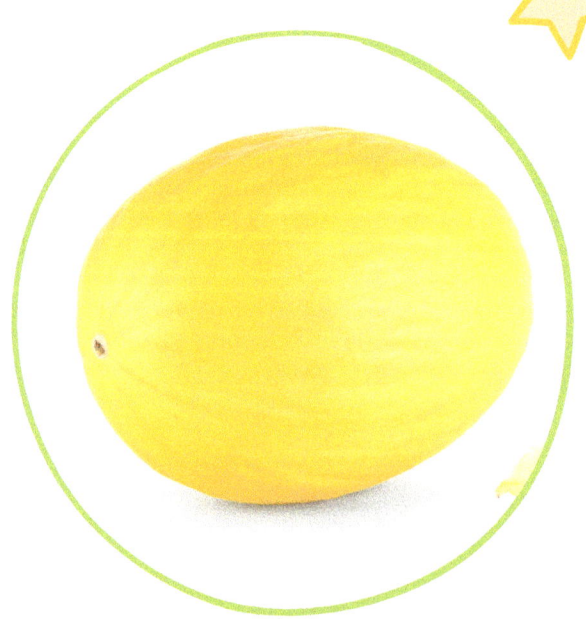

KIWANO | HORNED MELON
[KI-WAH-NOH] | [HAWRND MEL-UHN]

A melon with a bright yellow and orange rind that is an oval shape with spiky points. Kiwano melon has rich, jelly-like, lime green seeded flesh. This **variety** has a sweet and tart **flavor** that is best when chilled and can be used in both sweet and savory recipes.

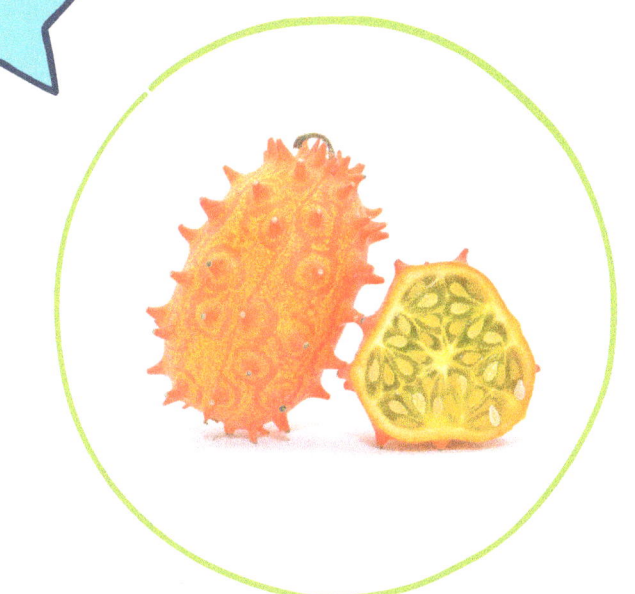

PIEL DE SAPO | SANTA CLAUS
[PE-EL DAY SAW-POH]
[SAN-TUH KLAWZ]

A small football shaped melon with a green to yellow wrinkled rind. Piel de Sapo melon has pale green to white flesh with a succulent **texture**, mildly sweet flavor, and light aroma. The more yellow on the rind, the sweeter the fruit.

WATERMELON
[WAW-TER-MEL-UHN]

There are over 1,200 known varieties of watermelon! The **thick**, hard rinds of watermelon vary from dark to pale green, solid to striped, and round to oval in shape. Watermelon flesh range in color from deep red to pink to yellow and seeds can be red, white, black, pink, or brown. Each bite of this juicy, refreshing, sweet melon is 92% water.

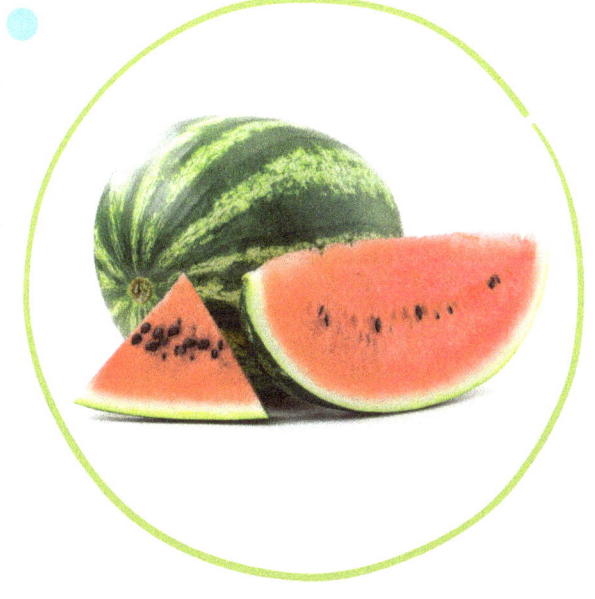

MIRACLE BERRY
MAGIC BERRY

[mir-uh-kuhl ber-ee] | [maj-ik-ber-ee]

cherry-like, mild, sweet, tasteless, tart

BERRY

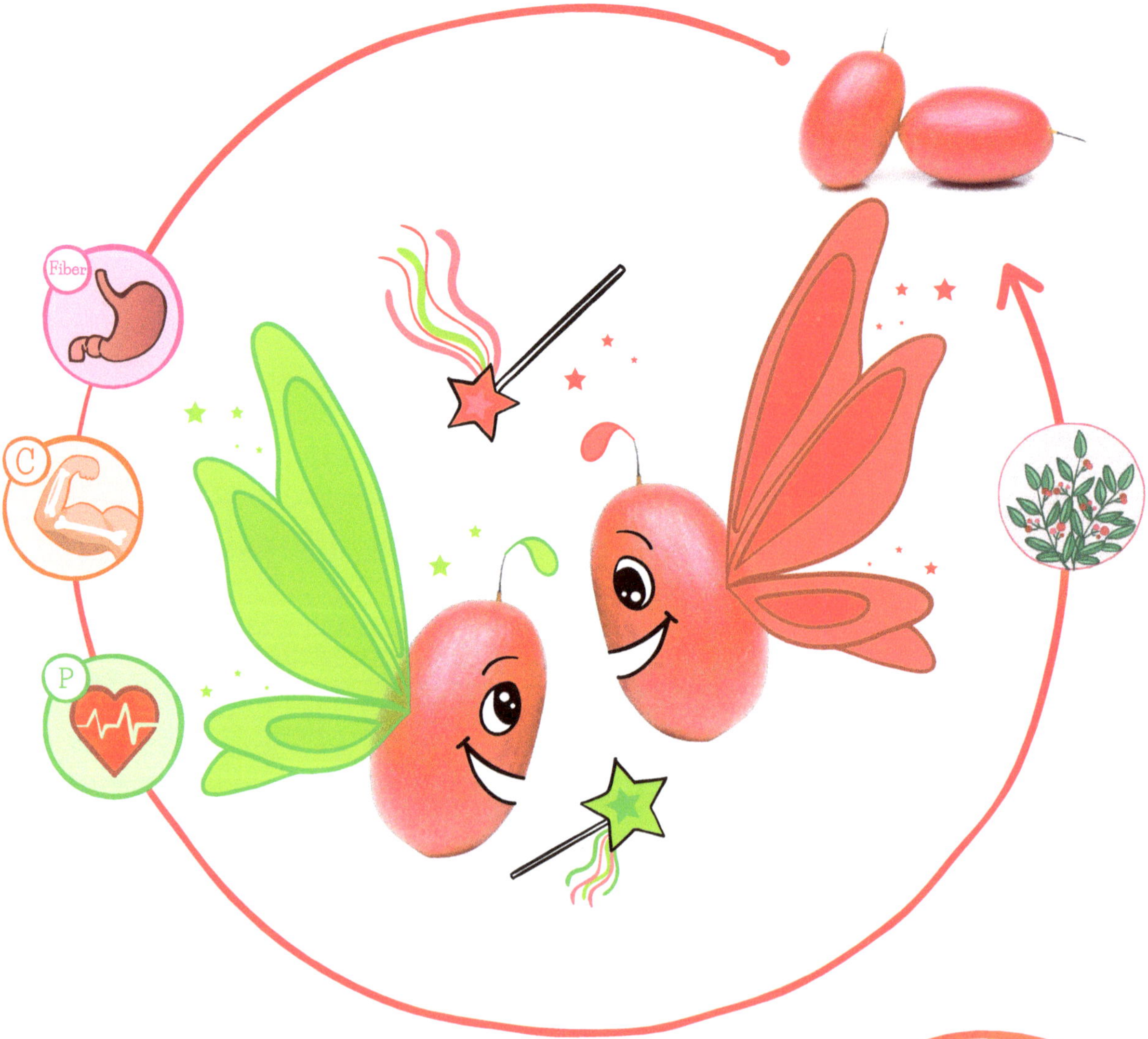

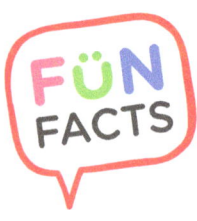

A substance called **miraculin** coats the taste buds when eating a miracle berry. Miraculin makes sour foods taste sweet and changes the perceived sweetness of foods. This means you can sample sour foods and they will taste sweet! The effects of miraculin can last up to 30 minutes until your **saliva** washes it away.

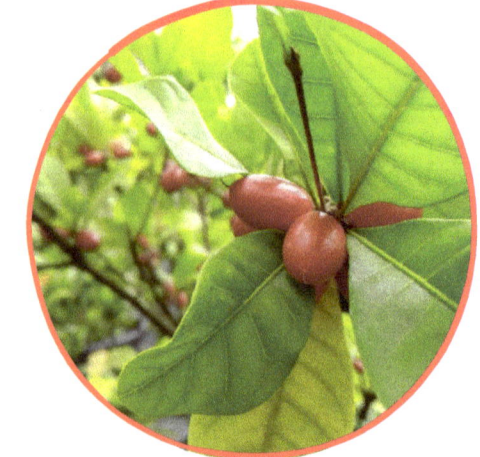

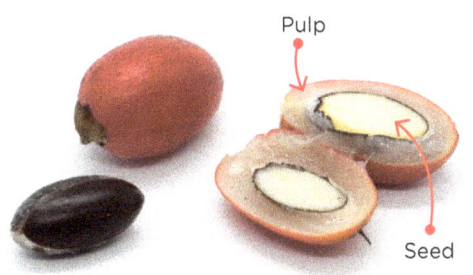
Pulp
Seed

PICK
Miracle berry are typically sold frozen, freeze-dried, **dehydrated**, or in tablet form because they **spoil** very quickly. For fresh miracle berry, pick bright red, **firm** fruit with a smooth surface.

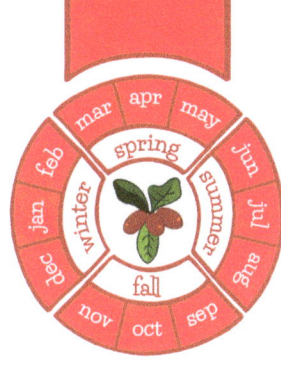

Availability varies

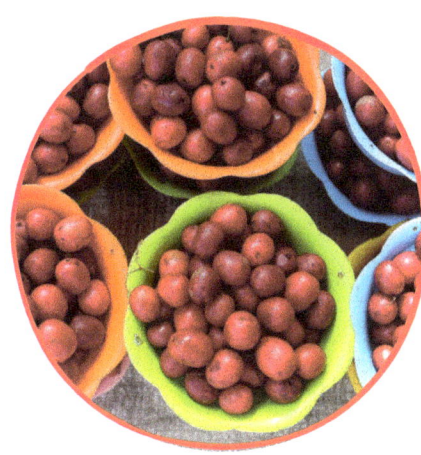

STORE
Keep fresh miracle berry at room **temperature** for up to 2 days or freeze in airtight containers for up to 1 month. Store per packaging.

Chefs may use miracle berries as part of a tasting menu to change the same dish from sour to sweet.

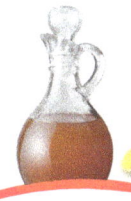

EAT
Clean the skin, bite in half, and remove the **seed** from the center.

Miracle Berry Taste Testing
Get your "My 5 Senses Worksheet," on page 25, out for this experiment! Collect a few sour items you want to use for taste-testing such as lemon wedges, vinegar, and sour candy. First, taste each item and document the **flavors** and how each makes your mouth feel. Next, place a miracle berry in your mouth and chew the **rind** and pulp off the seed. Keep the fruit **flesh** in your mouth for a full minute allowing the fruit and juice to coat your tongue. Then taste-test the foods again and record the difference! What did you notice? The effects of the miracle berry should last up to 30 minutes.

MIRACLE BERRY TIDBITS

Miracle berry is often eaten for fun at tasting parties where participants eat a berry and then taste a **variety** of tart and astringent foods.
lemon ⟶ lemonade
sour candy ⟶ sweet candy
vinegar ⟶ sweet vinegar

Miracle berry is used as a sweetener and to **flavor** food and drinks in West Africa where the berry originates. However, in the United States miracle berry is only used as a berry or supplement and not as a food additive or sweetener.

A Book of Fruits 109

ORANGE AND MANDARIN

[or-inj] | [man-duh-rin]

acidic, bright, juicy, sweet, tart

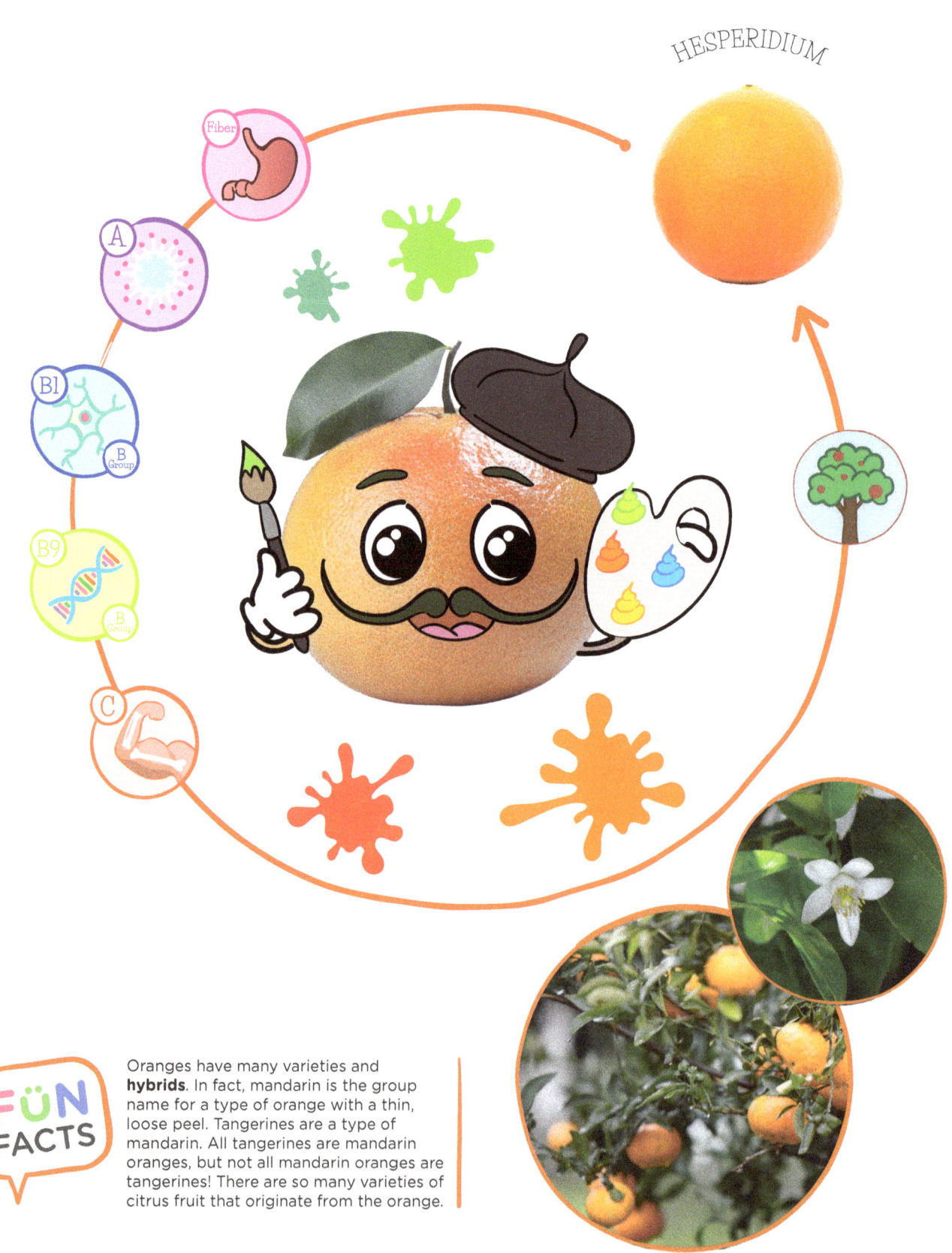

FUN FACTS

Oranges have many varieties and **hybrids**. In fact, mandarin is the group name for a type of orange with a thin, loose peel. Tangerines are a type of mandarin. All tangerines are mandarin oranges, but not all mandarin oranges are tangerines! There are so many varieties of citrus fruit that originate from the orange.

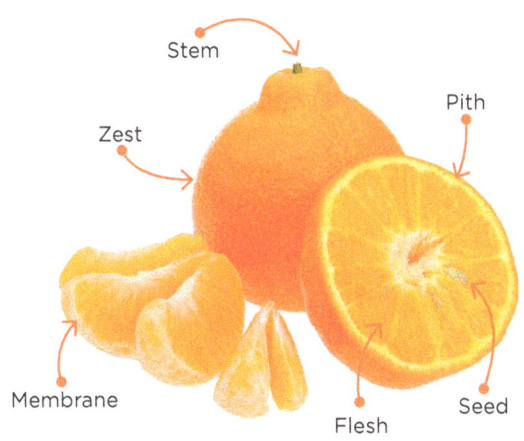

PICK
Pick semi-firm to **firm**, smooth-skinned fruit that feel heavy for their size and have a sweet aroma. Orange and mandarin varieties should be free of **bruises**, cuts, and soft spots. Colors, shapes, sizes, and **textures** differ depending on **variety**.

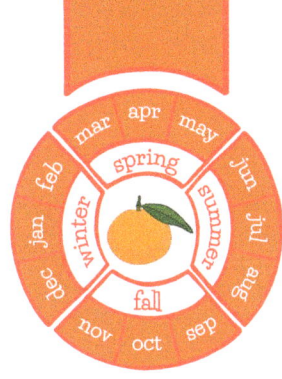

Varieties available year-round; Imported year-round

Peak Season
Varies based on variety

STORE
Keep oranges and mandarins at room **temperature** for up to 7 days. Refrigerate whole oranges and mandarins in a plastic bag for 2-4 weeks or peeled in airtight containers for 3-4 days. Freeze oranges and mandarins in airtight containers for 10-12 months.

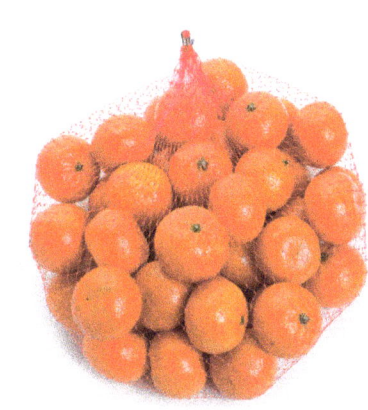

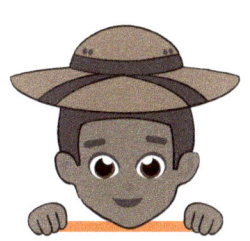

ORANGE TIDBITS

Orange and mandarin varieties developed both naturally in the wild and by **farmers** who **cultivated** new fruit based on selecting desired qualities, like seedless fruit.

EAT
Clean the skin, peel and eat, slice, or juice per recipe.

Citrus Vinaigrette
In a small jar with a lid, shake together 3 ounces of any fresh squeezed orange or mandarin juice, 2 tablespoons white balsamic vinegar, 2 tablespoons olive oil, 1 tablespoon Dijon-style mustard, 2 teaspoons honey, and a pinch of salt and pepper. Use over salads or as a **marinade**.

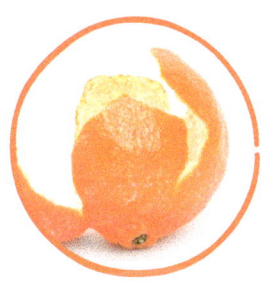

Zest is the outer part of the peel of a citrus fruit such as oranges and lemons. Zest provides a concentrated **flavor** and can be used as an additive or garnish in both savory and sweet dishes. To zest, grate the outermost skin of the whole citrus fruit.

A Book of Fruits 111

ORANGE AND MANDARIN VARIETIES

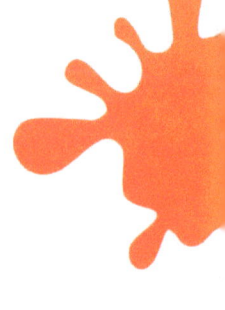

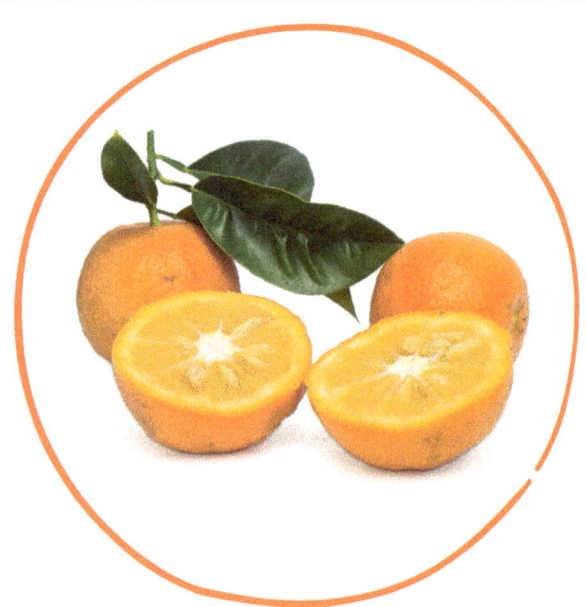

BITTER ORANGE | SEVILLE
[BIT-ER ORINJ] | [SUH-VIL]

Orange
The **rind** of this **variety** is orange in color. Bitter oranges, are small, round, and too sour to be eaten fresh. They are used for making marmalade, candied orange peel, and sauces. Another name for this variety is Seville. Seville is a city in Spain where this orange was originally **cultivated**.

BLOOD ORANGE [BLUHD OR-INJ]

Orange
The rind of this variety is orange, orange-red, red, or purple. Blood oranges are named for their deep red flesh. This seedless orange has a soft **membrane** and a sweet, rich, **zesty flavor** with a raspberry aftertaste that is best served fresh.

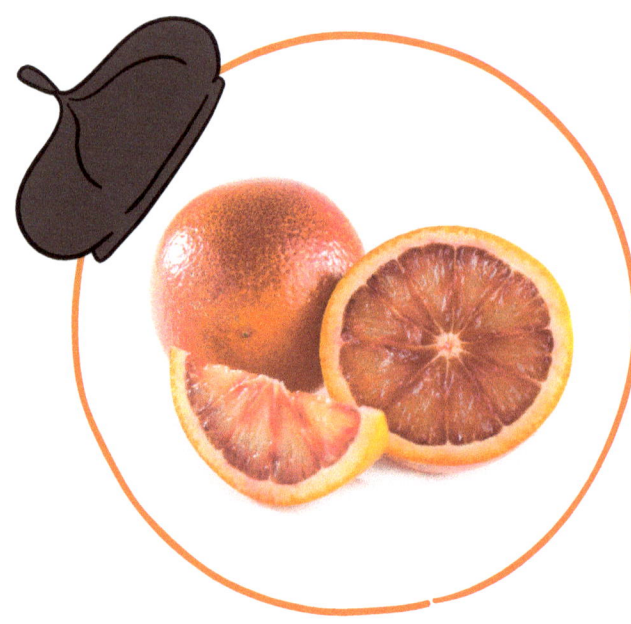

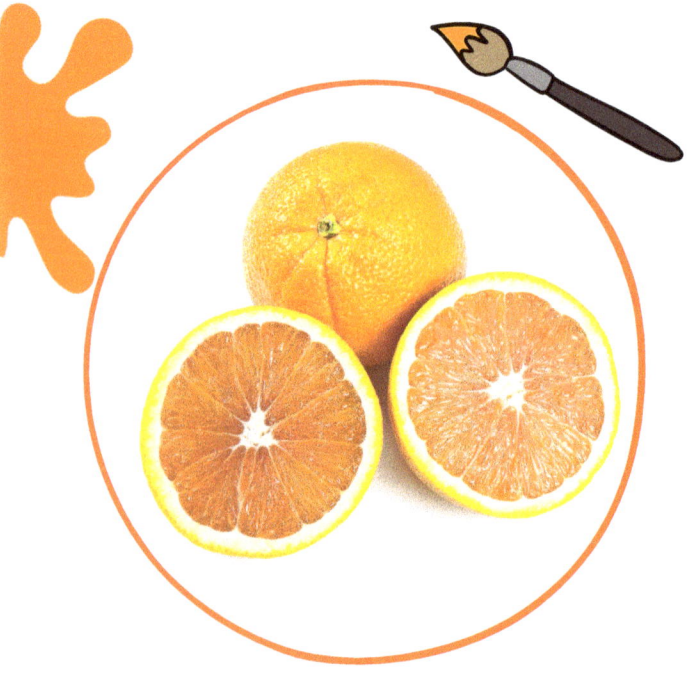

CARA CARA [KAIR-UH KAIR-UH]

Orange
The rind of this variety is bright orange. Cara Cara oranges are actually a variety of the Navel orange. They have pink, juicy, sweet, zippy flesh, and a floral aroma. The **flavor** is often described as a mix between a tangerine and a grapefruit and is considered sweeter than all other oranges. The few seeds and sweetness make this variety perfect for eating fresh and using in both sweet and savory dishes.

CLEMENTINES
[KLEM-UHN-TAHYN]

Hybrid: bitter orange + mandarin
The rind of this **hybrid** is a shiny orange color and is easy to peel. Clementines have a honey-like **flavor** and are the smallest mandarin variety. They are often called the "Christmas Orange" because they are widely available between November and January. Clementines are a seedless variety of mandarins when they are not grown around and pollinated by another seeded citrus. They are sometime sold under the name Cuties.

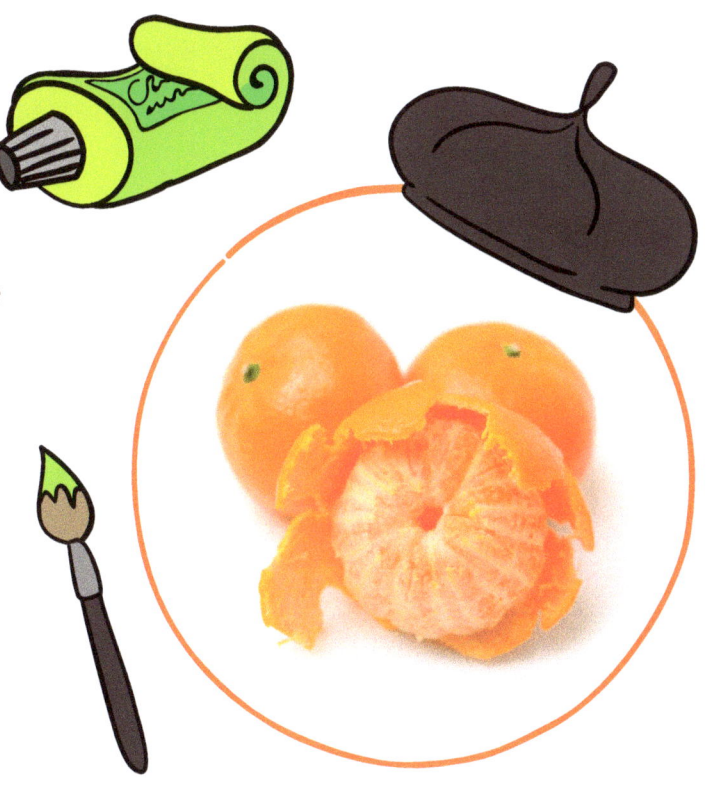

GRAPEFRUIT [GREYP-FROOT]

Hybrid: orange + pomelo
The rind of this hybrid is yellow with a tint of green or red skin. Grapefruit have juicy, sour to sweet flesh that varies in color from bright red, to pink, to white depending on variety. Grapefruit get their name from how they look in a grapefruit grove. They cluster together like a bunch of oversized grapes.

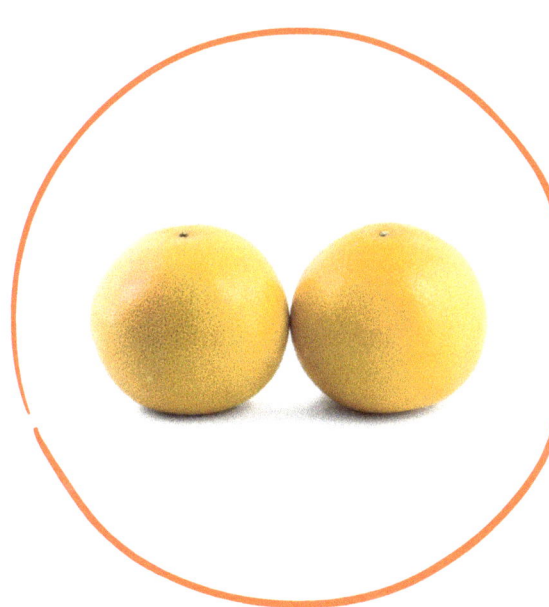

MANDARIN ORANGE
[MAN-DUH-RIN OR-JIN]

Mandarin
The rind of this variety ranges in color from green to orange when **ripe**. Mandarin Oranges may have seeds, are sweet, and easy to peel. The name Mandarin Orange refers to both the orange and to a family of orange varieties that includes clementines and satsumas.

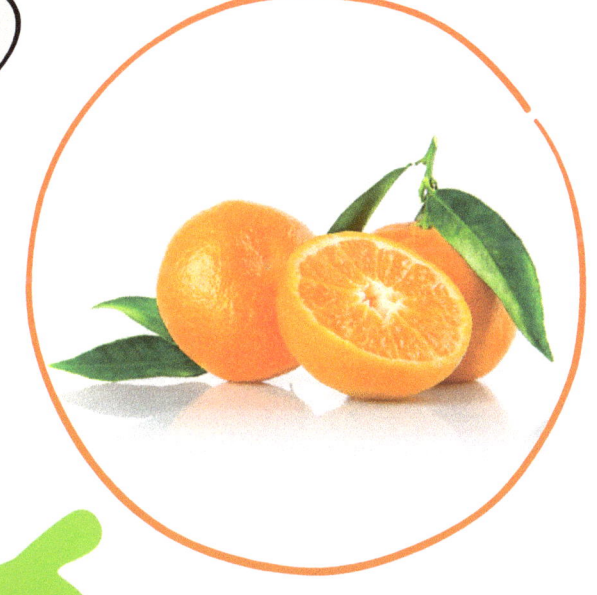

A Book of Fruits 113

ORANGE AND MANDARIN VARIETIES

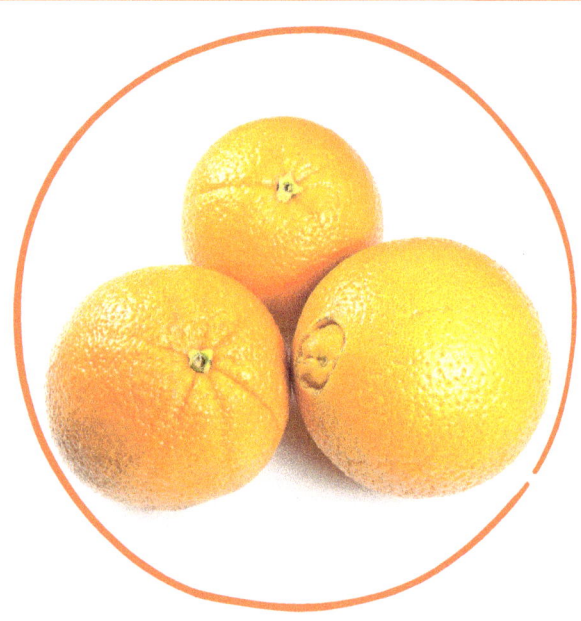

NAVEL ORANGE [NEY-VUHL OR-INJ]

Orange
This **variety** is orange in color inside and out. Navel oranges are mostly seedless, have **thick** rinds, and sweet and juicy flesh that is best served fresh. Navel oranges get their name from the bellybutton formation opposite the stem end. The bigger the navel in an orange, the sweeter the fruit.

SATSUMA [SAT-SOO-MUH]

Mandarin
The **rind** of this variety is light orange to dark orange and has a flattened sphere shape. Satsumas have extremely juicy, seedless flesh. They are known for their bright citrus aroma and loose skin that is easy to peel. This variety is often found in canned mandarin oranges.

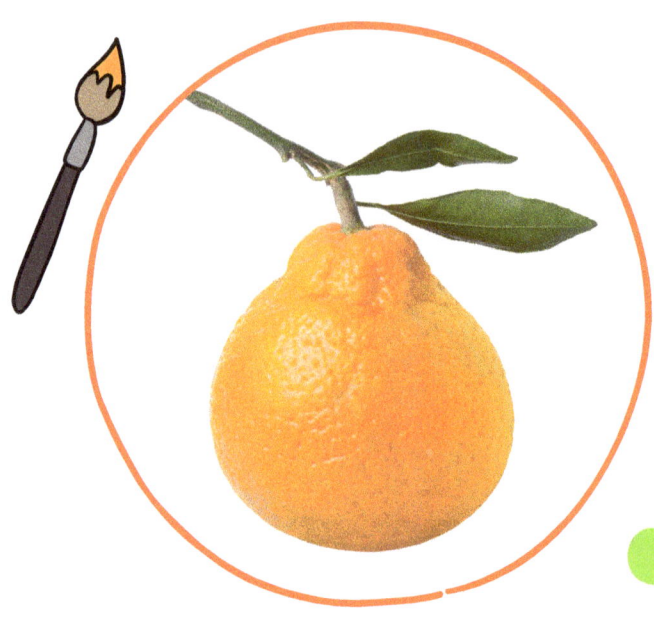

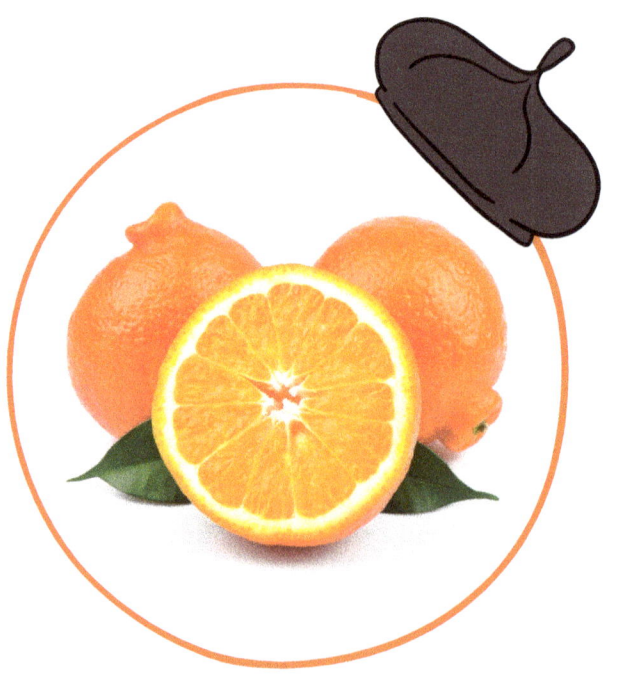

TANGELO [TAN-JUH-LOH]

Hybrid: mandarin orange + grapefruit or pomelo
The rind of this **hybrid** is a deep orange bronze and has the appearance of a large unsymmetrical orange. The most popular variety of a tangelo is the Minneola which has a knob on the stem end. Minneola have juicy, seeded flesh that can be either very sweet or very tart. They are best fresh or juiced.

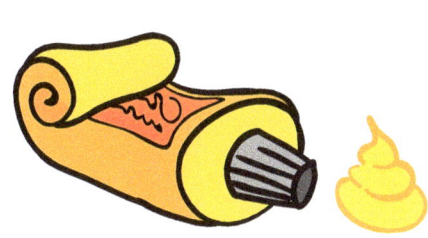

TANGERINE [TAN-JUH-REEN]

Mandarin
The rind of this variety is bright orange. Tangerines are smaller than an orange and heavily seeded. They have a sweet-tart, zippy **flavor** that is great fresh or juiced. The name tangerine originates from Tangier, Morocco. Tangier is the port where the very first tangerine fruit was shipped to Europe.

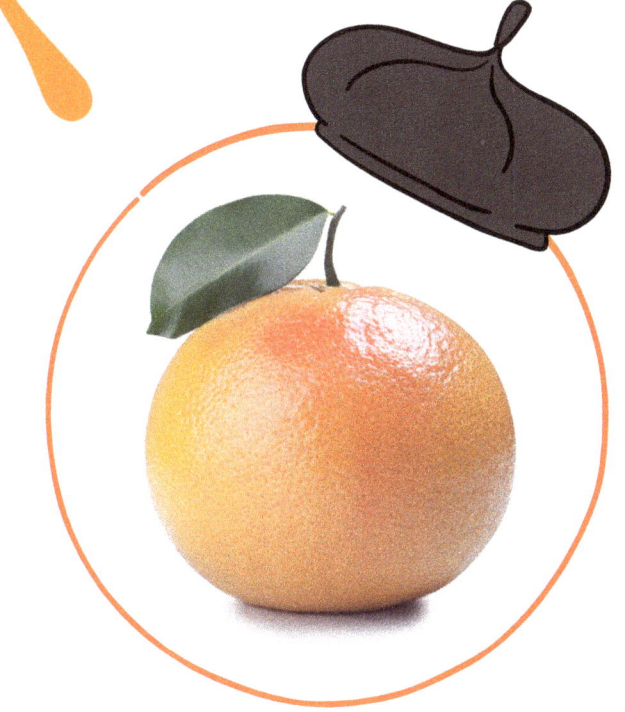

UGLI FRUIT [OO-GLI FROOT]

Hybrid: tangelo hybrid between a grapefruit + bitter orange + tangerine
The rind of this hybrid is light green to light orange. Ugli Fruit is fragrant and can be the size of an orange up to the size of a grapefruit. The mostly seedless, pinkish-orange or yellow-orange pulp is sweet, **zesty**, with a pungent flavor similar to an orange with honey. Ugli Fruit is a wild growing hybrid and gets its name from its lumpy, knobby, loose-fitting skin.

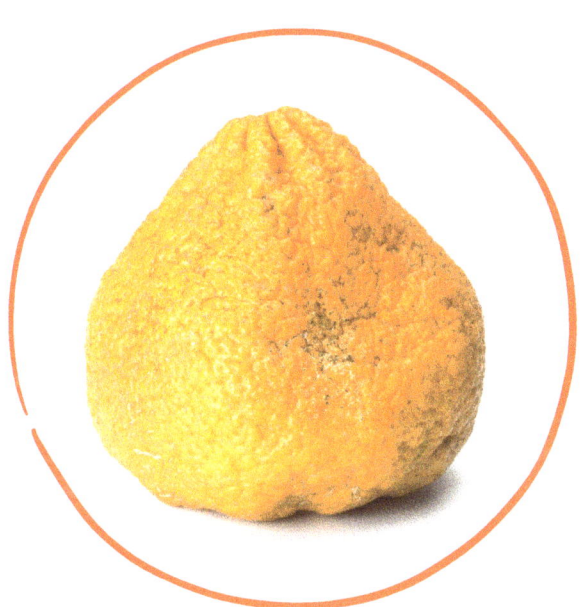

VALENCIA ORANGE [VUH-LEN-SHEE-UH OR-INJ]

Orange
The thin, smooth rind of this variety is light orange. Valencia oranges are the most widely grown orange and range in size from small to very large. They are slightly oval in shape, have seeds, and are sweet and very juicy. This is the primary variety used to make orange juice.

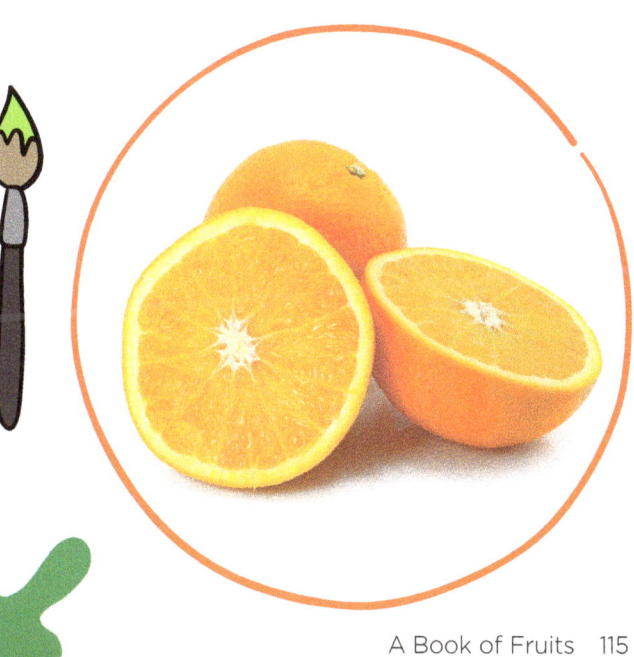

A Book of Fruits 115

PAPAYA

[puh-pah-yuh]

butter-like, juicy, musky, sweet, tender

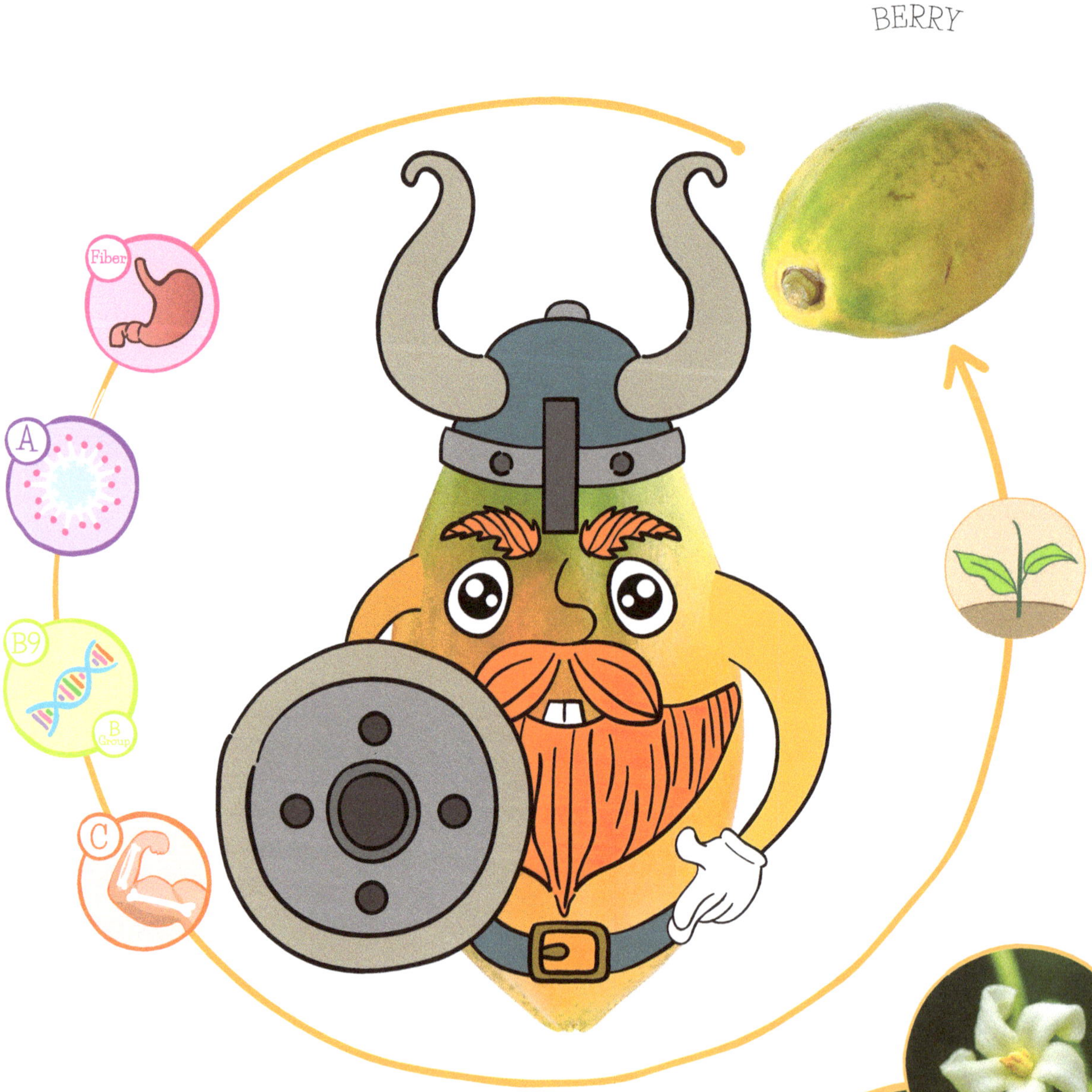

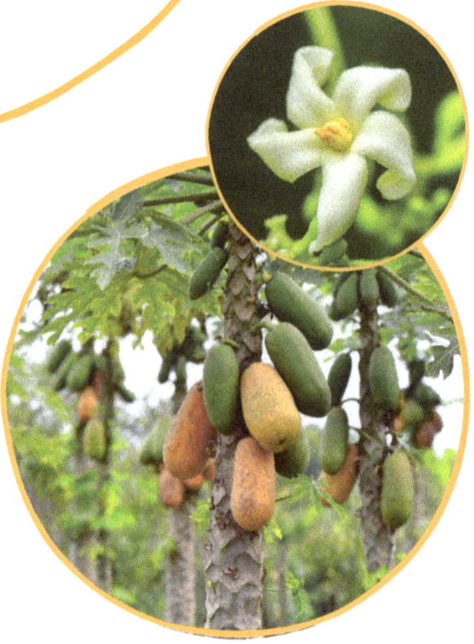

BERRY

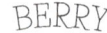

FUN FACTS

Unripe papayas are often eaten as a vegetable in savory dishes. Have you ever tried an unripe papaya?

Where Do Bananas Come From?

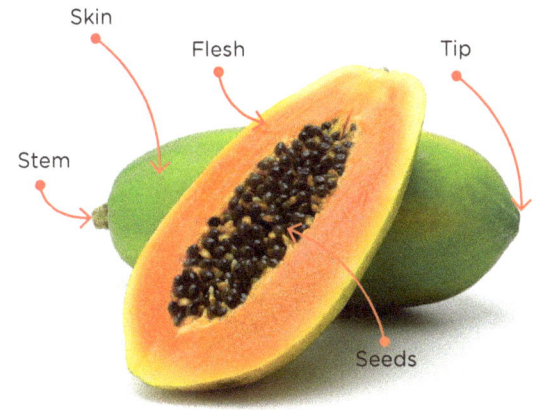

Skin, Flesh, Tip, Stem, Seeds

PICK
Pick yellow or yellow-orange fruit that are soft to touch, feel heavy for their size, and have a sweet aroma at the stem. Papayas should be free of **bruises**, mushy or hard spots.

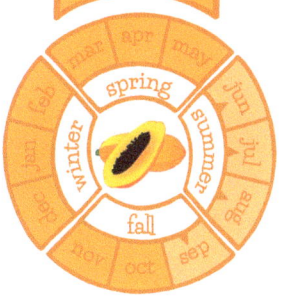

Available year-round; Imported year-round

Peak Season
June-September

STORE
Keep papayas at room **temperature** for up to 5 days or until **ripe**. Refrigerate whole papayas in a plastic bag for 5-7 days or cut-up in airtight containers for 3-4 days. Freeze papayas in airtight containers for 6-12 months. Dried papayas may be stored in airtight containers for 6-12 months.

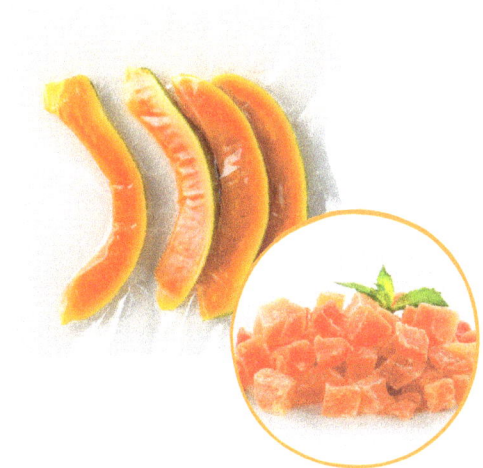

PAPAYA TIDBITS

Place unripe papayas in a paper bag to ripen more quickly

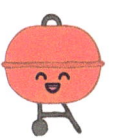
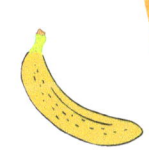

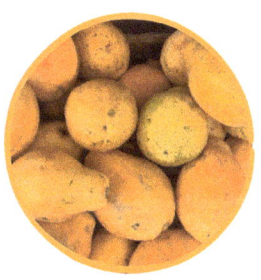

Do not refrigerate papayas until they are fully ripe. Allowing papayas to ripen at room temperature will result in more flavorful, juicy papaya.

EAT
Clean the skin, slice in half lengthwise stem to tip, and scoop out the **seeds**. Use a potato peeler or knife to slice off the skin and chop or slice per recipe.

Grilled Papaya
Preheat grill to medium heat. Slice peeled and deseeded papaya into 2 inch **thick** wedges and coat with olive oil. Place on the grill for 3-5 minutes each side until the skin starts to bubble. Combine 2 juiced limes with 2 tablespoons honey. **Drizzle** sauce over the top and garnish with toasted coconut.

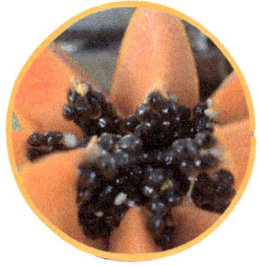

Black papaya seeds are crunchy and have a peppery **flavor** like mustard or watercress. Use them as a garnish or blend them into a dressing.

A Book of Fruits 117

PASSION FRUIT
GRANADILLA

[pash-uhn froot] | [gran-uh-dil-uh]

grainy, juicy, slimy, sweet, tart

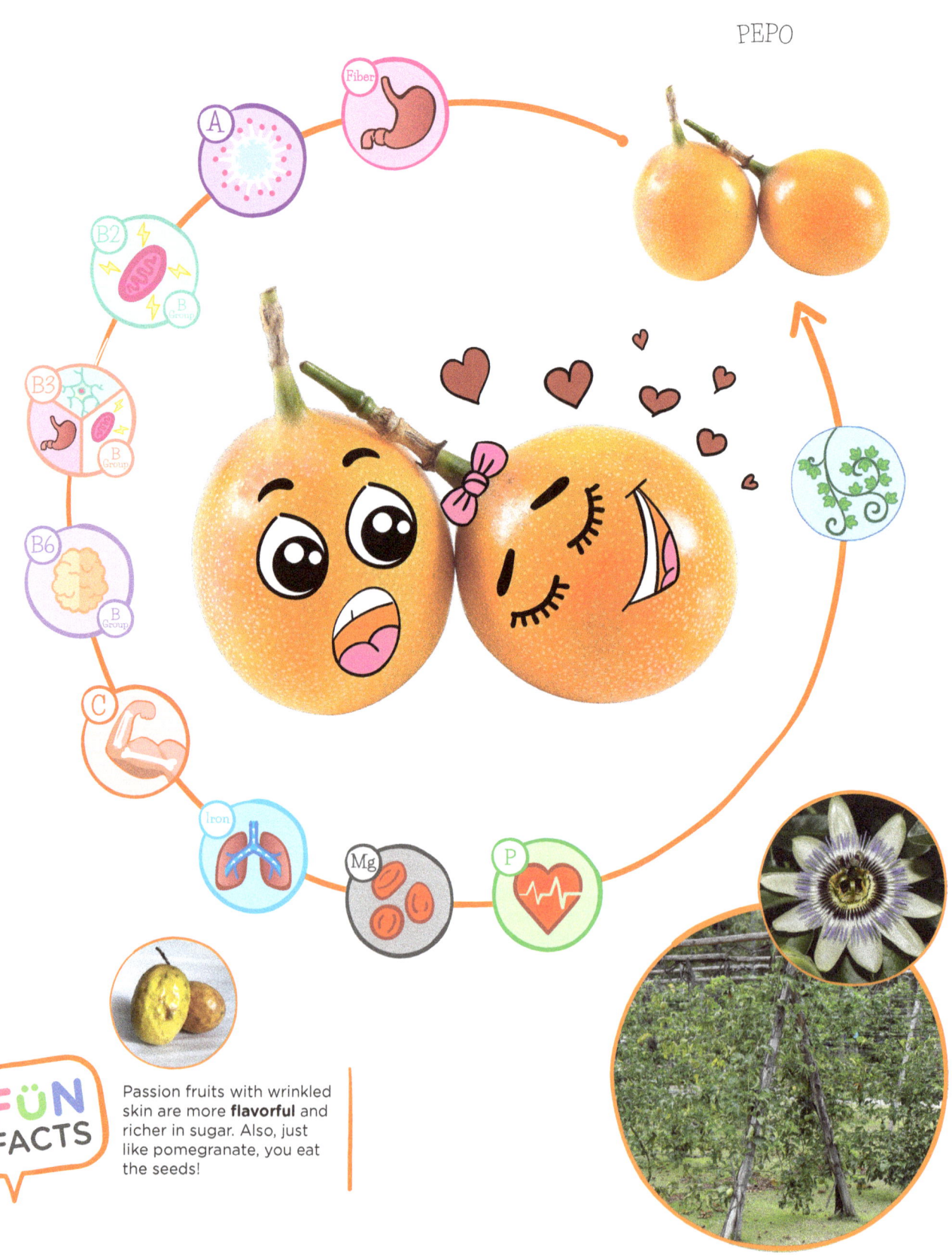

PEPO

FUN FACTS Passion fruits with wrinkled skin are more **flavorful** and richer in sugar. Also, just like pomegranate, you eat the seeds!

118 | Where Do Bananas Come From?

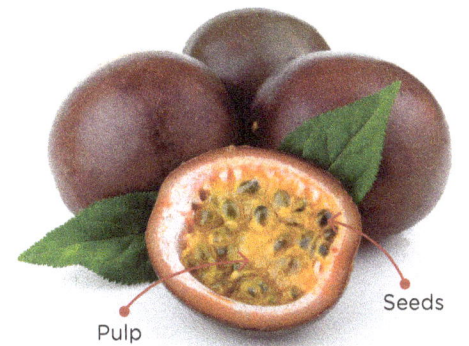

Pulp · Seeds

PICK
Pick deep purple, light yellow, or orange colored fruit with wrinkled skin, feel heavy for their size, and have a tropical aroma. Passion fruits should be free of mushy spots and **mold**.

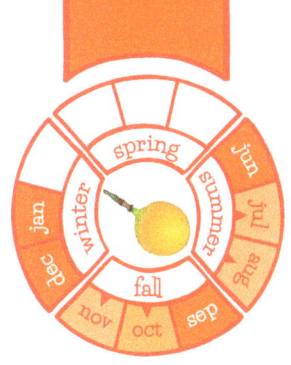

Available June to January;
Imported year-round

Peak Season
July-August;
October-November

STORE
Keep passion fruits at room **temperature** for up to 5 days or until **ripe**. Refrigerate whole passion fruits for 5-7 days or the **flesh** in airtight containers for 3-4 days. Freeze passion fruits in airtight containers for 6-8 months.

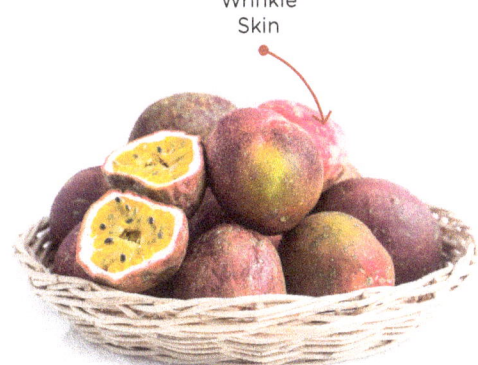

Wrinkle Skin

PASSION FRUIT TIDBITS

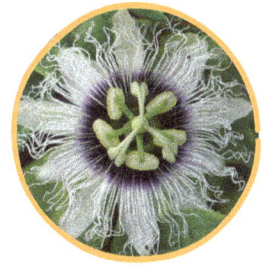

The name for the passion fruit flower was given by **missionaries** who used the flower as a **symbol** to share religious education.

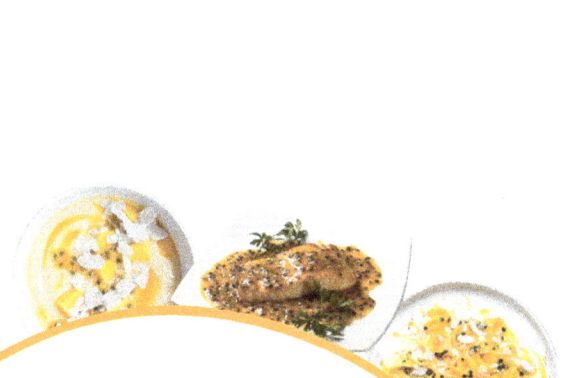

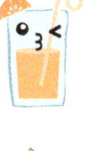
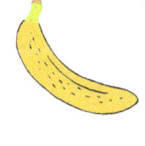
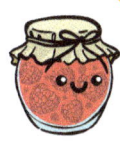

EAT
Clean the skin, cut in half, and scoop out the juicy, pulpy **seeds** with a spoon.

Passionfruit Popsicles
In a blender, combine 6 ounces passion fruit pulp, about 4 ripe fruit, 1 banana, 1 - 13.5 ounce can coconut milk, and 2 tablespoons honey (optional). Divide **puree** into popsicle molds and freeze overnight.

Makes about 6, 4 ounce popsicles

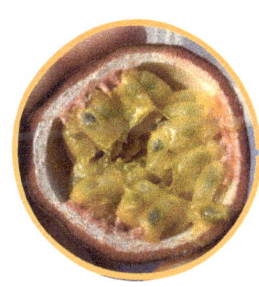

Passion fruit pulp is slimy and jelly-like while the seeds are crunchy and gritty.

A Book of Fruits

PAWPAW

[paw-paw]

creamy, fragrant, rich, sweet, tangy

BERRY

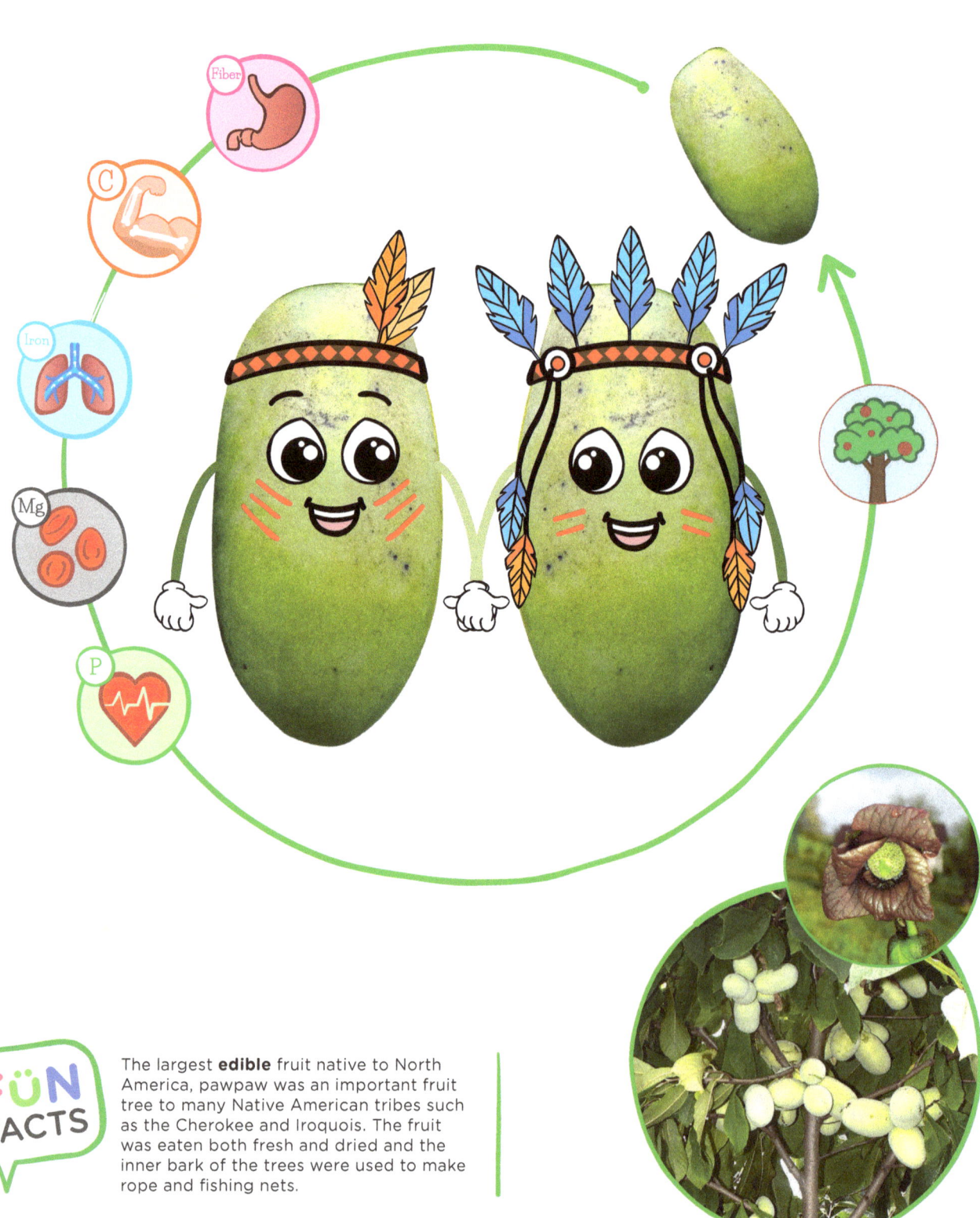

FUN FACTS: The largest **edible** fruit native to North America, pawpaw was an important fruit tree to many Native American tribes such as the Cherokee and Iroquois. The fruit was eaten both fresh and dried and the inner bark of the trees were used to make rope and fishing nets.

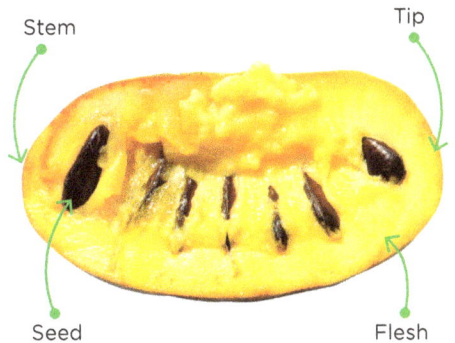
Stem · Tip · Seed · Flesh

PICK
Pick greenish yellow fruit that are soft to touch with a sweet floral aroma. Pawpaws should be free of **bruises** and mushy spots.

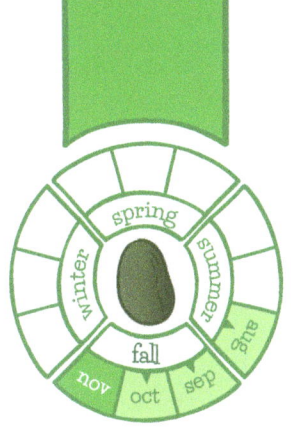

Available August to November;

Peak Season
August-October

STORE
Keep pawpaws at room **temperature** and eat within 3 days. Refrigerate pawpaws for up to 14 days. Freeze pawpaws in airtight containers for 10-12 months.

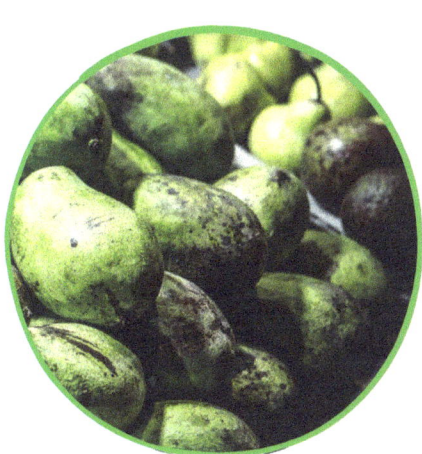

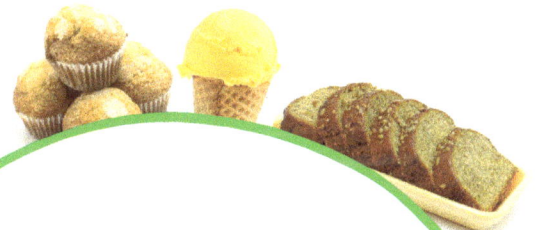

EAT
Clean the skin, slice in half stem to tip, spoon out the **flesh**, and remove the **seeds**.

Pawpaw Ice Cream
Combine 2 cups pawpaw pulp, 1 cup sugar, 1 teaspoon vanilla extract, 1/2 teaspoon cinnamon, and 1/4 teaspoon nutmeg in a blender until smooth. Mix in 2 cups cream, 2 cups milk, and pour into an ice cream maker. Follow manufacturer directions for ice cream machine.

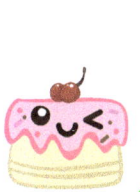
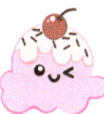
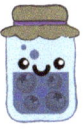
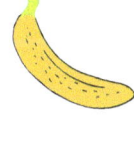

PAWPAW TIDBITS

The **flavor** of pawpaw is compared to a banana with hints of vanilla custard and mango.

***

Pawpaw is related to the cherimoya, guanabana, and custard apple.

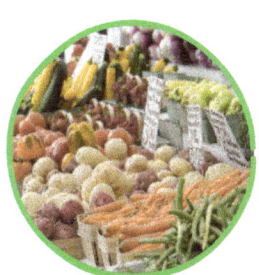

Look for pawpaw at a local **farmers** market versus a grocery store because they don't ship or store well.

A Book of Fruits 121

PEACH

[peech]

fuzzy, juicy, mealy, sweet, syrupy

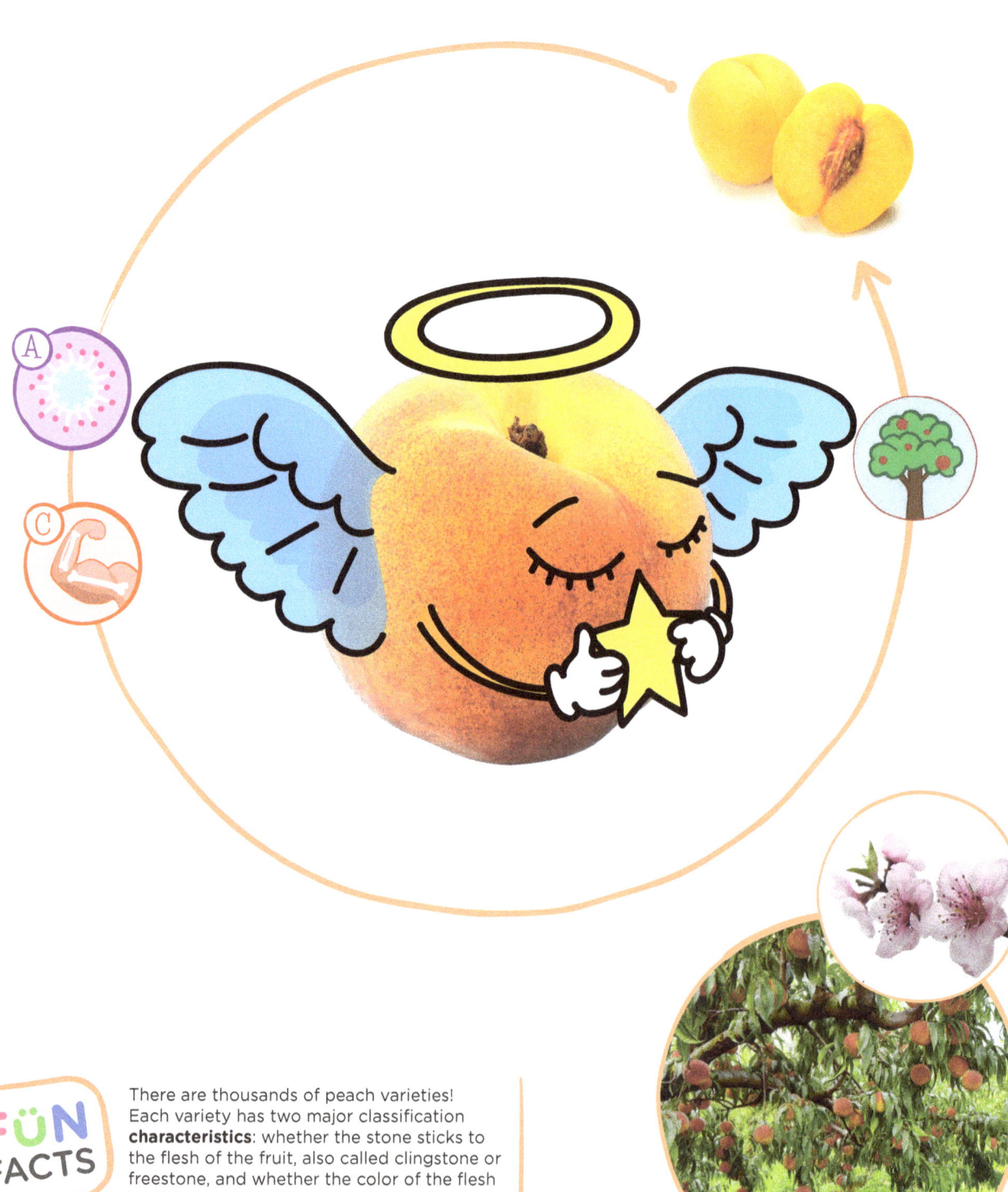

FUN FACTS: There are thousands of peach varieties! Each variety has two major classification **characteristics**: whether the stone sticks to the flesh of the fruit, also called clingstone or freestone, and whether the color of the flesh is white or yellow. For example, the O'Henry variety is a freestone peach with yellow flesh.

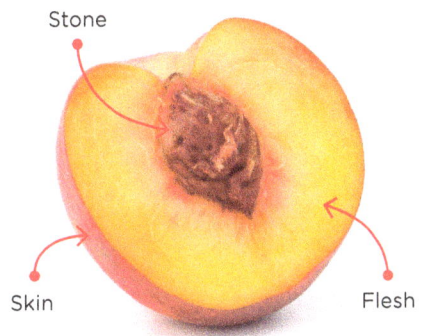

Stone · Skin · Flesh

PICK
Pick fruit that are soft to touch and smell sweet. Peach varieties a should be free of green coloring, **bruises**, and mushy spots. Colors, shapes, and **textures** differ depending on **variety**.

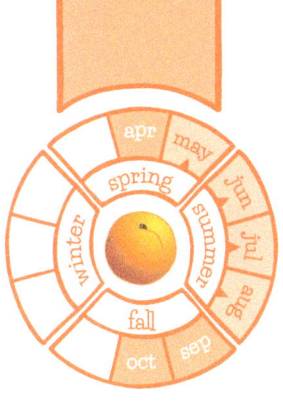

Available April to October; Imported year-round

Peak Season
May-August

STORE
Keep peaches at room **temperature** for up to 3 days or until **ripe**. Refrigerate whole peaches in plastic bags for 3-5 days or cut-up in airtight containers for 3-4 days. Freeze peaches in airtight containers for 10-12 months. Dried peaches may be stored in airtight containers for 6-12 months.

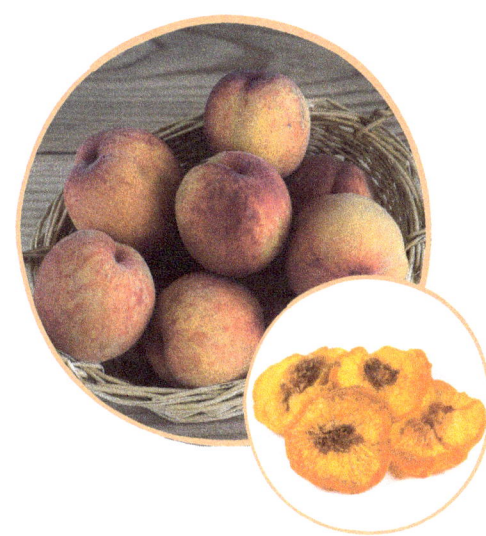

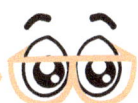

Place unripe peaches in a paper bag to ripen more quickly.

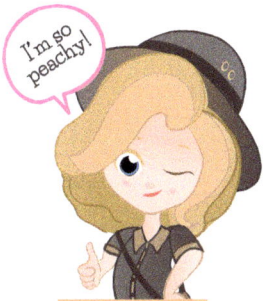

"I'm so peachy!"

PEACH TIDBITS

The word "peach" is often used to describe things being the very best. Have you ever used the phrase "I'm just peachy" or "You're a peach?"

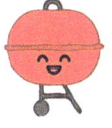
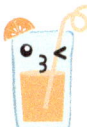
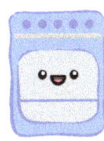

EAT
Clean the skin, slice or bite in half, and remove the **stone** from center. Eat, chop, or slice per recipe.

BBQ Peaches
Preheat grill to medium heat. Slice **firm**, freestone peaches in half and remove the stone. Coat with olive oil and place on the grill cut side down. Grill for 4-5 minutes and then flip and grill on the other side for 4-5 minutes until peaches are tender and soft. Serve with a scoop of vanilla ice cream and sprinkle with cinnamon.

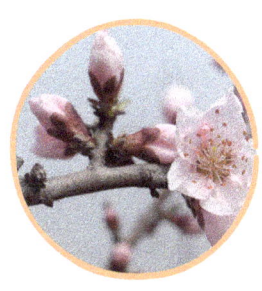

Peach blossoms are **edible**. They have a soft texture and a sweet aroma similar to honey and almond. Add them to sweet and savory dishes as a garnish, **steep** as a tea, or try in a jelly.

PEACH VARIETIES

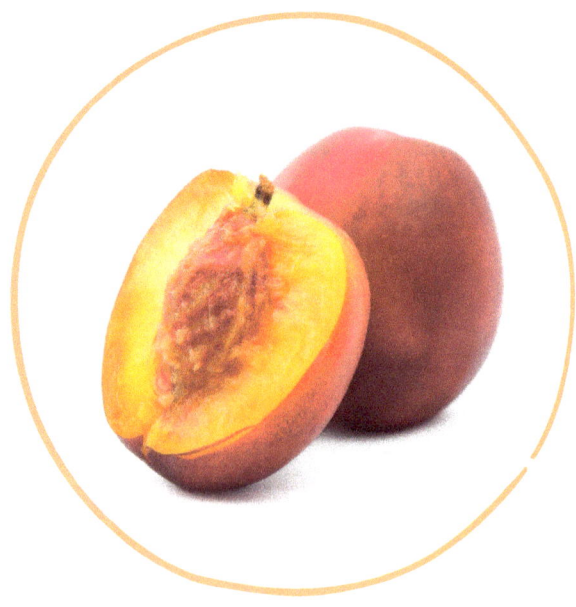

CLINGSTONE [KLING-STOHN]

A peach with extremely juicy, flavorful, and sweet flesh. Clingstone peaches get their name from the way their flesh is attached or **clings** to their **stone** making stone removal more difficult. Clingstone peaches have a soft texture and are great fresh or for baking and canning.

DOUGHNUT [DOH-NUHT]

A **mutation** of the peach resulted in a **variety** that is flattened with a shape similar to a doughnut. Doughnut peaches may be clingstone or freestone and have white or yellow flesh which influences the **flavor** and **texture** of the fruit.

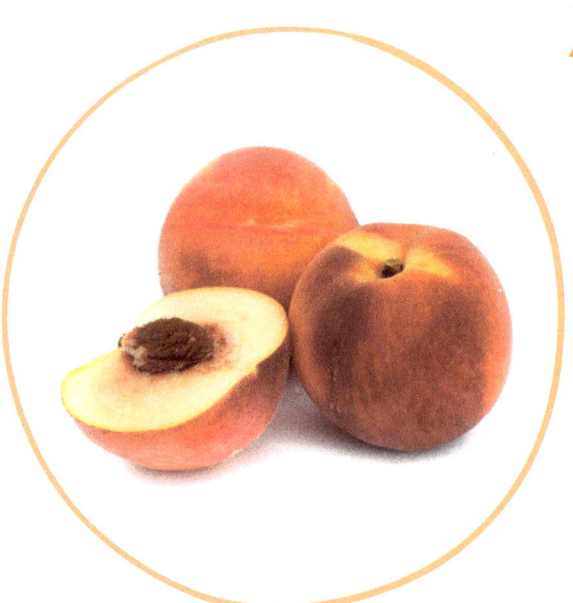

FREESTONE [FREE-STOHN]

A peach that is mildly juicy, sweet, and **firm**. The flesh of freestone peaches are separate or free from the stone making stone removal very easy. Freestone peaches are most popular for eating fresh because they are easy to **prepare**. They are also used for baking and preserves.

NECTARINE [NEK-TUH-REEN]

A mutation of the peach resulted in a variety that lacks velvety, fuzzy skin. Nectarines may be clingstone or freestone and have white or yellow flesh which influences the flavor and texture of the fruit.

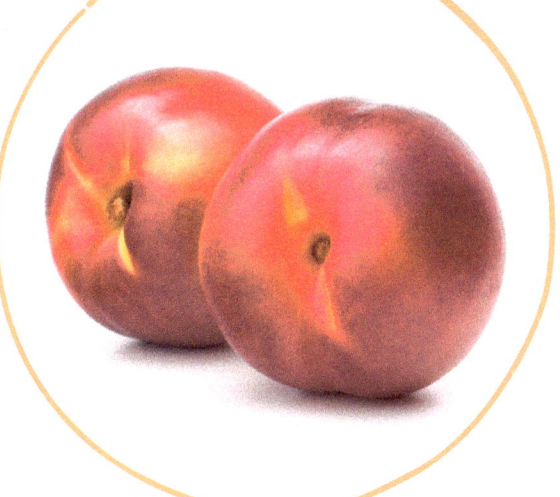

WHITE PEACH [WAHYT PEECH]

A peach with yellow, pink or red skin and white flesh. White peaches look very similar to yellow peaches on the outside; however, the white flesh is less acidic, smooth, succulent, and sweeter. Most peach trees in Asia produce fruit with white flesh.

YELLOW PEACH [YEL-OH PEECH]

A peach with yellow, pink or red skin and flesh ranging in color from yellow to an orange-yellow, yellow streaked with red, or yellow and red close to the stone. Yellow peaches look similar to white peaches on the outside, however yellow peaches are more acidic and have a juicy, sweet tang. Most peach trees in the United States produce fruit with yellow flesh.

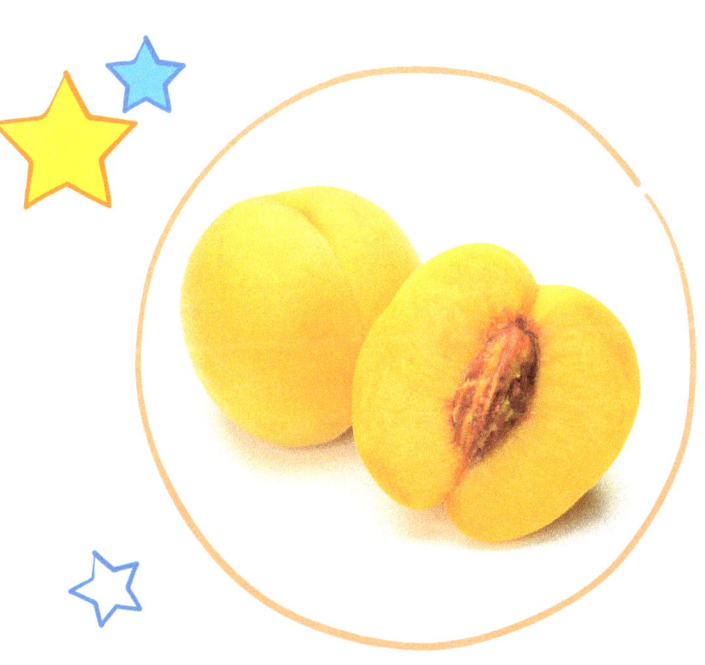

A Book of Fruits 125

PEAR

[pair]

gritty, juicy, soft, sweet, textured

POME

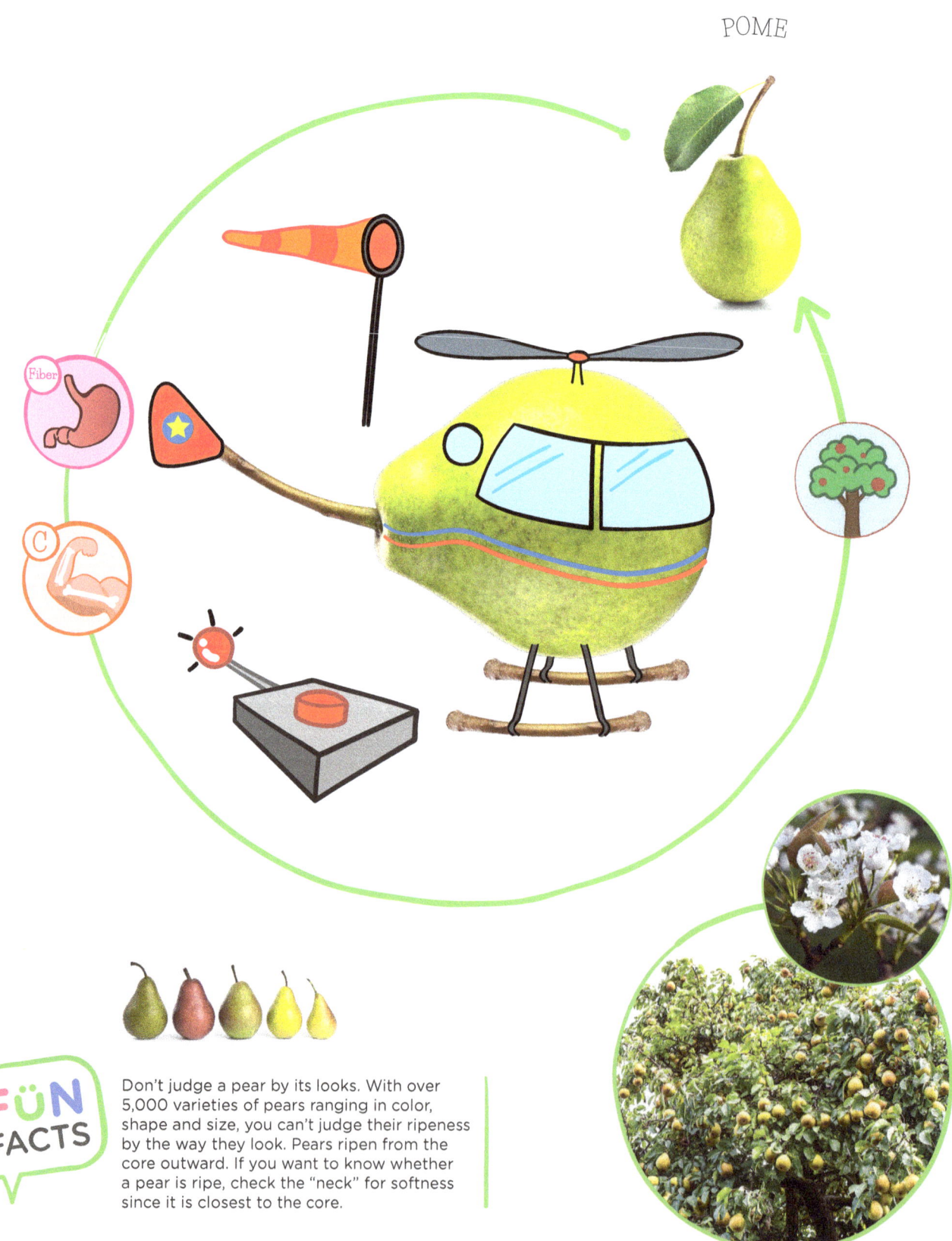

FUN FACTS Don't judge a pear by its looks. With over 5,000 varieties of pears ranging in color, shape and size, you can't judge their ripeness by the way they look. Pears ripen from the core outward. If you want to know whether a pear is ripe, check the "neck" for softness since it is closest to the core.

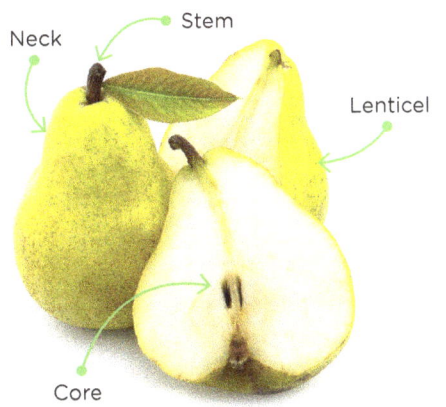

PICK
Pick **firm** fruit that are soft to touch at the "neck." The neck is between the stem and above the rounded body of the fruit. Pear varieties should be free of **bruises** and mushy spots. Colors, shapes, and **textures** differ depending on **variety**.

Available August to February; Imported year-round

Peak Season
Varies based on variety

STORE
Keep pears at room **temperature** for up to 4 days or until **ripe**. Refrigerate whole pears in plastic bags for 5-7 days or cut-up in airtight containers for 3-4 days. Freeze pears in airtight containers for 10-12 months. Dried pears may be stored in airtight containers for 10-12 months. Keep away from foods with strong odors.

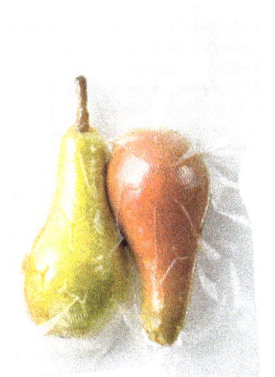

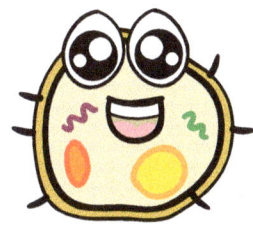

PEAR TIDBITS

When pears fully ripen on the tree, they can become gritty because of something called **stone cells**. Stone cells are the same material that make cherry stones and walnuts shells hard. Pears **harvested** before they ripen typically have a more even, smooth texture.

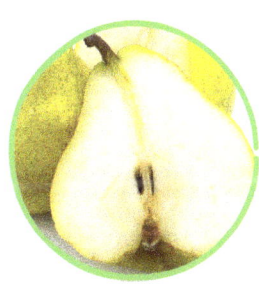

Pears are also known as "butter fruit" because they have soft, melting flesh with a smooth texture similar to butter when they are ripe.

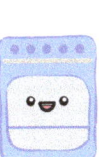
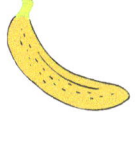

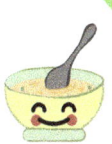

EAT
Clean the skin, remove the core, and chop or slice per recipe.

Stewed Pears
Core and chop 1 pound of all-purpose pears and place in a saucepan over medium heat. Add 2 tablespoons brown sugar, 2 tablespoons water, and a cinnamon stick. Cook fruit with the lid on for 10-15 minutes or until fruit softens. Once fruit softens, remove the lid and cook until the liquid has the consistency of a **thick** sauce. Serve over yogurt or waffles.

A Book of Fruits

PEAR VARIETIES

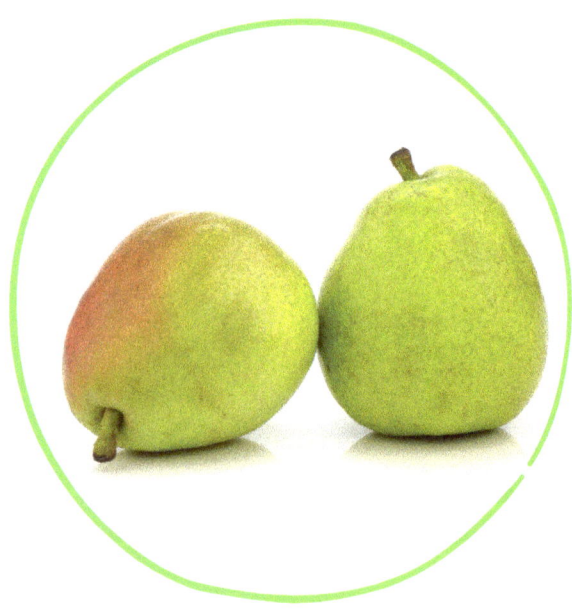

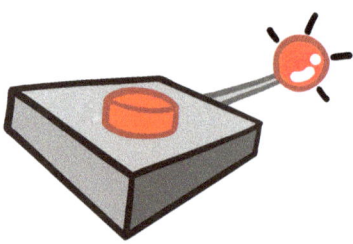

ANJOU [ON-JU]

A bright green or red pear with smooth, **firm** skin that is covered in **lenticels** or pores. Anjou pears are medium in size, egg-shaped with a large spherical body, and narrow "neck." The flesh of this **variety** is cream-colored, dense, and buttery with a slightly gritty texture and a sweet refreshing, tangy **flavor**. Anjou pears are considered an all-purpose variety and can be eaten in many ways from grilling, to sautéing, to baking, to fresh.

ASIAN PEAR | SAND PEAR
[EY-SHUHN PAIR] | [SAND PAIR]

A green yellow pear that has skin speckled with brown spots. Asian pears are round with a crisp **texture** that is juicy, slightly gritty, fragrant, and sweet. This variety is sometimes called an apple pear for its shape. They are **harvested** and eaten **firm**. Try them fresh.

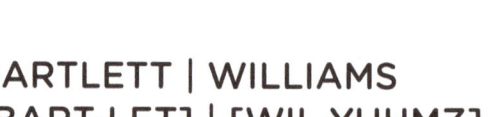

BARTLETT | WILLIAMS
[BART-LET] | [WIL-YUHMZ]

A yellow pear with a true pear shape. Bartlett pears are medium to large in size, very aromatic, juicy, and sweet. The musky ivory flesh of this variety has a tender grainy texture. Most pears do not change color when they ripen, however the Bartlett variety turns from green to yellow and are best eaten fresh or used for canning.

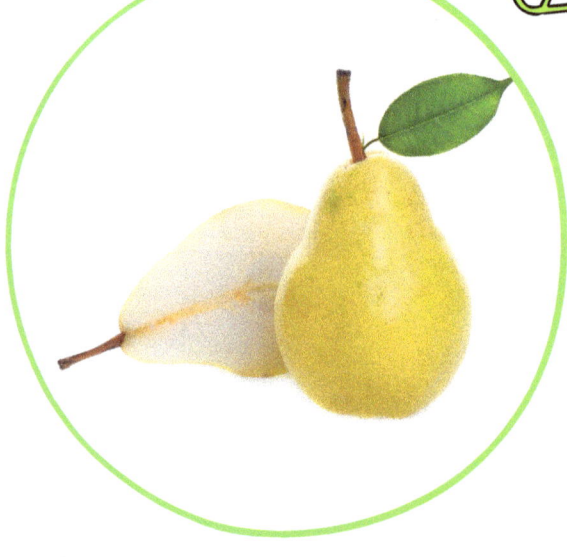

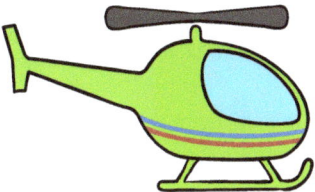

BOSC | KAISER ALEXANDER
[BAHSK] | [KAHY-ZER AL-IGZAN-DER]

A golden tan pear with **russeting** on the skin. Bosc pears are known for their shape, a rounded base with a long narrow neck. This variety is crisp and woodsy with a honeyed sweetness and aroma. The ivory flesh is firm and dense which helps them keep their shape and texture when cooked. Try baking, broiling, or poaching this pear.

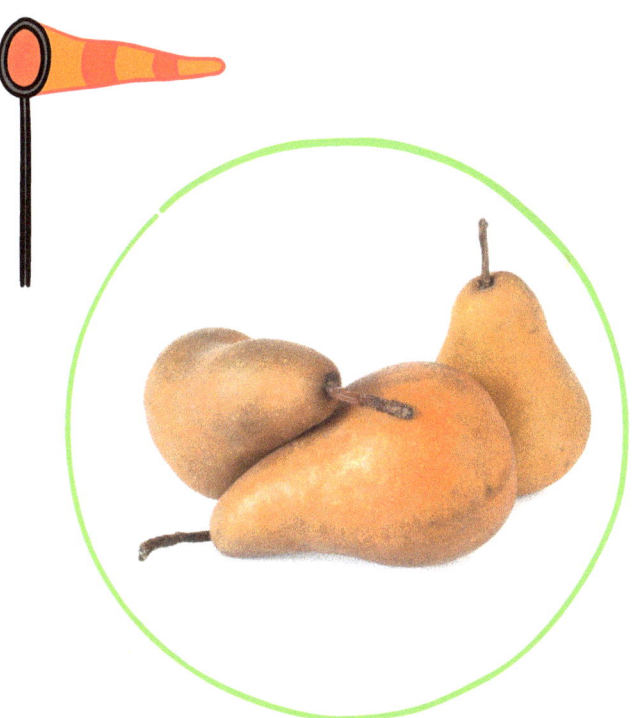

CONCORDE [KON-KORD]

A yellow-green pear with a red blush and golden russeting. Concorde pears are small to medium in size with a round base and a long, narrow, pointed neck. This variety has dense flesh that is sweet and floral with a vanilla flavor. They can be eaten crunchy and **firm** or left to ripen and soften. This all-purpose variety is slow to turn brown, after being sliced, so they are perfect in salads and keep their shape when cooked.

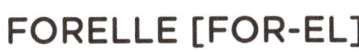

Russeting

FORELLE [FOR-EL]

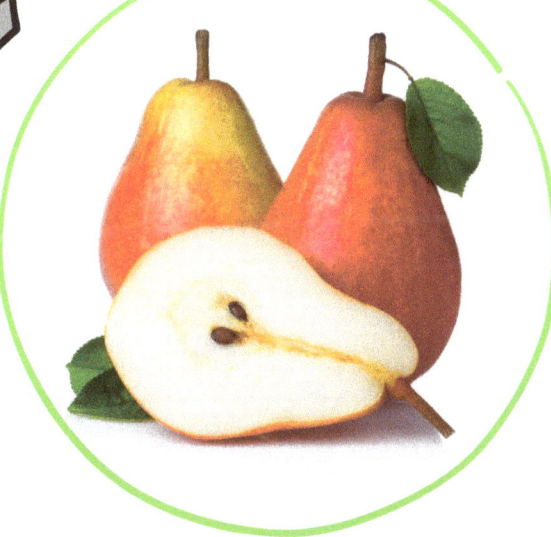

One of the most colorful pear varieties. Forelle pears change color from green to yellow when **ripe**, have a red blush, and are known for their red freckling called lenticels or pores. This small bell-shaped variety is crisp, tangy, and sweet. They are best enjoyed fresh.

A Book of Fruits 129

PERSIMMON

[per-sim-uhn]

astringent, honeyed, jelly-like, silky, spicy

BERRY

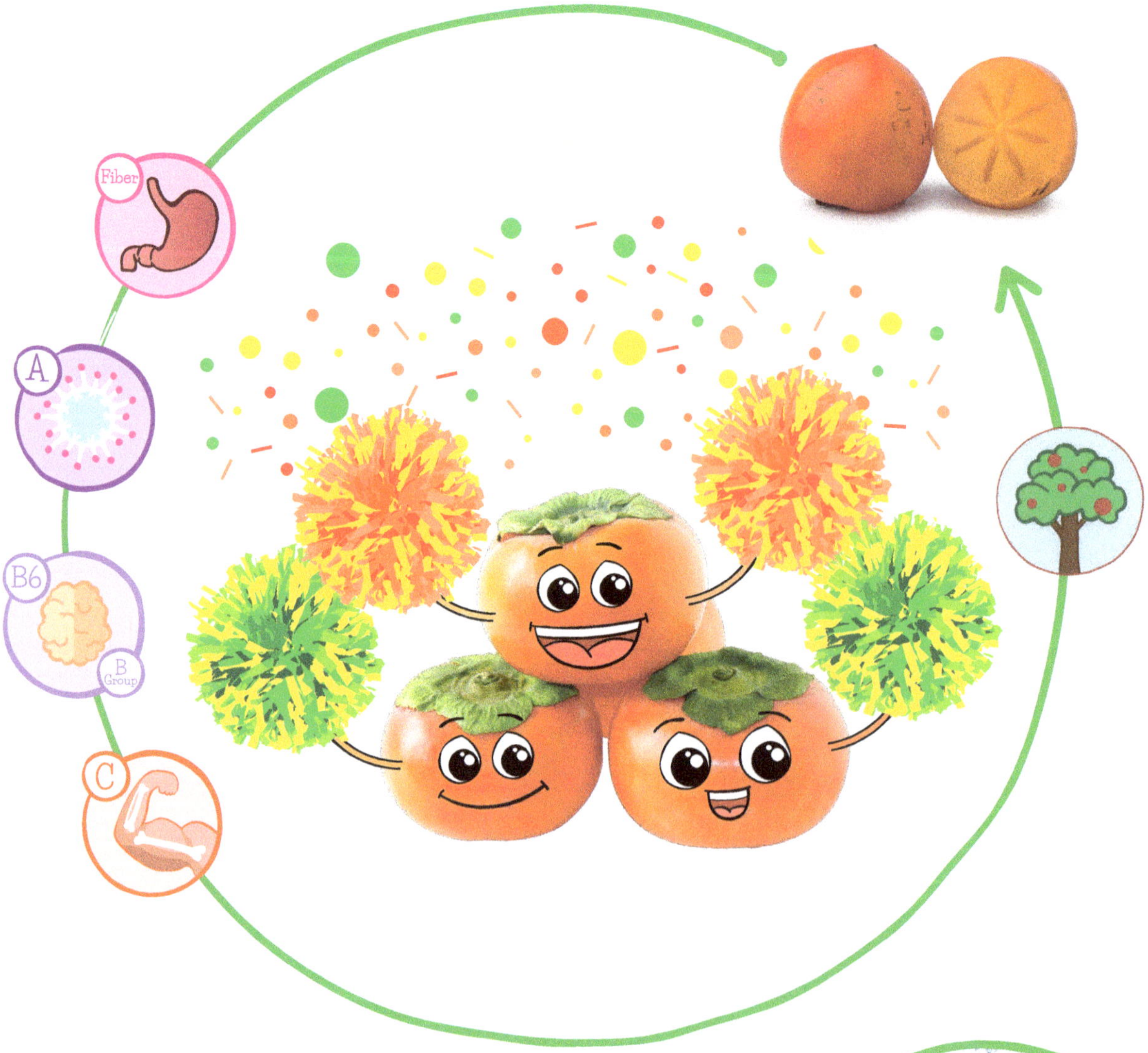

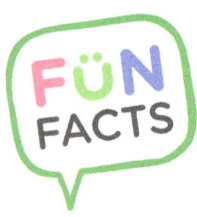

Persimmon trees are often used as edible landscaping. Edible landscaping is a gardening technique that uses fruit and vegetable plants and **herbs** rather than lawns or decorative trees and flowers. This promotes a cycle of growth and **harvest** rather than maintenance and results in food to eat.

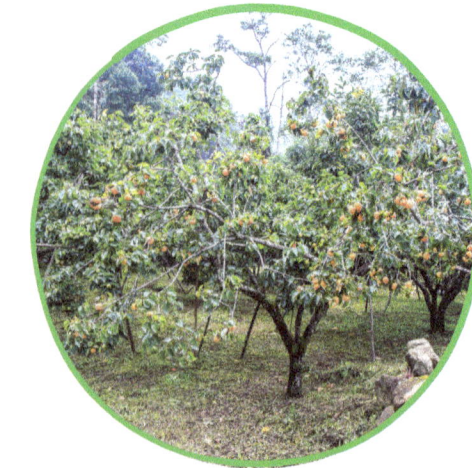

130 | Where Do Bananas Come From?

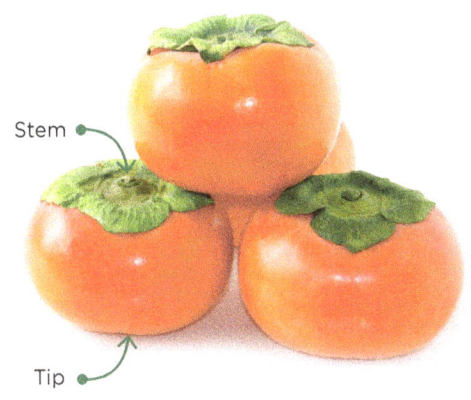

Stem

Tip

PICK
Pick shiny, orange, **plump**, smooth fruit that are soft to touch and heavy for their size. Persimmons should be free of **bruises** and mushy spots.

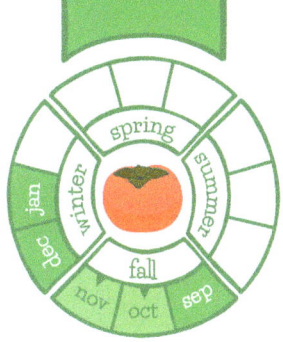

Available September to January; Imported September to February

Peak Season
October-November

STORE
Keep persimmons at room **temperature** for up to 4 days or until **ripe**. Refrigerate whole persimmons in a plastic bag for 2-3 days or cut-up in airtight containers for 3-4 days. Freeze persimmons in airtight containers for 10-12 months. Dried persimmons may be stored in airtight containers for 6-12 months.

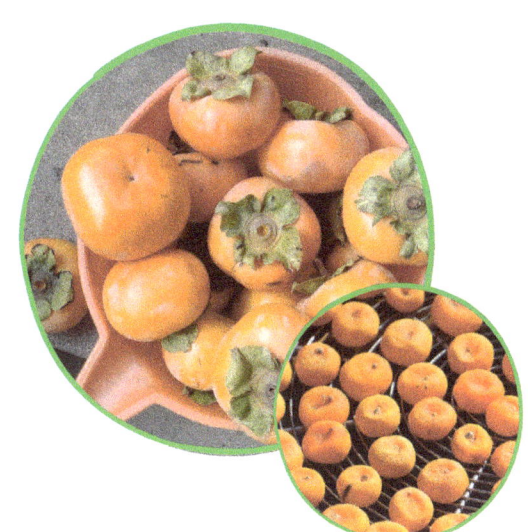

PERSIMMON TIDBITS

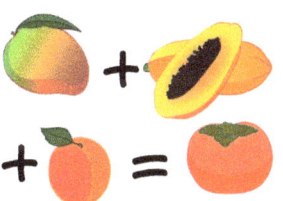

The **flavor** of the Fuyu persimmon **variety** is often compared to a mix of mango, papaya, and apricot.

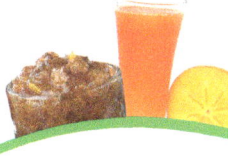

EAT
Clean the skin, slice in half from stem to tip, spoon out the **flesh** and remove the **seeds**.

Persimmon Bread
Preheat oven to 325 degrees F and **grease** a 1 pound bread loaf tin with butter. In a small bowl combine 1 1/2 cups flour, 1/2 cup chopped dried dates, 1/2 cup toasted walnuts, 1 teaspoon cinnamon, 1 teaspoon **zested** orange, 1/2 teaspoon nutmeg, and 1/2 teaspoon salt. In a large bowl blend 2 eggs, 1/2 cup brown sugar, 4 ounces canola oil, and 1 teaspoon vanilla extract. Finely chop 3 deseeded persimmons, about 1 cup of pulp, and combine with 1 teaspoon baking powder, then add to egg and sugar mixture. Next, add in flour mixture and stir until just combined. Spoon batter into bread loaf tin and bake in oven for 50-60 minutes or until a toothpick comes out clean.

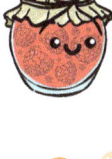
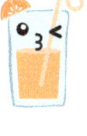

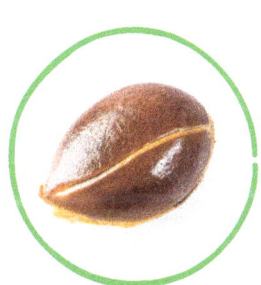

Persimmon seeds can be dried, roasted, and ground into a caffeine free coffee substitute and the leaves can be **steeped** as a tea.

A Book of Fruits

PHYSALIS
CAPE GOOSEBERRY

[fy-sal-is] | [keyp goos-ber-ee]

acidic, grape-like, juicy, tangy, tart

BERRY

FUN FACTS: Physalis are surrounded by a papery light brown husk called the **calyx** that looks like a lantern. Peel back the husk to reveal the fruit!

132 | Where Do Bananas Come From?

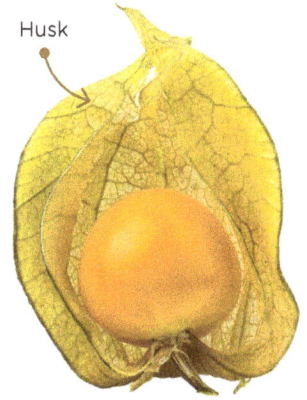
Husk

PICK
Pick yellow or orange, **firm** fruit with papery **husks**. Physalises should be free of mushy spots and **mold**.

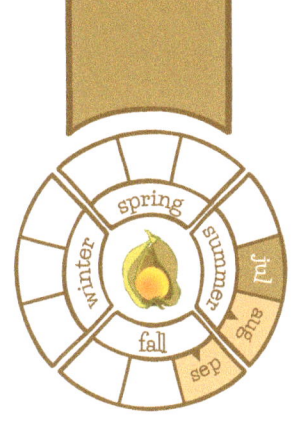

Available July to September; Imported year-round

Peak Season August-September

STORE
Keep physalises well-ventilated in a cool, dark place for up to 6 months. Freeze physalises in airtight containers for 10-12 months. Dried physalises may be stored in airtight containers for 6-12 months.

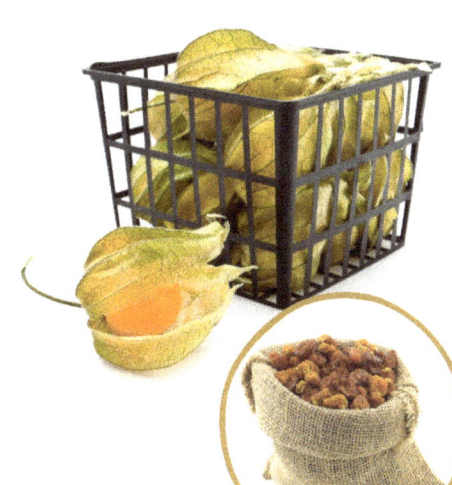

PHYSALIS TIDBITS

The **flavor** and **texture** is often compared to a cherry tomato crossed with pineapple, mango, and Meyer lemon.

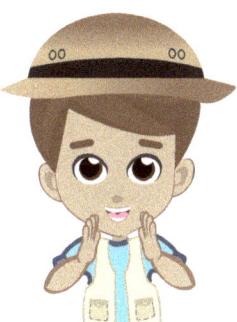

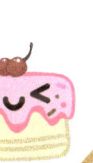
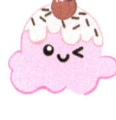
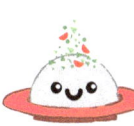

EAT
Remove the husk and clean just before eating or using.

Chocolate Covered Physalis
Gently pull back the papery husk of 1 dozen physalis, but do not remove the fruit. Hold each **berry** by the husk and clean under running water. Dry each fruit with a paper towel and place on a clean kitchen towel. Pour 1/2 cup semi-sweet baking chocolate chips in a microwave-safe bowl. Microwave chocolate for 30 seconds, stir, and then repeat until chocolate is mostly melted and only a few small pieces remain. Allow chocolate to sit at room **temperature** for 5 minutes and then dip each berry in the chocolate and place on a parchment paper lined plate. Let berries rest until chocolate has set.

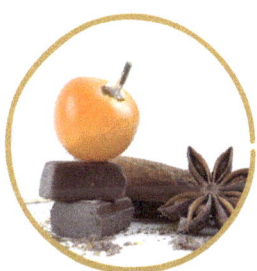

Physalis can be used in sweet and savory dishes. Try using them in a recipe that calls for tomatillo or dip them in chocolate for a sweet-tart treat.

PINEAPPLE

[pahy-nap-uhl]

acidic, fibrous, juicy, sweet, tart

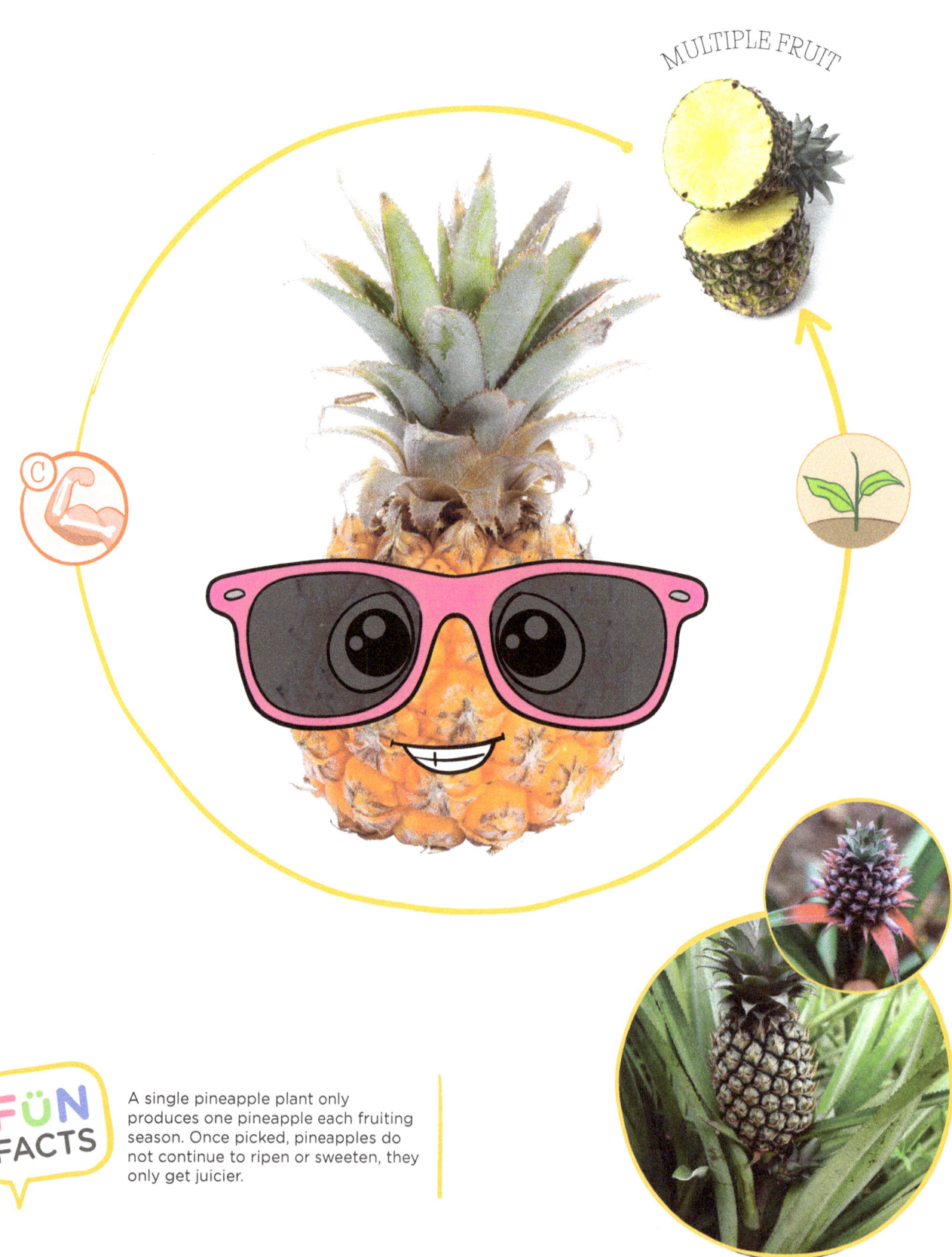

MULTIPLE FRUIT

FUN FACTS: A single pineapple plant only produces one pineapple each fruiting season. Once picked, pineapples do not continue to ripen or sweeten, they only get juicier.

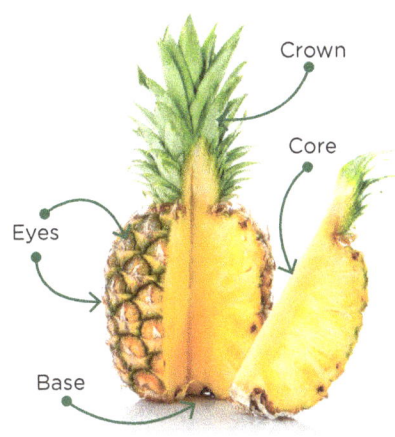

Crown
Core
Eyes
Base

PICK
Pick green to yellow-gold, **plump**, **firm** fruit with fresh green leaves that feel heavy for their size and have a sweet aroma. Pineapples should be free of dry looking skin, dirty leaves, soft spots, or a **fermented**, sour aroma.

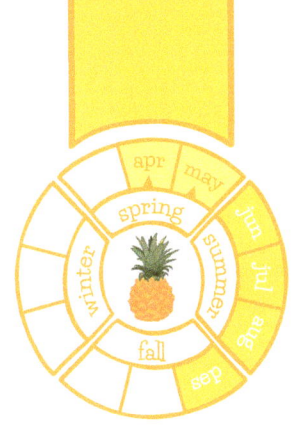

Available April to September; Imported year-round

Peak Season
April-May

STORE
Keep pineapples at room **temperature** for up to 2 days or until **ripe**. Refrigerate whole pineapples for 3-5 days or cut-up in airtight containers for 3-4 days. Freeze pineapples in airtight containers for 10-12 months. Dried pineapples may be stored in airtight containers for 6-12 months.

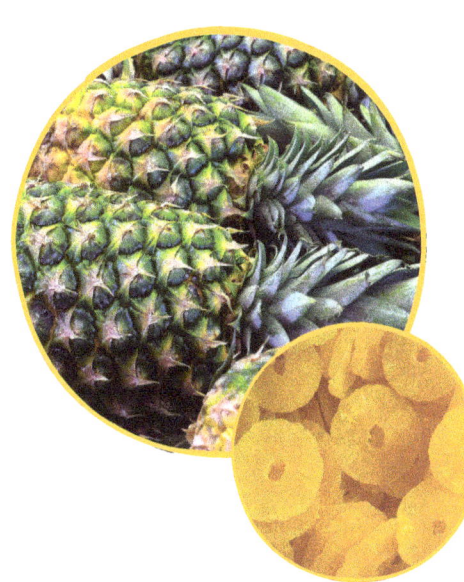

PINEAPPLE TIDBITS

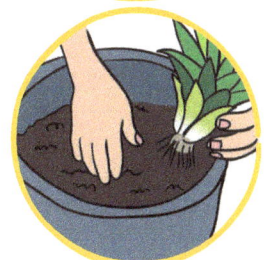

Try growing your own pineapple at home from fresh tops or **seedling** in the crown. Start by twisting off the crown of the fruit. Then pull out several of the lower leaves to **expose** the root. Next plant in a pot with soil and water. Watch it grow! It can take up to 2 years for your plant to fruit!

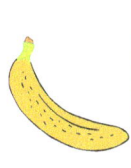
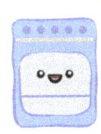
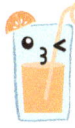

EAT
Clean the skin and slice off the crown and base of the fruit. Stand the pineapple up on one end and slice off the skin in a downward motion deep enough to remove the "eyes." Slice the pineapple in half lengthwise, crown to base, then in quarters. Slice off the tough center core of each quarter and chop the **flesh** into bite-sized pieces.

Grilled Cinnamon Pineapple
Preheat grill to medium-high heat. Peel, core, and slice pineapple into wedges. Whisk together 1/2 cup melted coconut oil, 1/2 cup brown sugar, and 1 teaspoon cinnamon. Coat pineapple wedges in coconut-cinnamon glaze and place on the grill 4-5 minutes per side. Pineapple should be tender and soft.

Plum

[pluhm]

chewy, juicy, sweet, tangy, tart

DRUPE

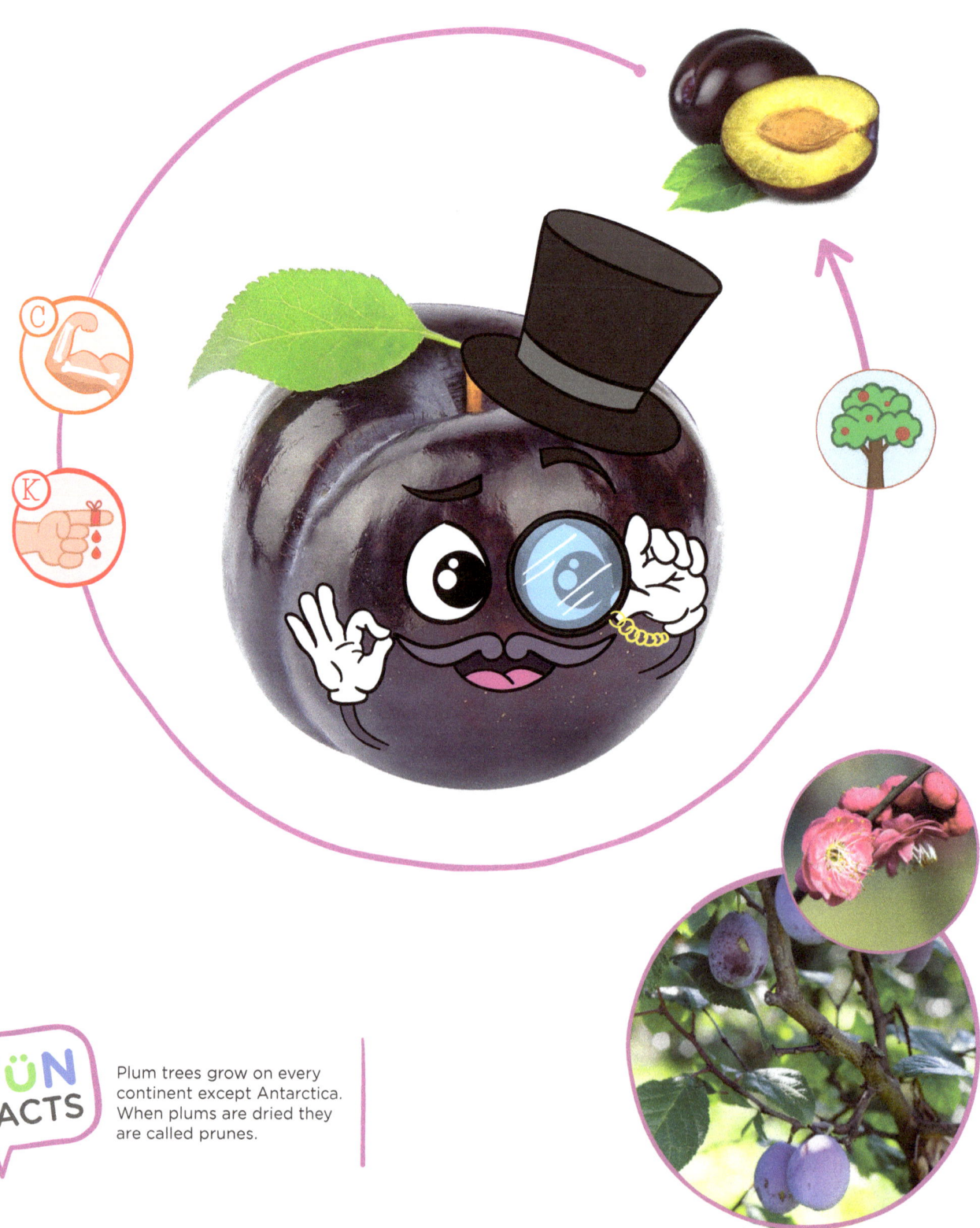

FUN FACTS: Plum trees grow on every continent except Antarctica. When plums are dried they are called prunes.

136 | Where Do Bananas Come From?

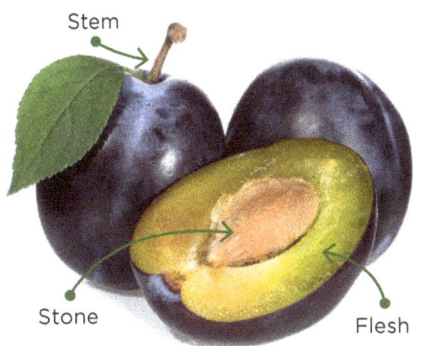

Stem · Stone · Flesh

PICK
Pick deep-colored, **plump**, smooth-skinned fruit that are soft to touch and feel heavy for their size. Plum varieties should be free of **bruises**, mushy spots, and wrinkled skin. Colors and sizes differ depending on **variety**.

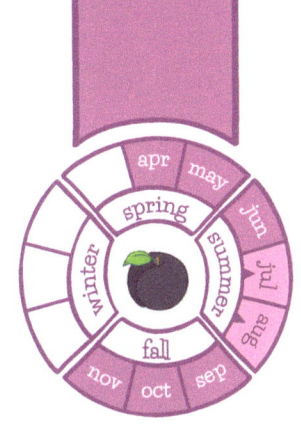

Available April to November; Imported year-round

Peak Season
July-August

STORE
Keep plums at room **temperature** for up to 3 days or until **ripe**. Refrigerate whole plums in plastic bags for 3-5 days or cut-up in airtight containers for 3-4 days. Freeze plums in airtight containers for 10-12 months. Dried plums, or prunes, may be stored in airtight containers for 6-12 months.

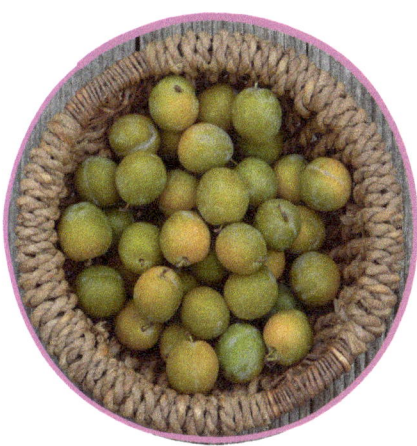

PLUM TIDBITS

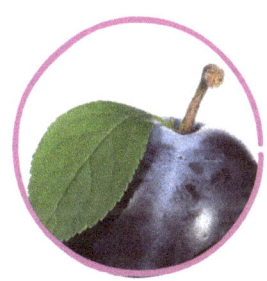

Plum skin should have a powdery **bloom**, a natural, protective, waxy coating.

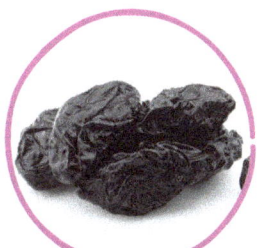

There are two major classifications of plums: Japanese plums and European plums. Japanese plums are fairly round and juicy. European plums are dense and more oval in shape. They are often dried to make prunes.

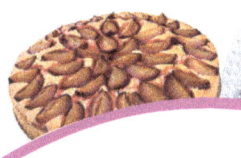
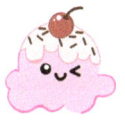
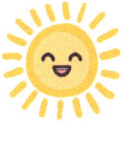
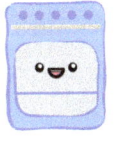

EAT
Clean the skin, slice or bite in half, and remove the **stone** from center. Eat, chop, or slice per recipe.

Honey Roasted Plums
Preheat oven to 375 degrees F and **grease** a 13 x 9 inch baking dish with butter. Quarter and de-stone 8 plums and place in a single layer in the baking dish. Whisk together 4 ounces orange juice, or about two medium oranges juiced, 2 tablespoons honey, 1 tablespoon orange **zest**, 1/2 teaspoon cinnamon, 1/4 teaspoon cardamom, and a pinch of pepper. Pour mixture over the plums and bake for 20 minutes or until the plums are tender and the sauce is bubbly. While plums are roasting, blend 1 - 15-ounce container ricotta cheese with 2 teaspoons vanilla extract and 2 teaspoons cinnamon. Serve roasted plums over a scoop of spiced ricotta cheese, **drizzle** with baking sauce, and garnish with chopped pistachios.

PLUM VARIETIES

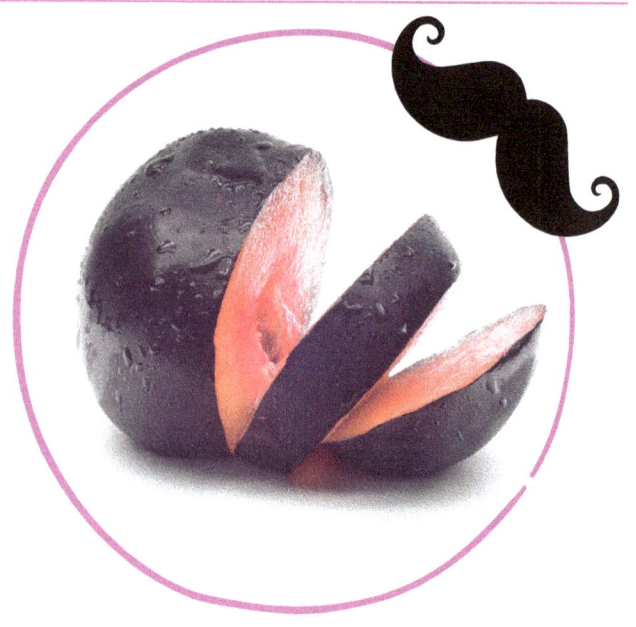

BLACK SPLENDOR [BLAK SPLEN-DER]

This black plum **variety** is named for its blue-black skin and dark red flesh. Black Splendor plums are larger than the average plum. This crispy, sweet-tart variety is great fresh, baked, or made into sauces.

GREENGAGE [GREEN-GEYJ]

This small green plum has skin that ranges from pale yellow-green to bright green with red speckling. Greengage plums are dense and have juicy orange flesh with a candy-like sweet **flavor**. They are best eaten fresh or as the main ingredient in desserts.

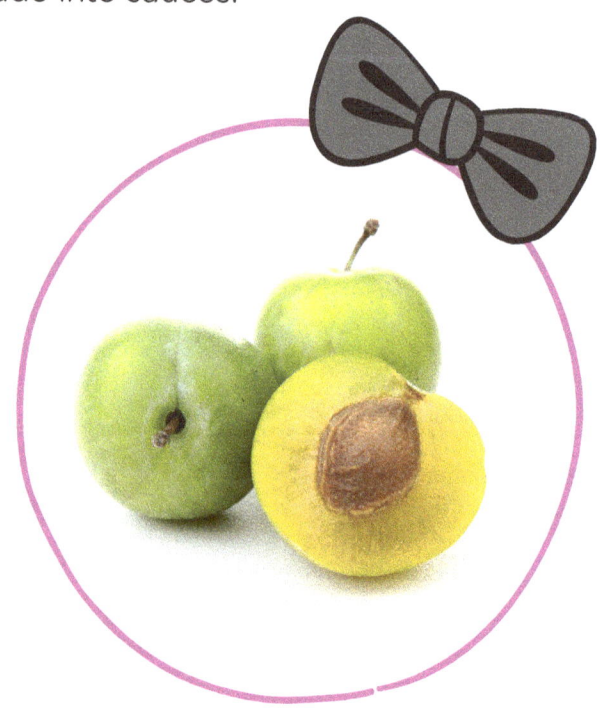

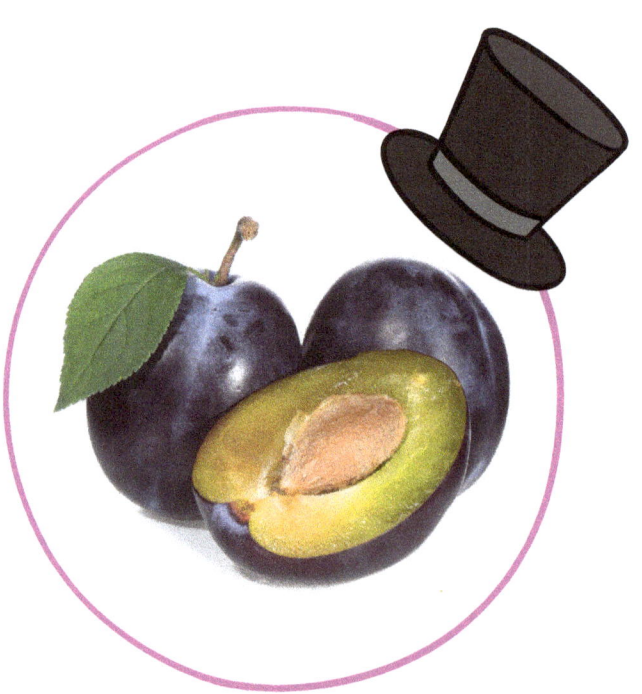

ITALIAN PRUNE | EMPRESS PLUM [IH-TAL-YUHN PROON] [EM-PRIS PLUHM]

This plum with purple-blue skin is an oval shape and has greenish-orange flesh that turns dark pink when cooked. Italian prune plums are rich, candy-like, and can be eaten fresh, baked, or preserved. They are typically grown to be dried into prunes.

MIRABELLE [MIR-UH-BEL]

This yellow plum is smaller than the size of a golf ball. Mirabelle plums are round, yellow, sweet, juicy, and crisp. The rich flavors of this variety are compared to apricots, golden raisins, and honey. They are often dried, used in baked goods, **fermented**, or made into jellies and jams.

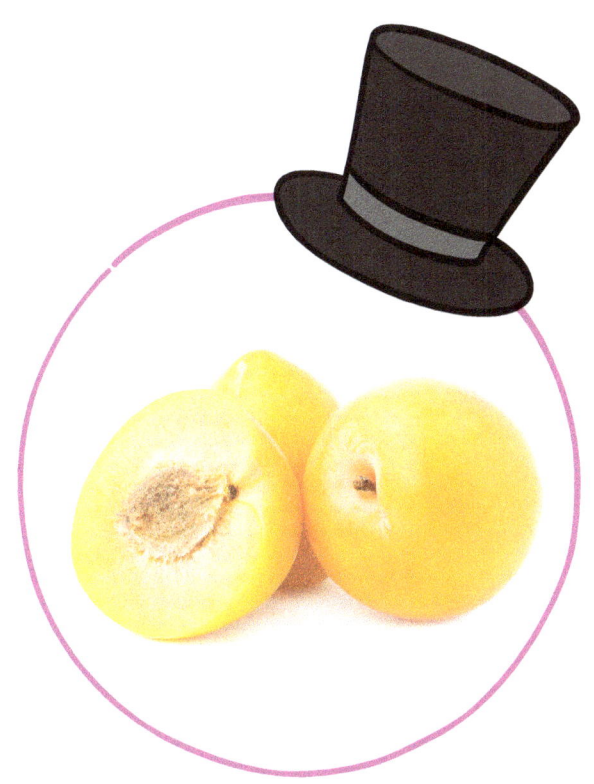

PLUOT | PLUMCOT
[PLEW-OTT] | [PLUHM-COTT]

Both pluots and plumcots are **hybrids** of the plum and apricot. The difference between the two is the percentage of each fruit that is represented in the hybrid. Pluots have more plum **characteristics** because they have more plum in their hybrid. Plumcots have equal characteristics of both fruit because they have equal quantities in their hybrid. There are many varieties within each hybrid.

SANTA ROSA
[SAN-TUH ROH-ZUH]

This medium to large, red plum with red and gold flesh is tender, sweet, and juicy. Santa Rosa plums can be used in both sweet and savory dishes. They can be eaten fresh, canned, and roasted.

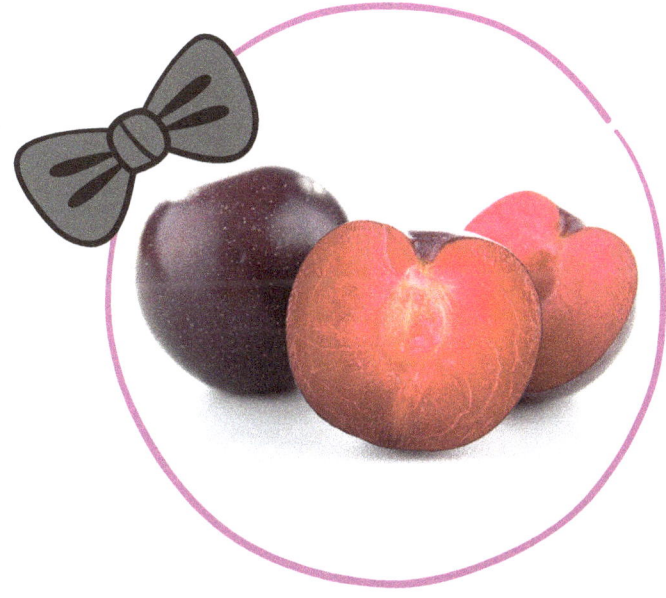

A Book of Fruits 139

POMEGRANATE

[pom-i-gran-it]

gritty, juicy, seeded, sweet, tart

BERRY

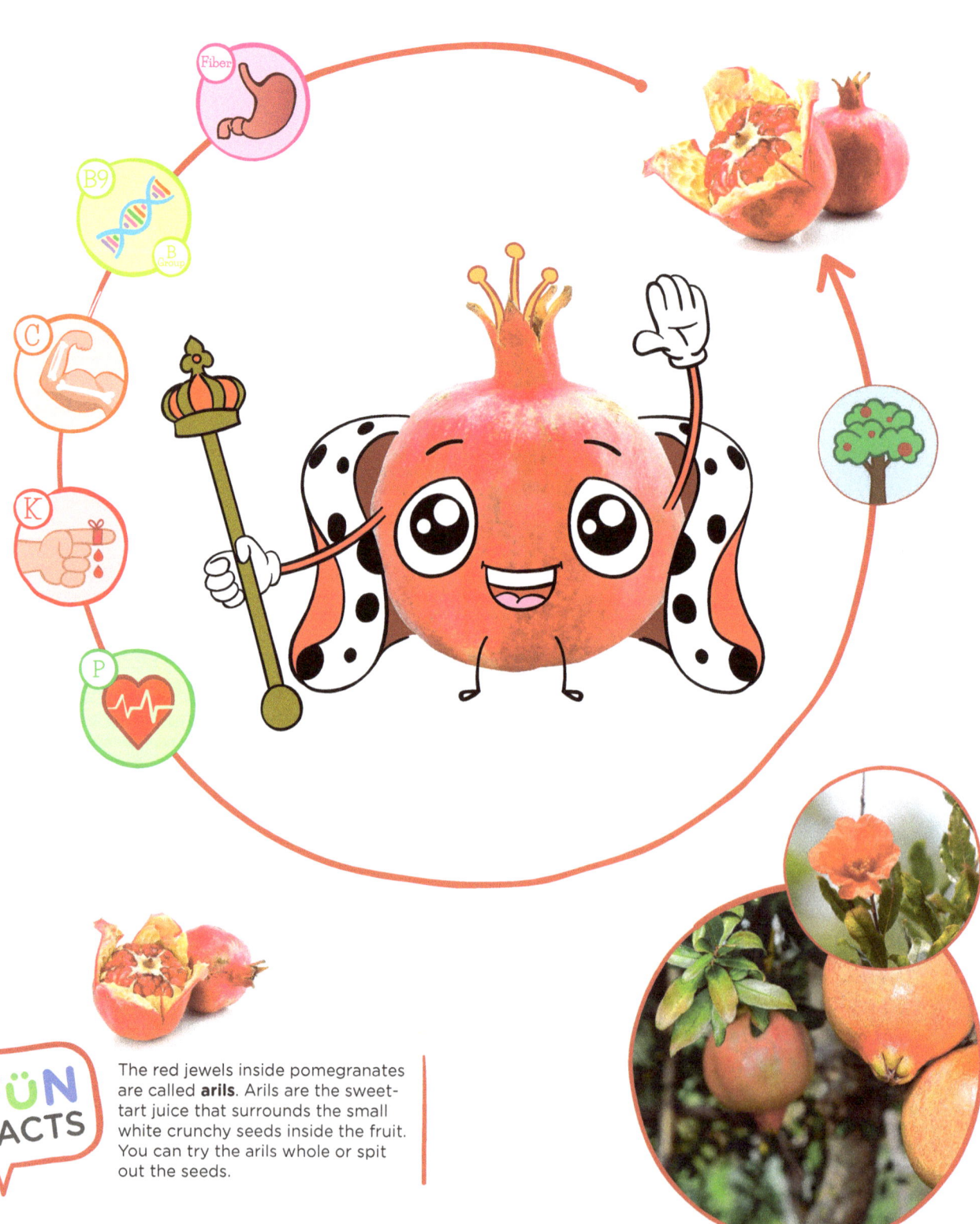

FUN FACTS: The red jewels inside pomegranates are called **arils**. Arils are the sweet-tart juice that surrounds the small white crunchy seeds inside the fruit. You can try the arils whole or spit out the seeds.

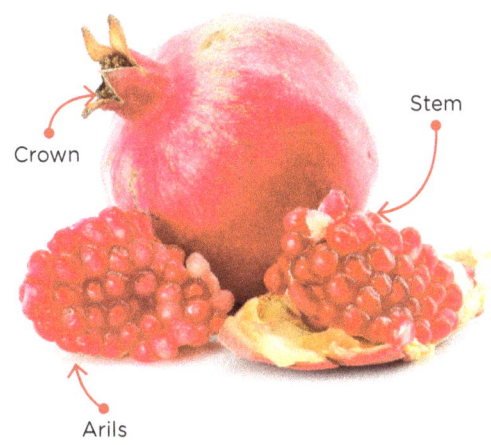

Crown · Stem · Arils

PICK
Pick deep-colored yellow to purple or pink to red fruit that are **plump**, round and feel heavy for their size. Pomegranates should be free of **bruises** and soft spots.

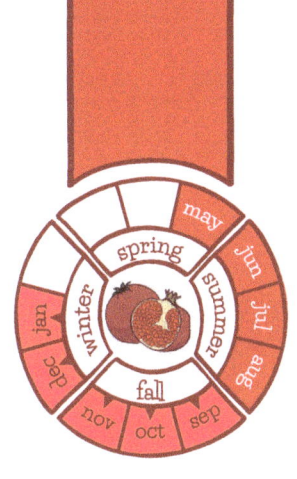

Available May to January; Imported year-round

Peak Season
September–January

STORE
Keep pomegranates at room **temperature** for up to 2 days. Refrigerate whole pomegranates in a plastic bag for 1-2 months or cut-up in airtight containers for 3-4 days. Freeze pomegranates in airtight containers for 10-12 months.

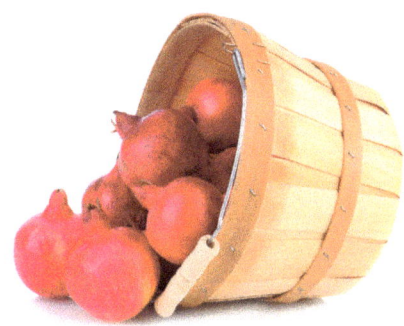

EAT
Clean the skin and slice off the crown and stem base of the fruit. Use a knife to **score** the skin into quarters from the crown to stem. Be careful not to cut into the fruit. Place the scored pomegranate in a bowl of water. Then break sections apart and massage the **seeds** out under the water.

Kale, Pear, and Pomegranate Harvest Salad
In a small bowl whisk together 4 tablespoons olive oil, 2 tablespoons orange juice, 1 teaspoon cinnamon, 1/4 teaspoon salt, 1/4 teaspoon pepper, 1/8 teaspoon ground clove. In a large bowl combine 1 pound fresh baby kale, 1 deseeded pomegranate, 6 peeled and sectioned clementines, 1 cored and chopped pear, and 1 cup toasted walnut pieces. Pour dressing over salad, toss, and serve.

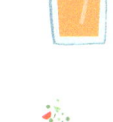
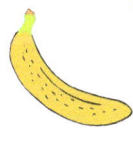

POMEGRANATE TIDBITS

Many scholars believe that the pomegranate was the forbidden fruit, not the apple, in the Garden of Eden.

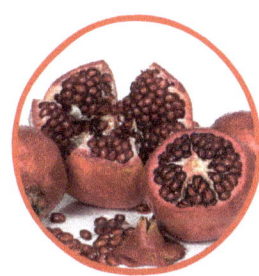

The name pomegranate comes from the Latin word pomum meaning "apple" and granatum meaning "having grains" or "seeded" translating to "apple with many seeds."

A Book of Fruits

POMELO
PUMMELO

[pom-e-lo] | [puhm-uh-loh]

acidic, bitter, juicy, pulpy, sweet

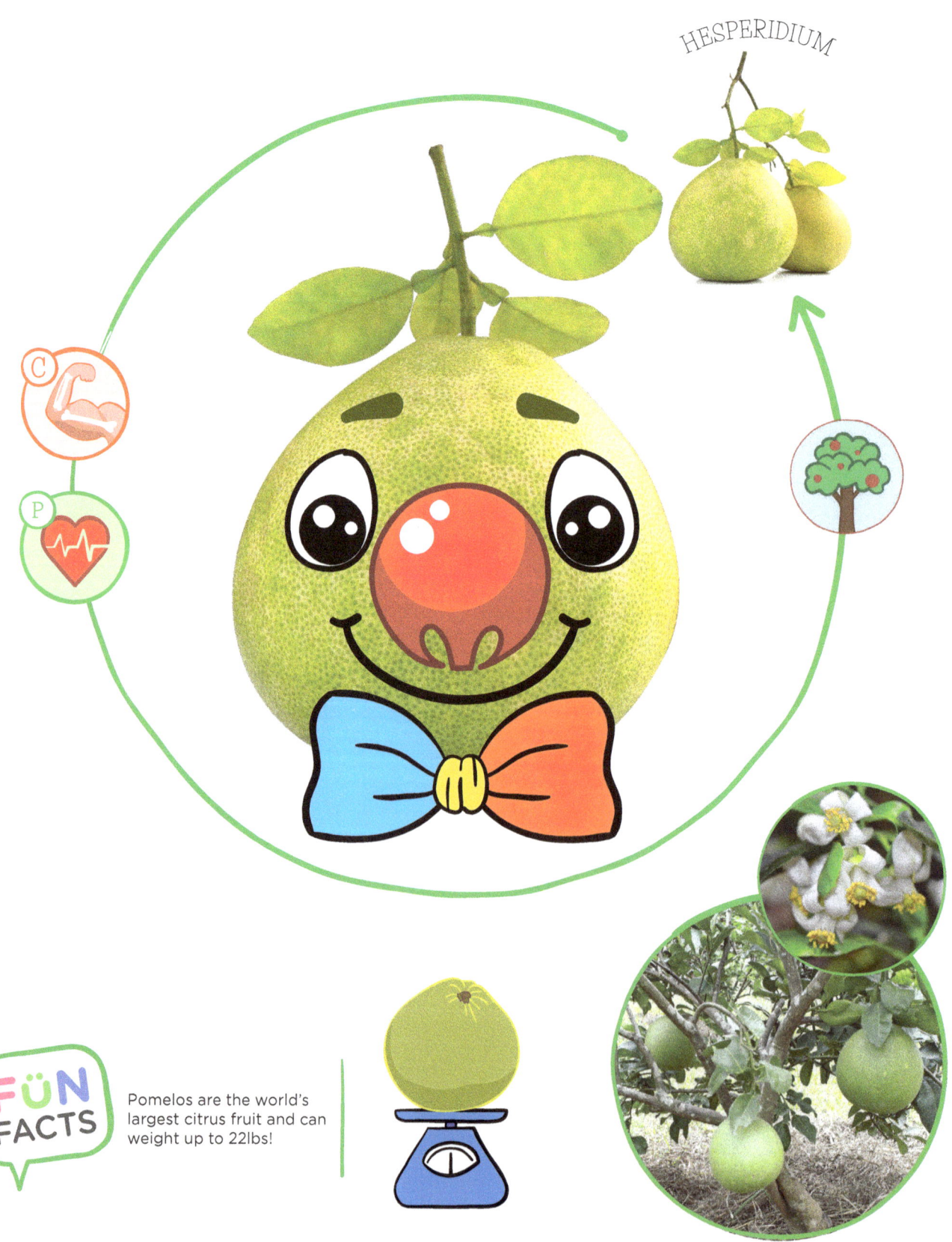

HESPERIDIUM

FUN FACTS Pomelos are the world's largest citrus fruit and can weight up to 22lbs!

142 | Where Do Bananas Come From?

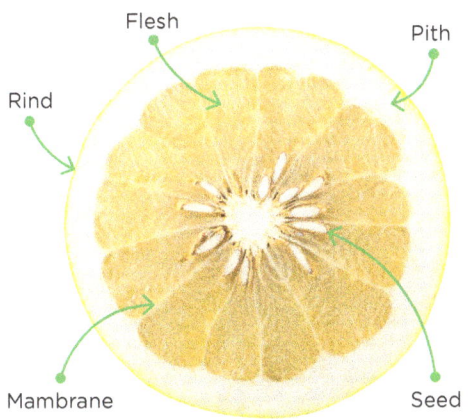

Rind • Flesh • Pith • Mambrane • Seed

PICK
Pick yellow-green, **firm**, smooth-skinned fruit that feel heavy for their size and have a floral aroma. Pomelos should be free of **bruises**, cuts, and soft spots.

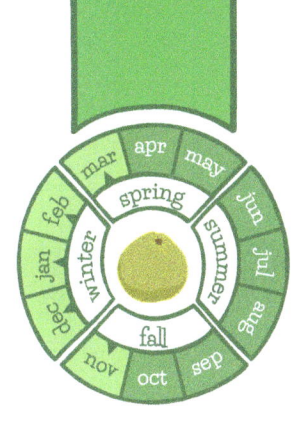

Varieties available year-round

Peak Season
November-March

STORE
Keep pomelos at room **temperature** for up to 7 days. Refrigerate whole pomelos in a plastic bag for 3-4 weeks or peeled in airtight containers for 3-4 days. Freeze pomelos in airtight containers for 10-12 months.

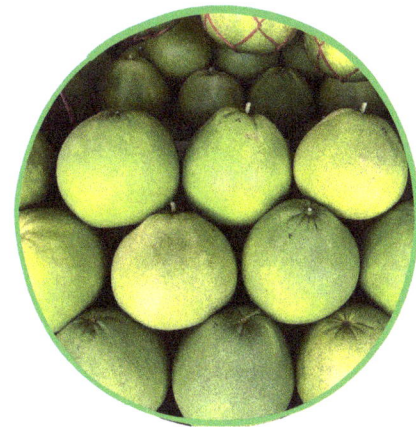

POMELO TIDBITS

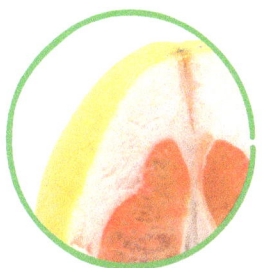

The peel and pith of a pomelo can grow up to 5 inches deep. The pith is the soft spongy **tissue** between the rind and the fruit flesh.

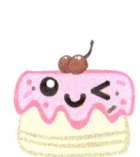

EAT
Clean the skin, peel the **rind**, and remove the **pith** and the **membrane** in between the **flesh**.

Candied Pomelo Rind
Peel a pomelo and remove the white spongy **pith**. Slice pomelo peel into thin strips, about 1/4 inch **thick**. Boil strips in a saucepan for 5 minutes, drain, rinse with cold water, squeeze the strips to remove the water, then repeat the boiling process 3 more times to reduce the bitterness. Next, combine the strips, 1 cup water, and 1 cup sugar in a saucepan. Bring to a boil and then reduce heat to a simmer and cook for an hour until the peel is **translucent**. Drain, roll each piece in sugar and allow to dry on a wire rack for 3 hours or until **firm**.

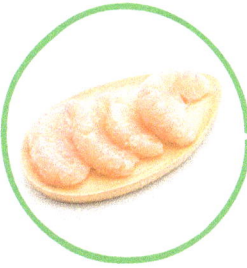

In Southeast Asia pomelo is eaten with salt because salt decreases our ability to taste bitterness and therefore makes the fruit taste sweeter.

***

Pomelo is a staple fruit in Vietnamese **cuisine** using both the flesh and the peel.

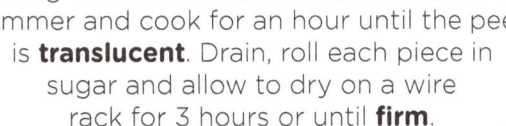

PRICKLY PEAR
CACTUS PEAR

[prik-lee pair] | [kak-tuhs pair]

grainy, juicy, refreshing, spongy, sweet-tart

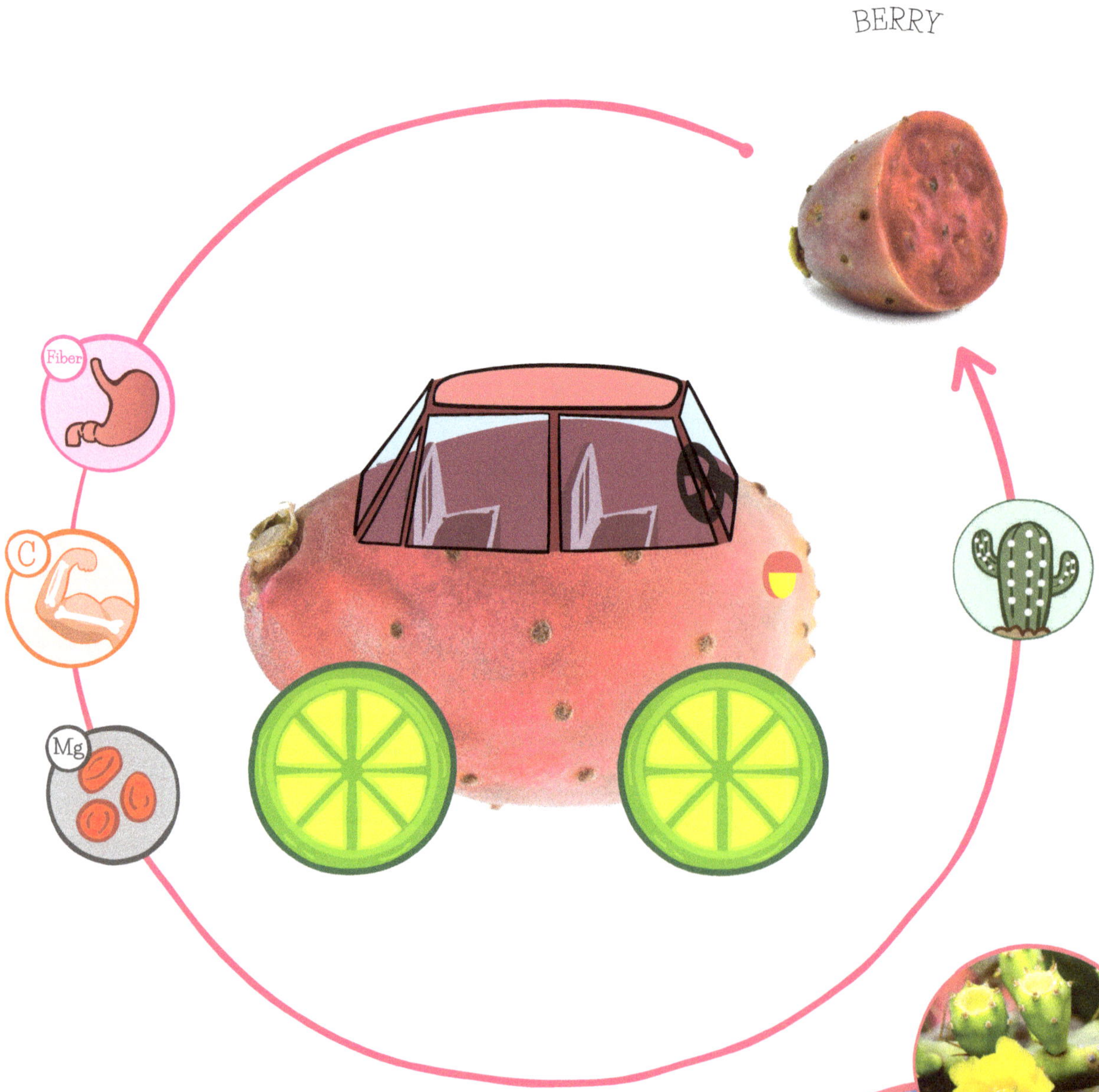

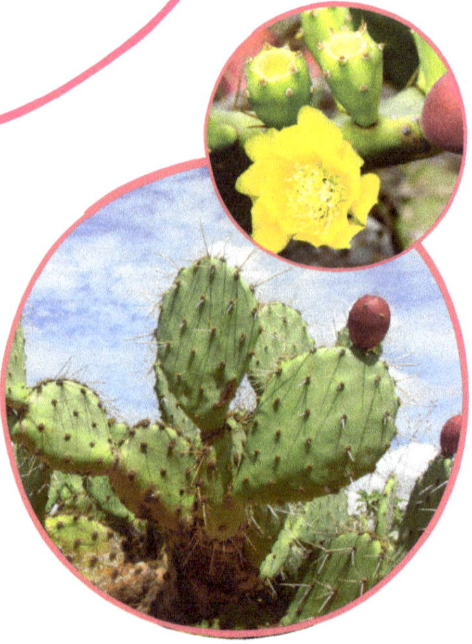

BERRY

FUN FACTS

Sharp and thorny hair-like **glochids** on the outside of the fruit make prickly pears look like they should not be eaten. Don't judge a fruit by its cover! Inside a prickly pear is vibrant, juicy, sweet-tart flesh. Do you see any thorns on the outside? If not, they may have been removed before they made it to you.

144 | Where Do Bananas Come From?

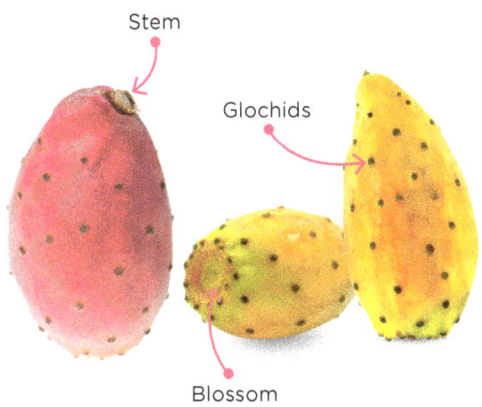

PICK
Pick deep-colored red or yellow fruit that are soft to touch. Prickly pears should be free of mushy spots and **mold**.

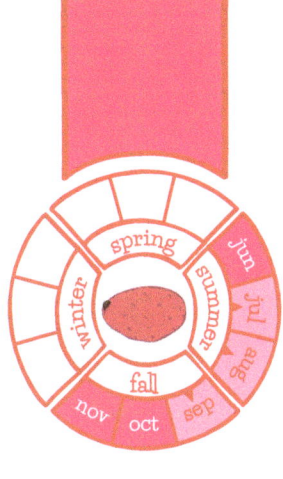

Available June to November; Imported year-round Peak Season July-September

STORE
Keep prickly pears at room **temperature** for up to 5 days. Refrigerate whole prickly pears in a plastic bag for 1-3 days or sliced in airtight containers for 3-4 days. Freeze prickly pears in airtight containers for 10-12 months.

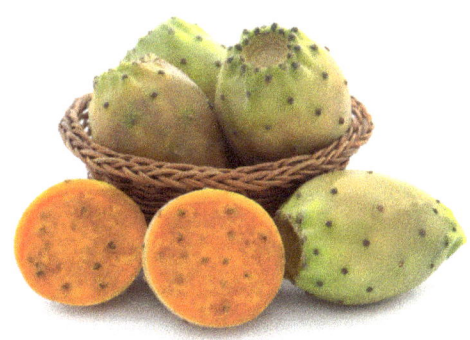

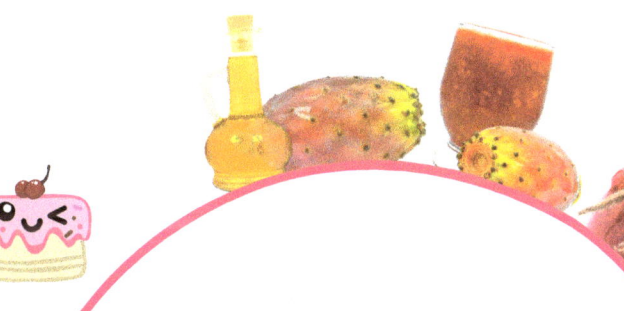

EAT
Clean the skin, slice off the blossom and stem ends of the fruit. Use a knife to **score** the skin from blossom to stem and then peel the skin off the **flesh**. Eat, chop, or slice per recipe.

Prickly Pear Juice
Blend the flesh of 4 prickly pears with 4 ounces water. Strain the **seeds** and pulp from the juice over a bowl and sweeten to taste with honey. Refrigerate in a glass jar up to 4 days.

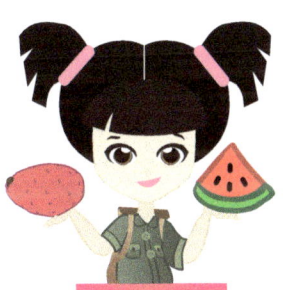

PRICKLY PEAR TIDBITS

The aroma of a prickly pear is similar to watermelon.

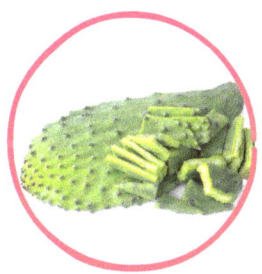

The cactus leaves or cactus pads are **edible** and used as a vegetable known as nopal cactus.

A Book of Fruits 145

RAMBUTAN

[ram-byu-tn]

acidic, aromatic, gelatinous, rich, sweet-sour

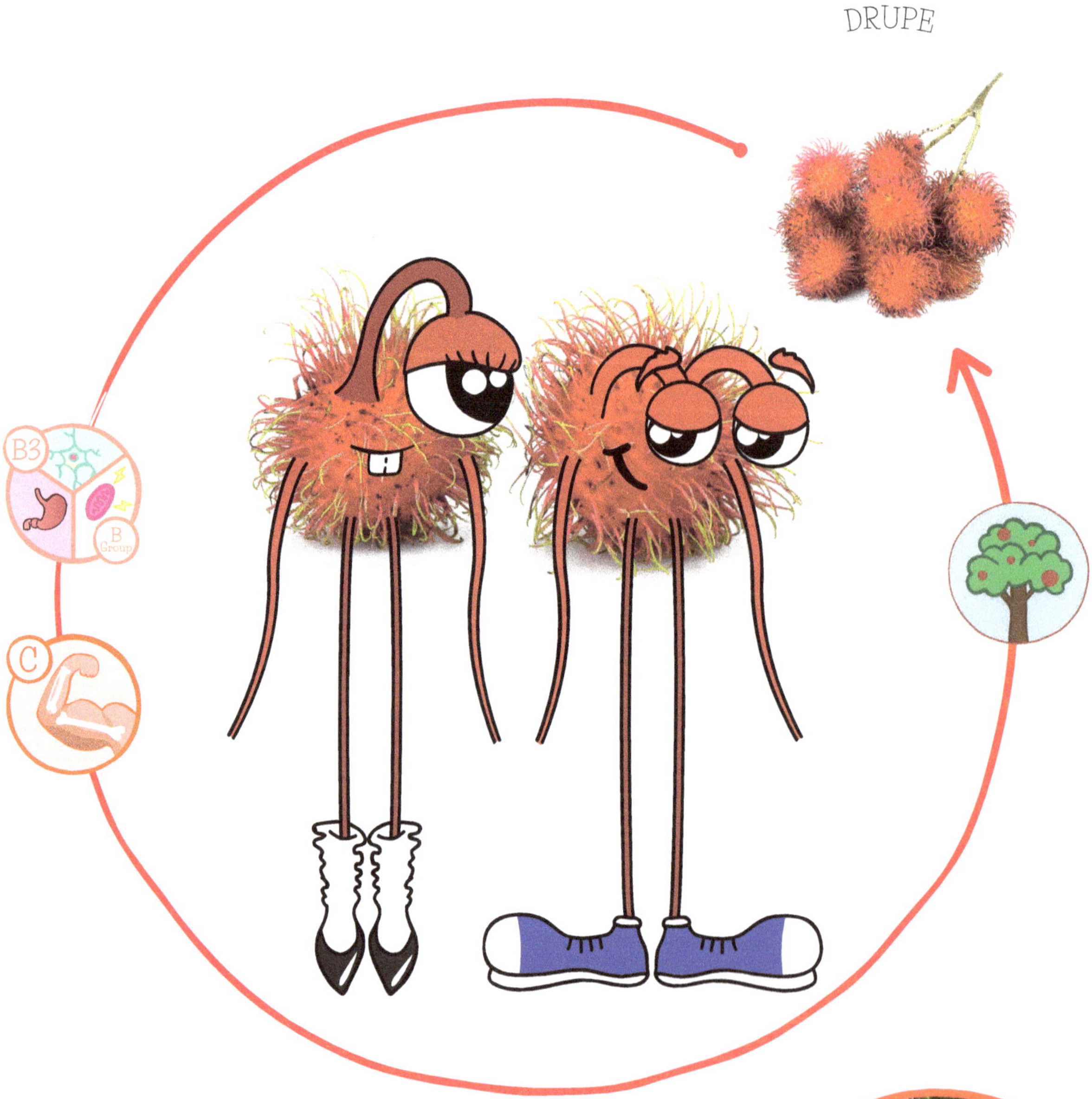

DRUPE

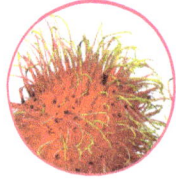

FUN FACTS: Rambutan are closely related to lychee fruit. However, it is easy to tell the two apart. Rambutan have red skin with soft, neon green, hairs all around them.

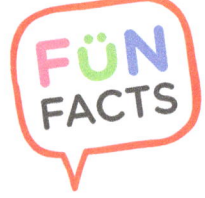
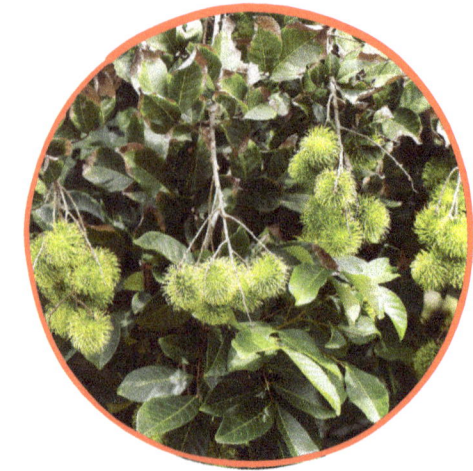

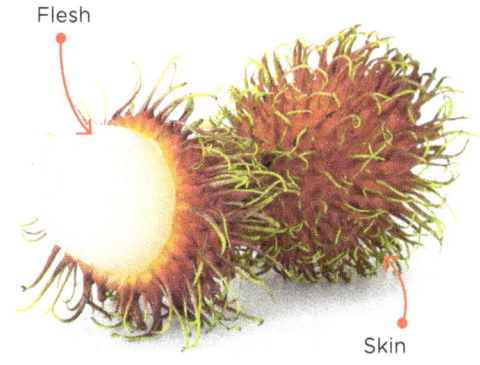

Flesh
Skin

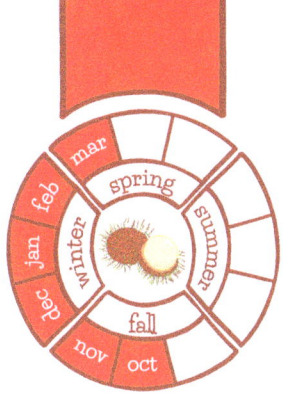

Available October to March

PICK
Pick red fruit with soft neon green hair that are **plump** and have a fresh aroma. Rambutans should be free of mushy spots and **mold**.

STORE
Keep rambutans at room **temperature** and eat within the first 2 days. Refrigerate rambutans in a **perforated** plastic bag for 7-14 days. Freeze rambutans in airtight containers for 10-12 months.

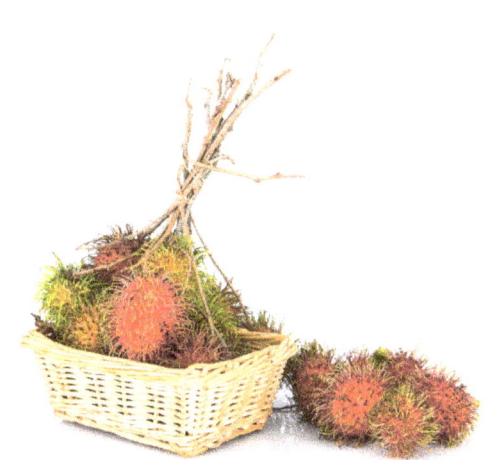

RAMBUTAN TIDBITS

Rambutan gets its name from the hair-like spikes on the skin surface from the Malaysian word for hair, "rambut."

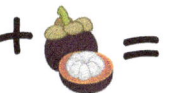 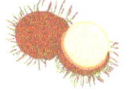

The **flavor** of rambutan is often compared to lychee, kiwifruit, and mangosteen.

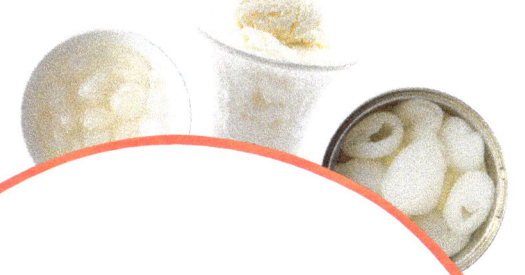

EAT
Clean the skin, pinch the hairy skin around the center, and pull the two ends apart to reveal the **fleshy** fruit. Slice or bite in half to remove the **stone** from the center. Eat, chop, or slice per recipe.

Fresh Rambutan
Peel the skin, pop the whole fruit into your mouth, and chew around the **seed**.

Raw rambutan seeds are **poisonous**; however, once roasted they can be eaten and have an almond-like flavor.

A Book of Fruits 147

RASPBERRY

[raz-ber-ee]

gritty, juicy, seeded, sweet, tart

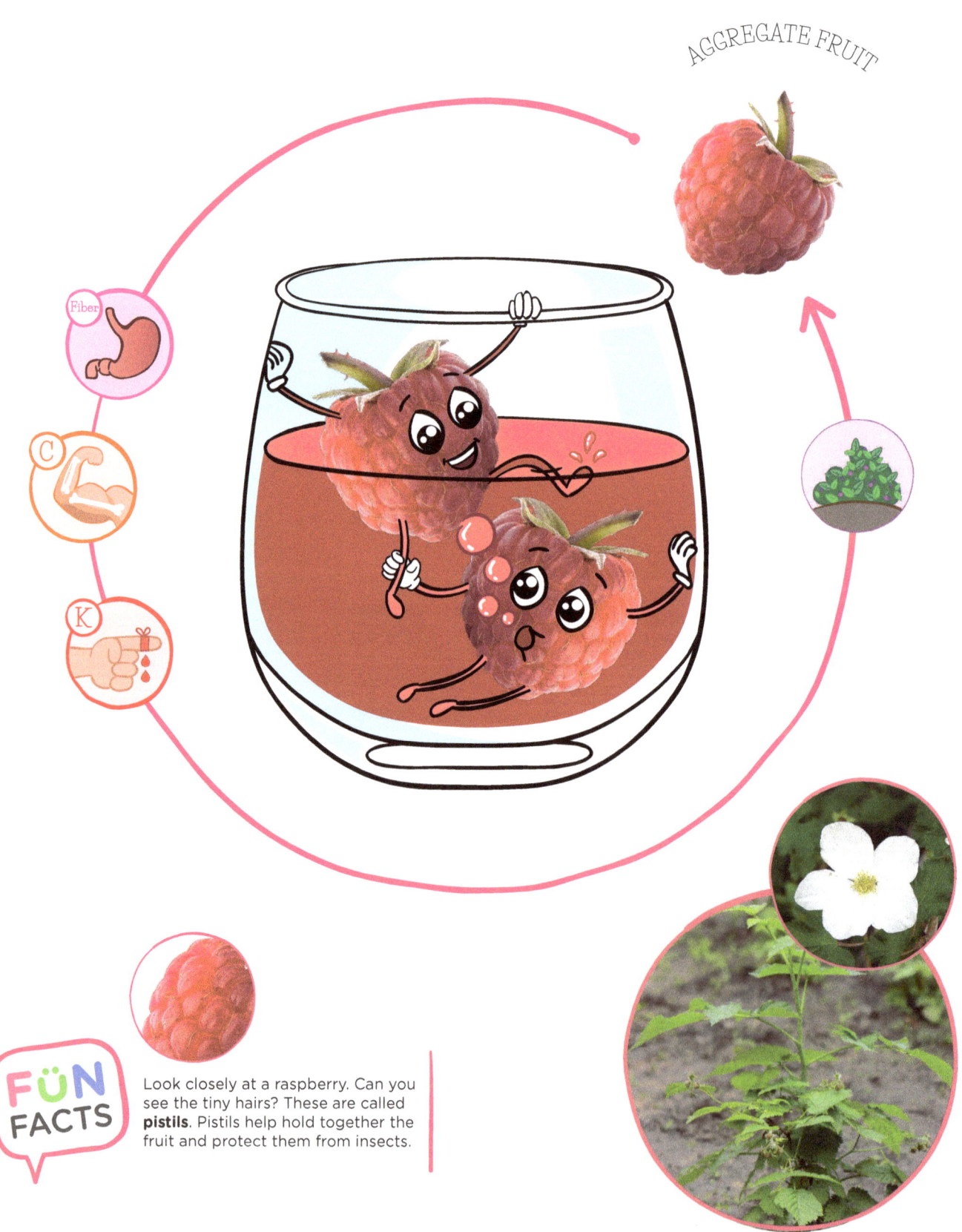

AGGREGATE FRUIT

FUN FACTS Look closely at a raspberry. Can you see the tiny hairs? These are called **pistils**. Pistils help hold together the fruit and protect them from insects.

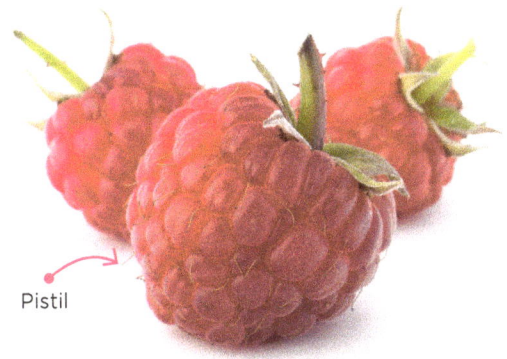
Pistil

PICK
Pick bright red, deep-colored fruit that are **plump**, **firm**, and dry. Check the bottom of the package to make sure there is not any juice or **mold** and that raspberries are not crushed.

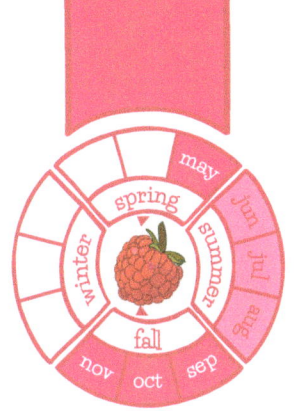

Available May to November; Imported year-round

Peak Season
June-August

STORE
Keep raspberries at room **temperature** and eat them the day they are picked or purchased. Refrigerate raspberries in their plastic container or place the berries loosely in a shallow container covered with plastic wrap for 2-3 days. Freeze raspberries in airtight containers for 10-12 months. Before storing raspberries, throw away any crushed or **moldy** fruit.

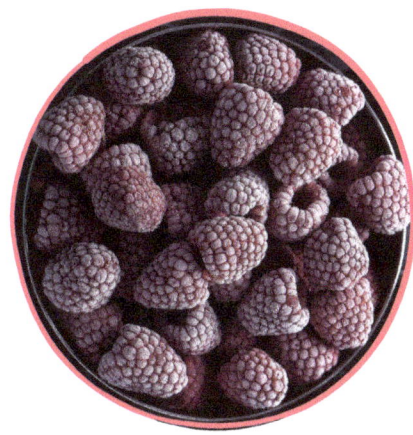

RASPBERRY TIDBITS

Raspberries are made up of around 100 tiny fruits called drupelets that come together to form one large fruit called an **aggregate fruit**.

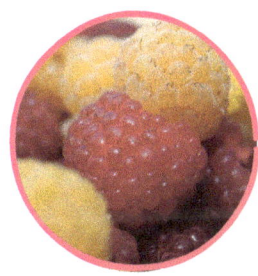

In addition to red, raspberries can also be black, yellow, and purple. Have you ever tried different colors of raspberries? What did you notice about the **flavors** and **textures**?

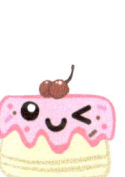

EAT
Clean just before eating or using.

Raspberry Fruit Leather
Preheat oven to 200 degrees F and line a baking sheet with **greased** parchment paper. **Puree** 4 cups raspberries, 4 ounces water, 3 tablespoons honey, and 1 tablespoon lemon juice until smooth. Pour fruit puree into a saucepan, bring to a simmer, and then reduce heat to low. Cook for 20-30 minutes until puree has **thickened**. Pour puree onto **prepared** baking sheet in a thin, even layer, and bake for 2.5-3 hours until the top of the fruit puree is no longer sticky. Allow fruit leather to cool completely, then peel from the parchment paper and slice into desired size.

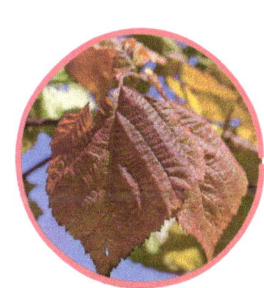

Red raspberry leaves are high in many **vitamin**s and **minerals**. They are included in **herbal** teas and have many **medicinal** uses.

A Book of Fruits 149

STAR FRUIT
CARAMBOLA

[stahr froot] | [kar-uhm-boh-luh]

crisp, floral, juicy, sweet, tart

BERRY

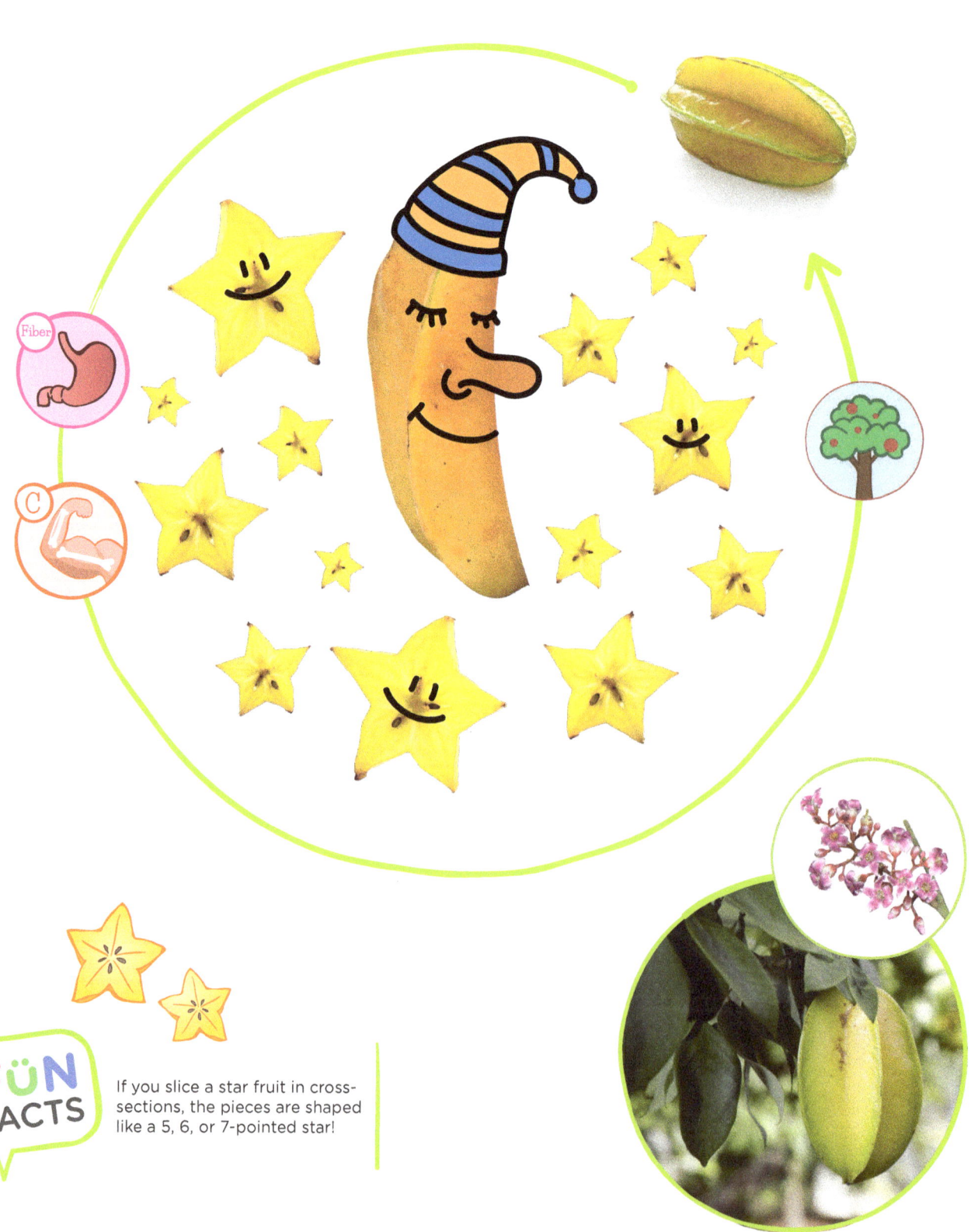

FUN FACTS: If you slice a star fruit in cross-sections, the pieces are shaped like a 5, 6, or 7-pointed star!

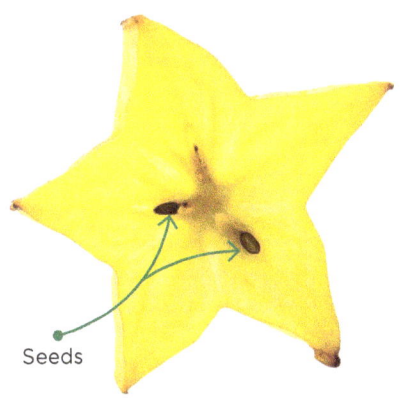
Seeds

PICK
Pick shiny, light to golden yellow fruit that are **firm** and have a floral aroma. Star fruits should be free of cuts, **bruises**, and brown shriveled edges.

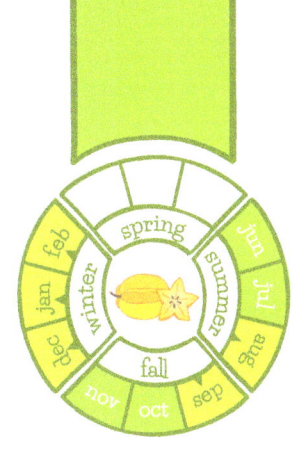

Available June to February; Imported year-round

Peak Season
August-September; December-February

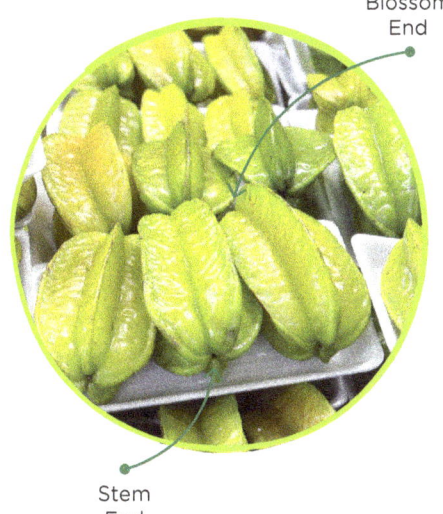
Blossom End
Stem End

STORE
Keep star fruits at room **temperature** for up to 5 days or until **ripe**. Refrigerate whole star fruits in a plastic bag for 5-7 days or sliced in airtight containers for 3-4 days. Freeze star fruits in airtight containers for 10-12 months.

STAR FRUIT TIDBITS

Star fruit trees fold in their leaves at night as a response the light or when the tree is shaken.

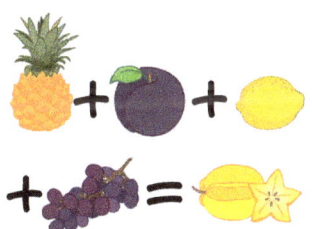

The **flavor** of a star fruit is often compared to a blend of pineapple, plum, and lemon. The **texture** of the flesh is similar to a grape.

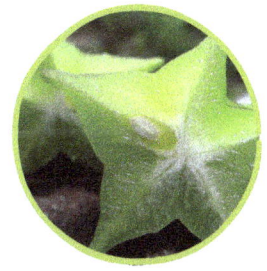

In China and India unripe, green star fruit are eaten as a vegetable.

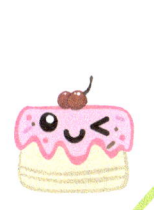
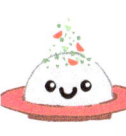
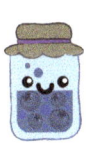
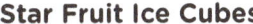

EAT
Clean the skin, slice off the blossom and stem end of the fruit. Eat, chop, or slice per recipe. Remove any **seeds**.

Star Fruit Ice Cubes
Clean the skin and slice around the center of the fruit to make star shaped pieces. Remove any seeds and freeze in a single layer on a parchment paper lined plate. Add to drinks as a cold garnish.

A Book of Fruits 151

STRAWBERRY

[straw-ber-ee]

floral, gritty, juicy, seeded, sweet

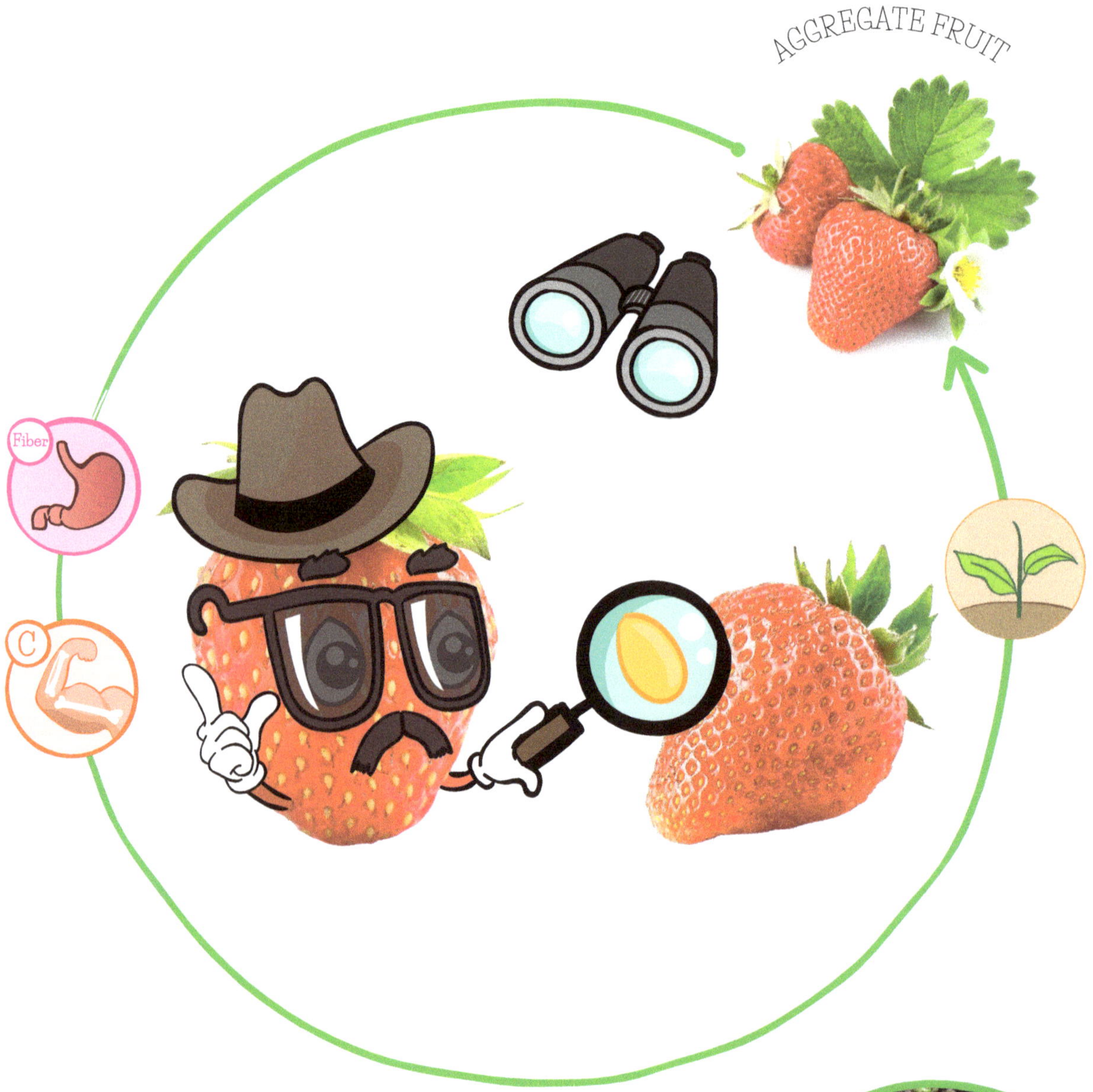

AGGREGATE FRUIT

FUN FACTS 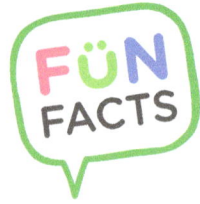 Strawberries are unlike other fruit because they bear their seeds on the outside of the fruit rather than the inside. Each strawberry has around 200 seeds! Can you count them all?

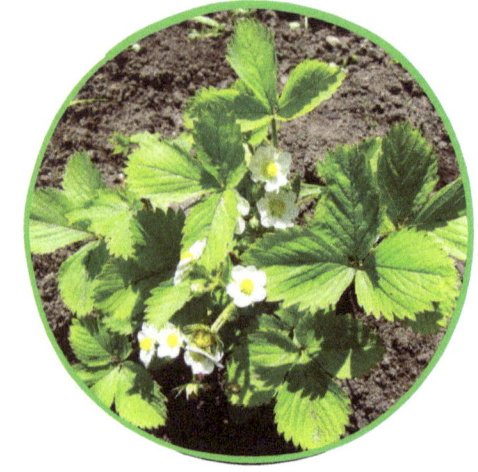

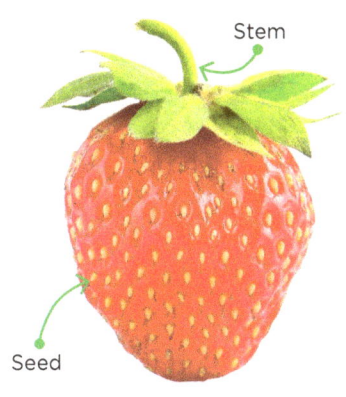

PICK
Pick bright red, evenly colored fruit with fresh green tops that are securely attached. Strawberry varieties should be **plump**, **firm**, and dry. Check the bottom of the package to make sure there is not any juice or **mold** and that strawberries are not crushed.

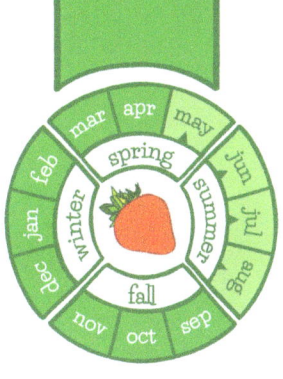

Varieties available year-round; Imported year-round

Peak Season
May-August

STORE
Keep strawberries at room **temperature** and eat them the day they are picked or purchased. Refrigerate strawberries in their plastic containers or place the berries loosely in shallow containers covered with plastic wrap for 3-7 days. Freeze strawberries in airtight containers for 10-12 months. Before storing strawberries, throw away any crushed or **moldy** fruit.

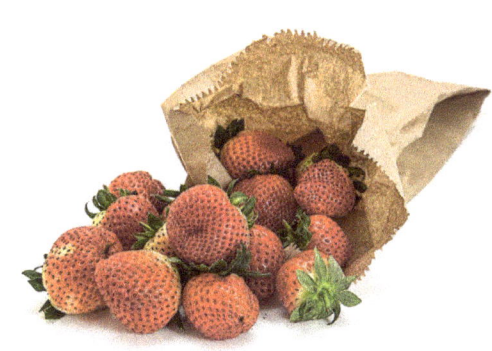

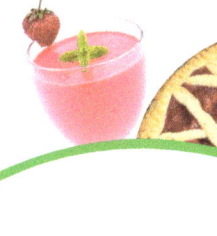

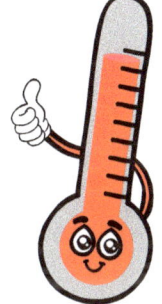

EAT
Clean just before eating or using. Eat, chop, or slice per recipe.

Cold Strawberry Soup with Pound Cake Croûtons
De-stem 2 pounds of strawberries. Combine strawberries, 2 cups Greek vanilla yogurt, and 4 ounces mango nectar in a blender until smooth and chill in the refrigerator for an hour. Preheat oven to 200 degrees F and line a baking sheet with aluminum foil. Chop 1 cup of pound cake into cubes and bake for 6 minutes, turning once to brown sides. Top soup with croutons and mint leaves.

STRAWBERRY TIDBITS

Strawberries taste their best at room temperature.

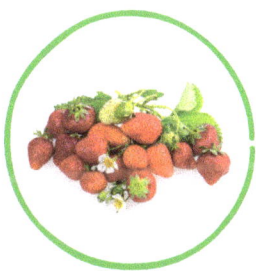

There are over 100 varieties of strawberries with different **flavors**, shapes, sizes, and best uses.

STRAWBERRY VARIETIES

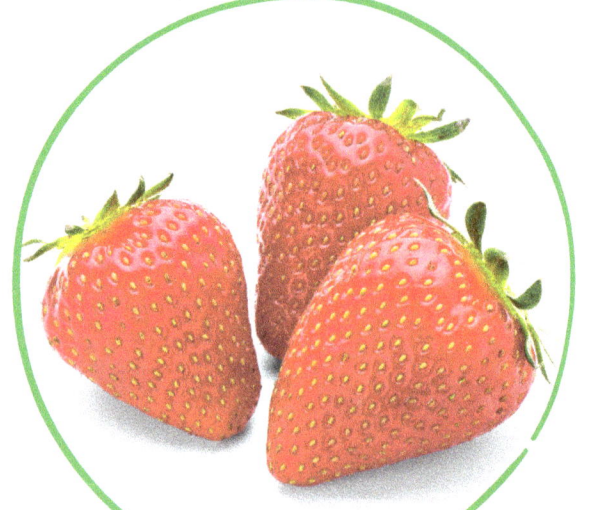

ALBION [AL-BEE-UHN]

A very large, **firm**, dark red strawberry with red flesh. Albion strawberries have a very sweet **flavor** and aroma. They are one of the only **varieties** that taste better chilled and are great fresh or sliced into salads.

ALLSTAR [AWL-STAHR]

A large, firm, glossy, orange-red strawberry. Allstar strawberries are known for having the perfect strawberry shape. The sweet and juicy Allstar is best enjoyed in fresh recipes or frozen.

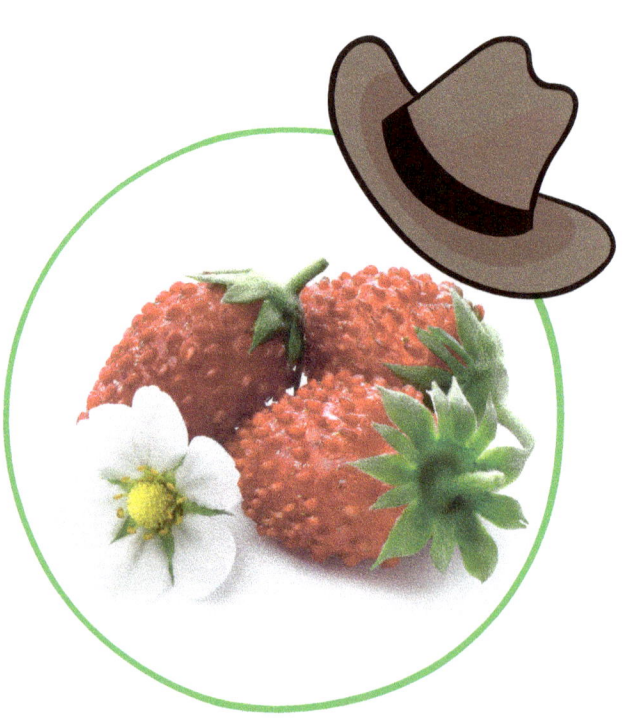

ALPINE [AL-PAHYN]

A tiny, sweet strawberry that may be small in size but is big in flavor. Alpine, or wild, strawberries are delicious to eat fresh, maybe even while picking them, or perfect for making into jam.

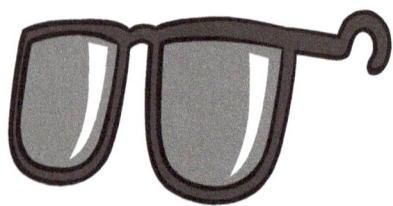

DIAMANTE [DEE-UH-MAHN-TEY]

A large, firm, bright, and shiny red strawberry that has a sweet flavor. Diamante strawberries are a popular variety for chocolate covered strawberries. They are also great fresh, in pies, and as preserves.

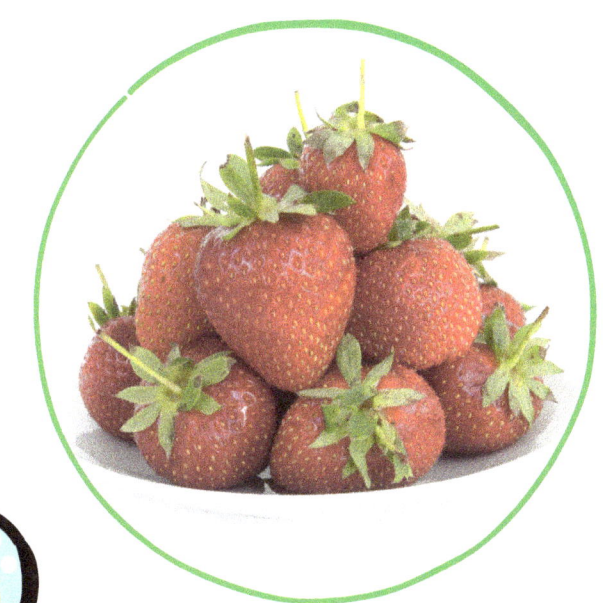

EARLIGLOW [UR-LEE GLOH]

A medium-sized, firm, aromatic strawberry that is well known for its rich flavor. Other strawberries are often compared to the Earliglow which is considered the **gold standard**. They are great fresh and used for canning.

HONEOYE [HUN-EE-OY]

A large, firm, bright orange-red to red, sweet strawberry. Honeoye strawberries are a common variety found in stores because they are known for their high **yield** of strawberries. Try them fresh, in jams, or frozen.

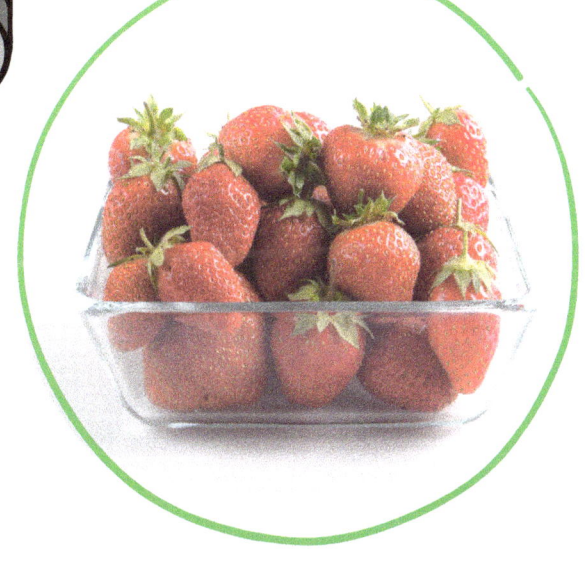

A Book of Fruits 155

TAMARILLO
TREE TOMATO

[tam-uh-ree-yoh] | [tree tuh-mey-toh]

astringent, bitter, piquant, sweet-tart, tangy

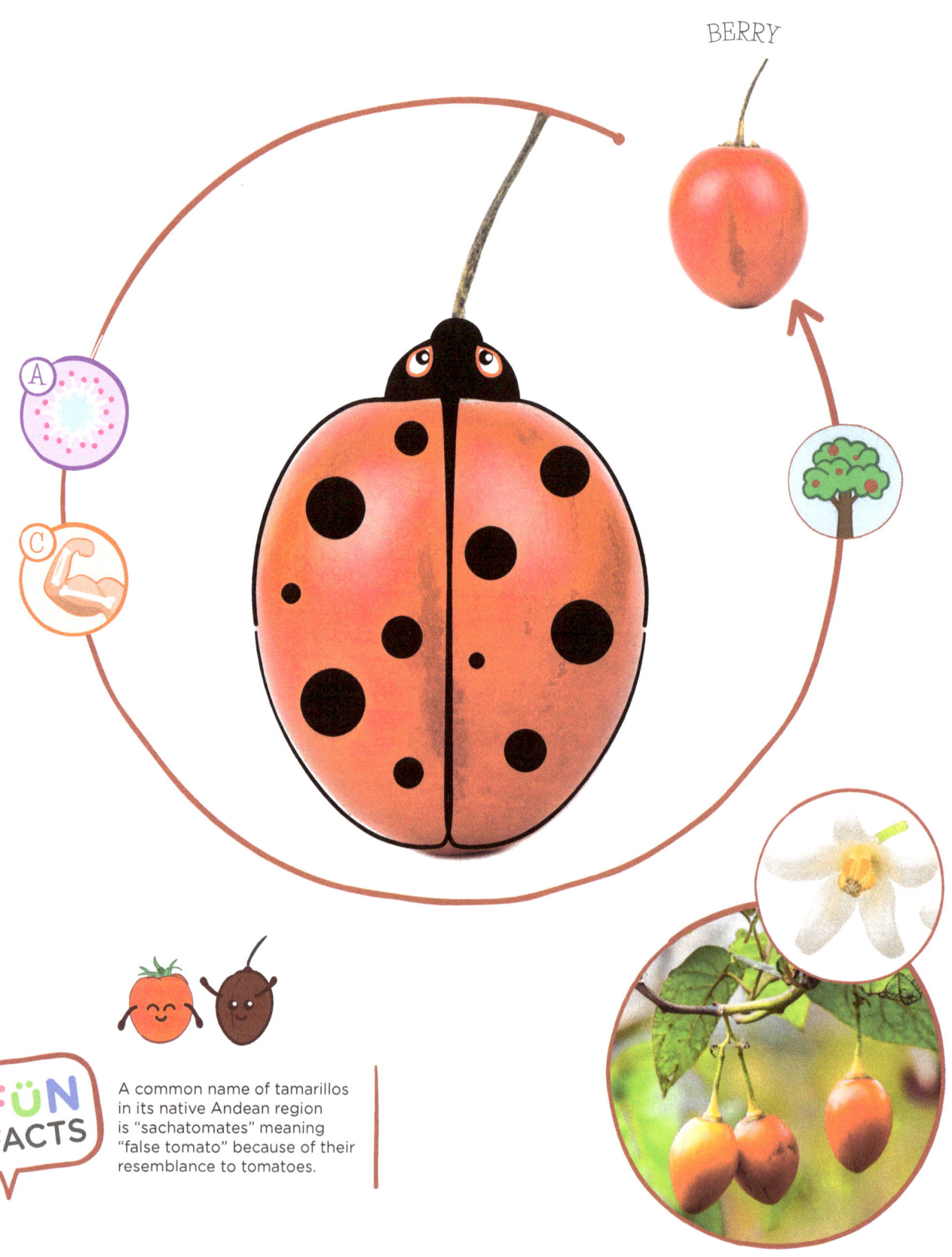

BERRY

FUN FACTS: A common name of tamarillos in its native Andean region is "sachatomates" meaning "false tomato" because of their resemblance to tomatoes.

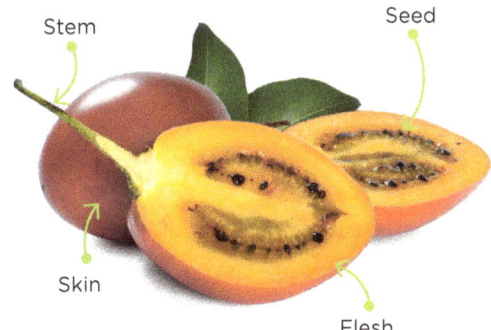

PICK
Pick glossy, golden yellow or red fruit that are **firm** but slightly soft to touch and feel heavy for their size. Tamarillos should be free of mushy spots and **mold**. Avoid Tamarillos with a sour aroma.

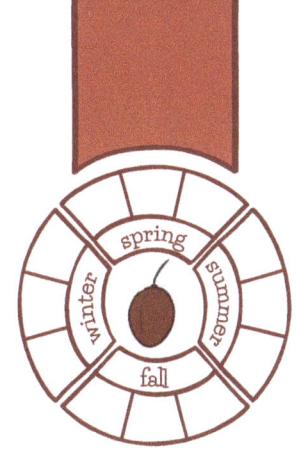

Available imported December-February

STORE
Keep tamarillos at room **temperature** for up to 3 days or until **ripe**. Refrigerate whole tamarillos in a plastic bag for 7-10 days or cut up in airtight containers for 3-4 days.

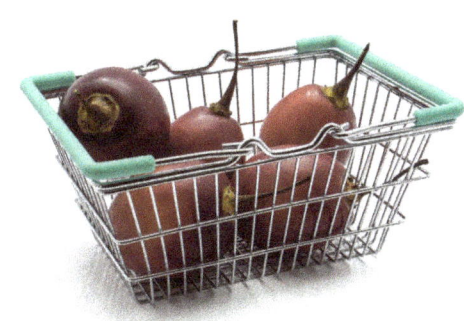

TAMARILLO TIDBITS

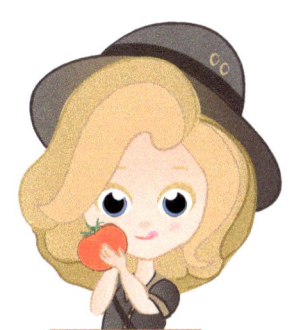

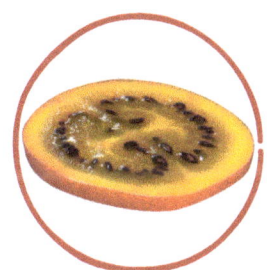

Tamarillos have more firm flesh and larger **seeds** than tomatoes.

EAT
Clean the skin and eat, chop, or slice per recipe.

Stewed Tamarillos
Boil 2 cups water with 1 cinnamon stick and 1 teaspoon of whole cloves for 5 minutes. Add 5 tamarillos and boil until their skin loosens about 2 minutes. Remove the tamarillos from the water, peel the fruit, then place them back into the water. Add 1/2 cup sugar, reduce heat to a simmer and cook until the liquid **thickens**, and fruit is the consistency of jam. Cool and store in a glass container for up to 1 month. Serve on bread or crackers.

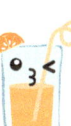
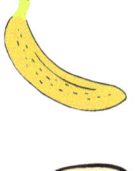

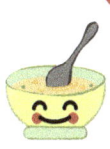

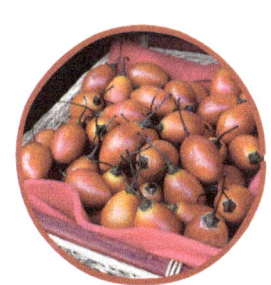

Tamarillos are often blended with water and sugar to make a refreshing juice or mixed with chili peppers to make hot sauce.

A Book of Fruits 157

Descriptive Words

Descriptive words help us identify qualities about foods and explain what we like or dislike about something we eat.

When you sit down for a meal or snack, take a moment to think about how it looks, how it smells, how it sounds, how it feels in your mouth, and how it tastes using your 5 senses. It's like your very own experiment every time you eat!

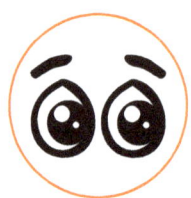

SEE
What colors or **textures** do you SEE?

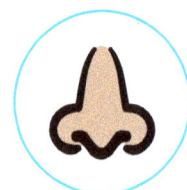

SMELL
What does it SMELL like?

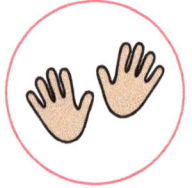

FEEL
How does it FEEL when you hold it or eat it?

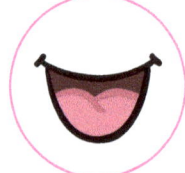

TASTE
How does the flavor TASTE?

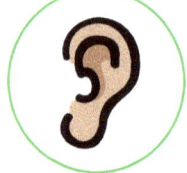

HEAR
What sound do you HEAR when you touch or take a bite?

	WORD	DESCRIPTION	SENSE(S)
1	Acidic	bitter, sharp, sour	Taste
2	Ambrosial	delicious, fragrant, sweet	Smell · Taste
3	Aroma; aromatic	scent, smell, odor	Smell
4	Astringent	mouth-puckering, sharp	Taste
5	Bitter	acidic, harsh, sharp, sour	Taste
6	Bland	flavorless, mild	Taste
7	Bright	acidic, sharp, tart, giving out or reflecting light, shiny appearance	See · Taste
8	Burnt	charred, crunchy, overcooked	Feel · See · Smell · Taste · Hear
9	Buttery	creamy, rich, smooth, velvety, feels similar to butter	Feel · Taste
10	Chewy	leathery, sticky, tough	Feel
11	Complex	multiple aromas, flavors, or textures	Feel · Smell · Taste
12	Creamy	smooth, velvety	Feel
13	Crisp(y)	crunchy, firm, snappy	Feel · Hear
14	Crunchy	brittle, crisp, loud	Feel · Hear
15	Delicate	fine texture, light or subtle taste, tender	Feel · Taste
16	Dense	compact, heavy, thick	Feel
17	Distinctive	unlike other flavors or textures, unique qualities	Feel · Taste
18	Dry	free of liquid or moisture	Feel · See · Taste
19	Earthy	feels, smells, or tastes similar to soil	Feel · Smell · Taste
20	Exotic	different, unusual, unfamiliar	See · Taste
21	Fibrous	stringy, thick, tough	Feel
22	Firm	hard, solid, stiff	Feel
23	Flavorful; flavorsome	having a lot of flavor	Taste
24	Flesh(y)	pulpy, soft, thick	Feel
25	Floral; flowery	smells or tastes similar to a flower	Smell · Taste
26	Fluffy	airy, light	Feel · See · Taste
27	Fragrant	sweet smell or scent, perfumed	Smell
28	Fresh	new, peak of ripeness, unspoiled	Feel · See · Smell · Taste
29	Fruity	varies and can mean citrusy, sweet, or tangy	Smell · Taste
30	Fuzzy	fibrous, furry, or hairy coating	Feel · See
31	Gelatinous	gluey, gummy, jelly-like, sticky	Feel · See · Taste
32	Glossy	glazed, polished, shiny	See

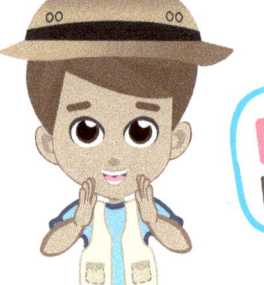

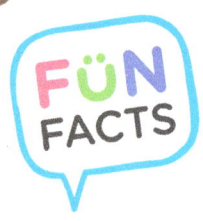

FUN FACTS

When a food feels, looks, smells, or tastes similar to another food you can say it is "like" another food or add a "y" at the end of the word. Such as butter-like, celery-like, or honey-like and citrusy, lemony, watery.

WORD	DESCRIPTION	SENSE(S)
33 Grainy	coarse, granular, gritty	Feel · See
34 Gritty	coarse, grainy, granular, rough	Feel · See · Taste
35 Hard	firm, solid	Feel
36 Herbal	smells or tastes similar to an herb	Smell · Taste
37 Honeyed	feels, looks, smells, or tastes similar to honey	Feel · See · Smell · Taste
38 Intense	sharp, strong, powerful	Smell · Taste
39 Juicy	full of juice or liquid, succulent	Feel · Hear · See
40 Knobby	lumpy surface, rounded	See
41 Light	contains air, does not make you feel full quickly, lacks a strong color, smell, or taste	Feel · See · Smell · Taste
42 Mealy	crumbly, dry, grainy	Feel · See
43 Meaty	dense, thick, taste or texture similar to meat	Feel · Taste
44 Melting	dissolve, liquify	Feel · See · Smell · Taste
45 Metallic	looks, smells, or tastes similar to metal	See · Smell · Taste
46 Mild	bland, free of a strong smell or taste	Smell · Taste
47 Milky	creamy, feels, looks, smells, or tastes similar to milk	Feel · See · Taste
48 Moist	slightly damp or wet	Feel · See
49 Mushy	may feel spoiled, soft, wet	Feel
50 Musky	fragrant odor, natural scent, pungent	Smell · Taste
51 Nutty	tastes similar to nuts	Taste
52 Odor	aroma, musk, scent	Smell
53 Peppery	hot, pungent, spicy, smells or tastes similar to pepper	Smell · Taste
54 Piney	looks, smells, or tastes similar to pine	See · Smell · Taste
55 Piquant	flavorful, tangy, zesty, pungent in smell or taste	Smell · Taste
56 Plump	fleshy, full, round	Feel · See
57 Pulpy	fibrous, fleshy, soft	Feel · See
58 Pungent	bitter, hot, peppery, sharp, powerful smell or taste	Smell · Taste
59 Refreshing	cool, fresh, or different	Feel · Smell · Taste
60 Rich	creamy, dense, fatty, full-flavored, heavy, strong and pleasant smell or taste	Feel · Taste · Smell
61 Robust	hearty, powerful, rich	Feel · See · Smell · Taste
62 Rotten	bad, moldy, spoiled	Taste · See · Smell
63 Rough	bumpy, textured, uneven surface	Taste · See · Feel
64 Rubbery	elastic, flexible, tough, similar to rubber	Feel · See
65 Savory	delicious smell or taste, having a salty or spicy quality without sweetness, well-seasoned	Taste · Smell
66 Seeded	having seeds	Feel · Hear · See
67 Shrivel	shrink, wither, wrinkle	Feel · See
68 Silky	glossy, smooth, soft, similar to silk	Feel · See
69 Skunky	aromatic, smells or tastes spoiled	Smell · Taste
70 Slimy	gooey, slippery, wet, feels similar to slime	Feel · See
71 Smooth	even, flat, uniform consistency	Feel · See
72 Soft	smooth, easy to press	Feel · See
73 Sour	acidic, bitter, tart, similar to lemon or vinegar	Feel · Smell · Taste
74 Spicy	aromatic, hot, peppery, pungent, strongly flavored	Smell · Taste
75 Spongy	airy, light, soft, feels similar to a sponge	Feel · See
76 Starchy	feels or tastes similar to other high starch foods such as potatoes or rice	Feel · Taste
77 Sticky	glue-like, syrupy, tacky, viscous	Feel · See
78 Stinky	unpleasant smell	Smell
79 Subtle	delicate, faint, light	Smell · Taste
80 Succulent	delicious, juicy, yummy	Feel · See · Smell · Taste
81 Sugary	sweet, honeyed, similar to sugar	Feel · See · Smell · Taste
82 Sweet	smells or tastes similar to sugar or honey	Smell · Taste
83 Sweet-Sour	both sweet and sour	Feel · Smell · Taste
84 Sweet-Tart	both sweet and tart	Feel · Smell · Taste
85 Syrupy	luscious, moist, thick or sweet similar to syrup	Feel · See · Smell · Taste
86 Tacky	gluey, gummy, sticky	Feel · Hear · See ·
86 Tang(y)	aromatic, flavorful, sharp, strong	Smell · Taste
88 Tart	acidic, sharp, sour	Feel · Taste
89 Tasteless	without flavor	Taste
90 Tender	delicate, soft	Feel
91 Textured	touchable or visual quality or characteristic	Feel · See
92 Tough	dense, fibrous, hard	Feel
93 Tropical	aromas and flavor similar to those found in the tropics	Smell · Taste
94 Velvety	delicate, smooth, soft	Feel
95 Vibrant	bright, colorful, zesty, zippy	See · Smell · Taste
96 Watery	feels, looks, or tastes similar to water	Feel · See · Taste
97 Waxy	shiny, sticky, similar feel and look to wax	Feel · See
98 Wrinkly	bumps, creases, or folds on a surface	See
99 Zesty	pungent, seasoned, sharp, spicy, tart	Smell · Taste
100 Zippy	fresh, invigorating	Taste

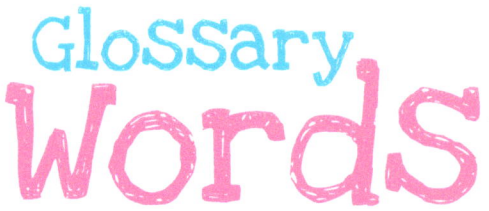
Glossary Words

A glossary helps us learn definitions of new or unusual words found in the book. Anytime you see a **bold** word throughout the book, you can find the definition here.

WORD	PHONETIC	DEFINITION
Aggregate Fruit	[ag-gray-gate froot]	a flower with several ovaries that come together to form a single fruit (e.g., strawberry)
Antioxidant(s)	[an-ti-ox-i-dant]	nutrients found in food that fight off sickness
Aril	[ar-il]	a fleshy seed covering that encourages animals to eat a fruit and helps spread seeds
Bacteria	[bak-teer-ee-uh]	very small living organisms that are everywhere and can either be harmful and make you sick or helpful and keep you healthy
Berry	[ber-ee]	fleshy soft-skinned fruit with several seeds (e.g., grapes)
Bloom	[bloom]	a natural, protective, waxy coating made by fruit to protect the skin, retain moisture, and keep fruit fresher longer
Brine	[brahyn]	a mixture of salt and water often used to preserve or add flavor to food
Bruise	[brewz]	damage to an area of a fruit, vegetable, or plant by being handled roughly that leaves a mark on the skin
Calyx	[kay-licks]	blossom or flower end of fruit
Capsule	[kap-suhl]	a type of simple, dry, fruit with two or more sections that bear seeds
Carbon dioxide (CO2)	[car-bon di-ox-eyed]	a substance or gas created by people and animals breathing out that is used by plants for energy
Cauliflory	[kaw-li-flawr-ee]	flowers and fruit that grow from the trunk of a tree rather than on the overhanging branches which allow animals that cannot climb or fly to eat them and pollinate or spread seeds
Cell	[sell]	the basic structural and functional unit of all living things or the smallest unit of life
Celsius	[sel-see-uhs]	a measurement of temperature
Characteristic	[kar-ik-tuh-ris-tik]	a feature or quality
Classified	[klas-uh-fahyd]	arrange or organize as belonging to a specific group or category
Climate	[klahy-mit]	weather conditions in a place or region
Cling	[kling]	stay attached
Clot	[klot]	thickened and partly solid blood that stops bleeding when you get cuts and scrapes
Cream	[kreem]	the result when butter and sugar are mixed until creamy, fluffy, and smooth which creates air pockets that help baked goods rise
Cuisine	[kwi-zeen]	a style of cooking usually associated with a specific culture or geographic location
Cultivate	[kuhl-tuh-vate]	prepare and work to raise or grow plants
Currency	[kur-uhn-see]	a form of payment or money
Cutting	[kuht-ing]	a root, stem, or leaf, cut from a plant and used for growing another plant
Dehiscent	[di-his-uhnt]	split open or burst when fruits are ripe
Dehydrate; dehydrator	[dee-hahy-dreyt]	to remove water from plant tissue; an appliance that removes water
Digestion; digestive system	[dih-jes-chuhn]	how the body breaks down food and gets nutrients and energy from food
Dissolve	[dih-zolv]	a reaction that occurs when a solid is mixed with a liquid and the solid becomes part of the liquid
Diverse	[dih-vurs]	having various kinds or forms
DNA	[d-n-a]	the instruction manual for your body on how your body works including the way you look

WORD	PHONETIC	DEFINITION
Drift	[drift]	movement from wind or ocean current
Drizzle	[driz-uhl]	pour a small amount of liquid onto or over something
Drupe	[droop]	fleshy fruit that surrounds a seed, also known as a stone or pit (e.g., plum)
Edible	[ed-uh-buhl]	safe to eat
Effervescent	[ef-er-ves-uhnt]	giving off bubbles or bubbling
Electrolyte(s)	[ih-lek-truh-lahyt]	minerals that balance the amount of fluid in your body (e.g., sodium, potassium, and chloride)
Energy	[en-er-jee]	a usable source of nutrition that can come from food and enables human, animals, and plants to function
Ethylene	[eth-uh-leen]	a gas that is naturally released when fruits ripen and helps soften fruit
Expose	[ik-spohz]	lay open or uncover
Fahrenheit	[far-uh n-hahyt]	a measurement of temperature; labeled as degrees F in this book
Farm; farming or farmed; farmer	[fahrm]	land used for growing crops such as fruits and vegetables; the process of growing crops; people who work to raise crops
Ferment	[fur-ment]	a process of changing food using microorganisms such as helpful bacteria
Firm	[furm]	a solid surface or structure; not soft when pressed
Flavor	[fley-ver]	a characteristic or quality of how something tastes
Flesh	[flesh]	the edible, soft, pulpy portion of a fruit, vegetable, or plant
Flourish	[flur-ish]	to grow or develop well
Forage	[for-ij]	to search for food
Gas	[gas]	a substance like air that does not have a fixed shape such as a solid or a liquid
Glochid	[gloh-kid]	a sharp and thorny hair-like thorn
Gold standard	[gohld stan-derd]	a point of reference for the highest quality that other things are compared
Grease	[greese]	a thin layer of fat or oil
Harvest	[hahr-vist]	the season when crops are gathered; to gather crops
Helpful bacteria	[help-fuhl bak-teer-ee-uh]	support digestion and fight harmful bacteria
Herb; herbal	[urb]	a plant or a part of a plant that is used to give flavor or scent to food
Hesperidium	[hes-puh-rid-ee-uhm]	a special family of berries with a leathery outer skin or rind and a divided, fleshy interior (e.g., orange)
Horticulture; horticulturist	[hawr-ti-kuhl-cher]	the science of growing fruits, vegetables, and flowers; an expert in the science of growing plants
Husk	[huhsk]	a dry layer that covers some seeds and fruits
Hybrid	[hahy-brid]	the final product of two plants of different varieties
Immune system	[im-u-n sis-tem]	the structures and processes in your body that protects your body and fights off sickness
Imported	[im-pohr-ted]	to bring a product to another country to be sold
Indehiscent	[in-di-his-uhnt]	does not split open or burst when fruits are ripe
Invasive species	[in-vey-siv spee-sheez]	a plant that is new to an environment that grows and spreads quickly damaging local plants
Lenticel	[len-tuh-sel]	a pore or opening of outer plant tissue that allows for fluid or gas exchange
Marinade	[mar-uh-neyd]	a seasoned sauce used to prepare food for cooking by coating it until the flavors are absorbed and the food is more tender
Mature	[muh-toor]	fully grown
Medicinal	[muh-dis-uh-nl]	used as medicine
Membrane	[mem-breyn]	thin piece of tissue in a fruit, vegetable, or plant
Mineral(s)	[min-er-uhl]	substances that occur naturally in certain foods and have different jobs in the body to help you grow healthy and strong
Miraculin	[mir-ach-u-lyn]	a substance found in the miracle berry that makes sour foods taste sweet
Missionaries	[mish-uh-ner-ees]	people sent by a church into an area to share religious beliefs
Mold; moldy; molding	[mohld]	a substance that grows on the surface of damp or rotting foods that can cause them to spoil

WORD	PHONETIC	DEFINITION
Multiple Fruit	[muhl-tuh-puhl froot]	multiple small flowers, each with their own ovary, that come together to form into one large fruit as they grow (e.g., pineapple)
Mutation	[myoo-tey-shuhn]	a change in one or more characteristics of an original plant that causes a new type of plant to grow
Nervous system	[nur-vuhs sis-tem]	the structure of nerves in your body that sends messages for controlling movement and feeling between the brain and the other parts of your body
Nutrient	[nu-tree-uhnt]	a substance found in food that our bodies use to grow, run, and play
Nocturnal	[nok-tur-nl]	active at night
Ovary; ovaries	[ov-air-e]	the part of a flower that makes seeds
Oxygen	[ok-si-juhn]	a colorless, odorless, and tasteless element that makes up the air we breathe and is vital to all living things
Parthenocarpy	[pahr-thuh-noh-kahr-pee]	to grow new fruit without seeds through "cuttings" of a root, stem, or leaf
Pepo	[pee-poh]	a family of berries with a hard-outer skin or rind (e.g., watermelon)
Perforated	[pur-fuh-rey-tid]	pierced with a hole or holes
Phloem	[flo-em]	part of a plant that carries sugar and nutrients to all parts of fruit such as the "strings" of a banana
Photosynthesis	[foh-tuh-sin-thuh-sis]	how plants make energy or food; plant + sun + water + nutrients from soil + carbon dioxide = energy or sugar and oxygen
Phytonutrient(s)	[fi-toe-new-tree-ent]	helpful parts of plants that keep us from getting sick
Pistil	[pis-til]	part of a flower that turns into a fruit once pollinated
Pit	[pit]	hard, stone-like shell that surrounds a single seed in the center of fruit, also called a stone (e.g., plum)
Pith	[pith]	soft, white, spongy tissue that surrounds citrus fruit
Plump	[pluhmp]	full, rounded shape
Poisonous	[poi-zuh-nus]	a substance that is harmful and can make you sick
Pollen	[pol-en]	a yellow, powder-like substance that flowers make to help grow new seeds
Pollination	[pol-in-a-tion]	the process of transporting pollen, through insects such as bees, animals, or by the wind, to other flowers to help grow new seeds
Prepare	[pre-pair]	to make or create something to eat
Probiotic	[proh-bahy-ot-ik]	helpful bacteria that support digestion and fight harmful bacteria
Processed	[pro-ses-ed]	to change food from one form into another form by preparing it in a special way
Pome	[pohm]	fleshy fruit that surrounds a seeded core (e.g., apple)
Puree	[pur-ray]	food blended into a thick pulp or paste
Rind	[rahynd]	the tough, outer skin of some fruit that is usually removed before the fruit is eaten
Ripe	[rahyp]	a fully grown and developed fruit or vegetable that is ready to be eaten
Rooting hormone	[root-ing hawr-mohn]	plant growth hormones that help to stimulate a plant cutting to grow new plants
Russeting	[ruhs-it-ing]	a brownish, roughened area on fruit that occurs naturally based on variety or weather conditions
Saliva	[suh-lahy-vuh]	watery fluid in the mouth that helps with tasting, chewing, swallowing, and digestion
Score	[skohr]	to make light cuts on the surface of food
Scurvy	[skur-vee]	a sickness from not eating enough vitamin C that causes teeth to loosen and skin to bruise easily
Seasonal	[see-zuh-nl]	produce that is grown during a particular time of the year due to varying climates (the four seasons are winter, spring, summer, and fall)
Seed; seedling	[seed]	a small object formed by a plant from which a new plant can grow
Self-Pollinate	[self pol-in-ate]	seedlings created without the help of insects, animals, or the wind
Simple Fleshy Fruit	[sim-puhl flesh-ee froot]	a flower with a single ovary forms a fruit and are grouped into categories based on how they grow (e.g., apple)
Spoil	[spoy-el]	to lose freshness and become rotten or bad and can no longer be eaten
Stain	[stay-en]	to leave a mark on something that is not easily removed
Steep	[steep]	to soak in water

WORD	PHONETIC	DEFINITION
Stone	[stow-en]	hard, stone-like shell that surrounds a single seed in the center of a fruit (e.g., plum)
Stone Cells	[stow-en sells]	thickened plant cells that form naturally causing fruit tissue to become gritty
Submerged	[suhb-murj]	under the surface of water
Symbol	[sim-buhl]	an image used to represent a word or a group of words
Symmetrical	[sim-et-ree-cal]	to look even in size and form; the same all over
Technology	[tek-nol-uh-jee]	science or knowledge put into use to solve problems
Temperature	[tem-per-uh-cher]	a measurement that indicates how hot or cold something is and can be measured using a thermometer in degrees Fahrenheit or degrees Celsius; Fahrenheit is labeled as degrees F in this book
Texture	[teks-cher]	the visual or physical qualities of a surface that you can see, feel, and touch
Thick; thicker; thickens; thicken	[thik]	dense; measurement; a liquid with a firm consistency; not flowing freely
Thrive	[thrahyv]	to grow or develop well
Tissue	[tish-oo]	a material that forms parts of a plant
Transform	[trans-fawrm]	to change the form, appearance, or structure of something
Translucent	[trans-loo-cent]	when an object is not completely clear, but light can pass through
Variety; Varieties	[vuh-rahy-i-tee]	a number or collection of different things in the same general category
Vinaigrette	[vin-uh-gret]	a dressing or sauce made from a mixture of oil, vinegar, and seasonings
Vitamin(s)	[vahy-tuh-min]	substances that naturally occur in certain foods and have different jobs in the body to help you grow healthy and strong
Viticulture	[vit-i-kuhl-cher]	a branch of horticulture that is the art and science of growing and harvesting grapes
Yield	[yield]	the amount or quantity produced
Zest; zesting	[zes-ting]	the outer peel of a citrus fruit that has a concentrated flavor; a food flavoring ingredient prepared by shaving or grating the colorful outer skin of citrus fruit

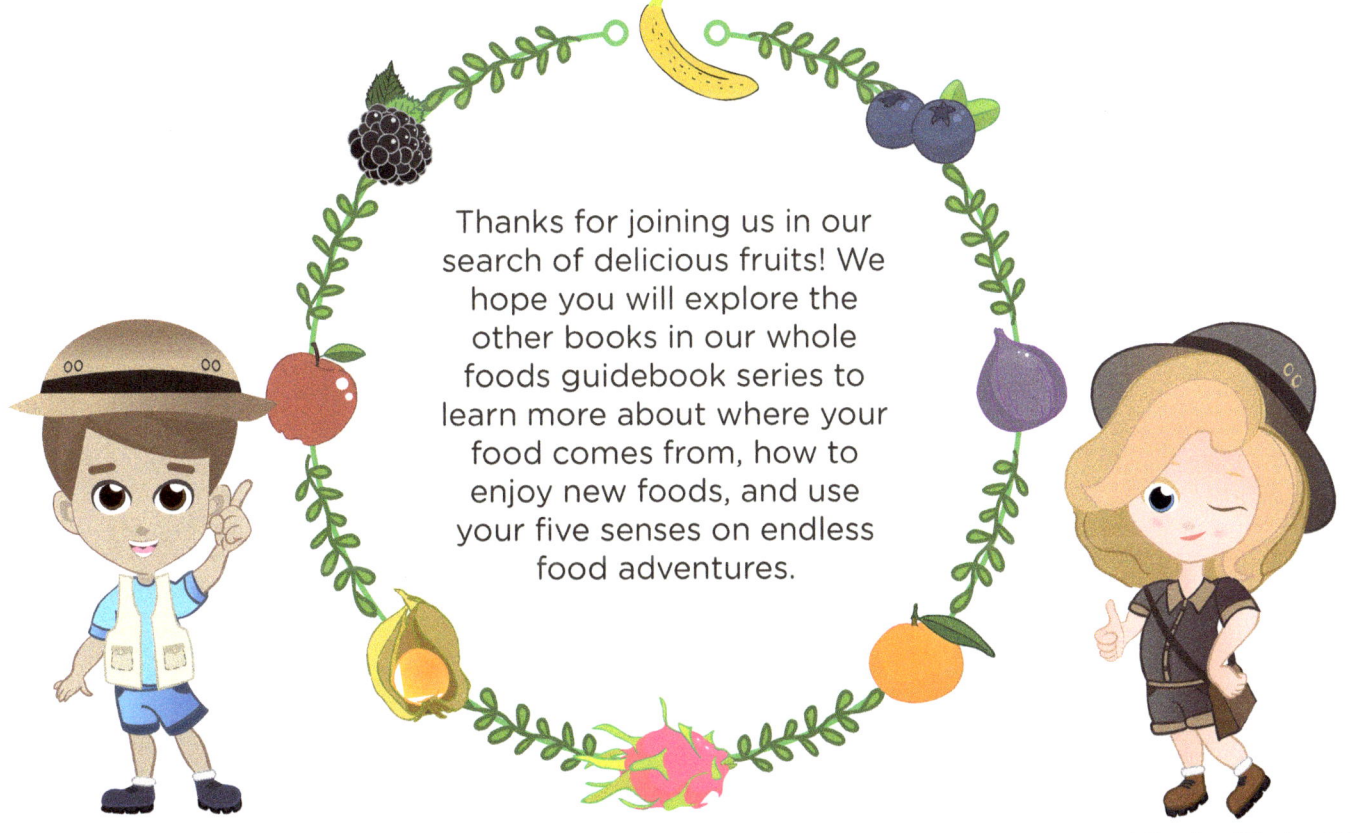

Thanks for joining us in our search of delicious fruits! We hope you will explore the other books in our whole foods guidebook series to learn more about where your food comes from, how to enjoy new foods, and use your five senses on endless food adventures.

www.ingramcontent.com/pod-product-compliance
Lightning Source LLC
Chambersburg PA
CBHW040124130526
44591CB00040B/2932